A History of Pharmacy in South Dakota

by

Harold H. Schuler

This book traces the history of the pharmacy profession within the Dakota Territory and the state of South Dakota from 1861 to 2003. It describes the evolution of practice from Kirk G. Phillips' 1876 Deadwood drug store, located in a dirt-floor log house, to the professional pharmacies of today.

It outlines the change in educational requirements from no high school and two years of apprentice training to the 2003 six-year Doctor of Pharmacy degree offered by South Dakota State University's College of Pharmacy. The change from a pharmacist compounding prescriptions with a mortar and pestle to dispensing life-saving manufactured drugs is reviewed.

A History of Pharmacy in South Dakota demonstrates how the practice of pharmacy has progressed to the point where the pharmacist has become a vital member of the professional health care team and how it got there.

Harold H. Schuler

Library of Congress Control Number: 2004093188

ISBN: 1-57579-283-4

Printed in the United States of America
Pine Hill Press, Sioux Falls, SD 57106

Acknowledgments

I would like to thank Cliff Thomas who encouraged me to write the history of pharmacy in South Dakota. I also appreciate that the Board of Directors of the South Dakota Pharmacists Association, at an early 2002 meeting, authorized me to proceed and use the Association's historical records. Executive Directors Robert Coolidge, Tobi Lyon, and Bob Overturf were very helpful in locating and supplying me with SDPhA research materials. Executive Director Dennis M. Jones, of the SD Board of Pharmacy and Dean Brian Kaatz, SDSU College of Pharmacy, also supplied me with extensive material. I would also like to thank the many pharmacists who sent me photographs and letters about their pharmaceutical experiences. Especially helpful was the use of old photographs located at the College of Pharmacy, SDPhA office, and Robert Kolbe Collections of Sioux Falls.

In early 2004, after two years of research and writing, I completed a draft text of *A History of Pharmacy in South Dakota.* I would like to thank Dean Brian Kaatz, SDSU College of Pharmacy; Executive Director Dennis M. Jones, Board of Pharmacy; SDPhA President Monica Jones; and Association Historical Committee member Cliff Thomas, who reviewed the text and provided me many helpful suggestions. I would also like to thank the SDPhA Board of Directors for agreeing to publish this book, as well as Carveth Thompson and Cliff Thomas who helped to make possible its publication. My wife, Leona R. Schuler and our daughter Lynda L. Schuler, deserve a special thanks for helping me with the proofreading.

I would like to dedicate this book to the 5,300 pharmacists who were licensed in South Dakota since 1890. To read about their hopes, as well as their hardships, was an exciting adventure. This history is an account of what they did to build and promote the pharmacy profession in South Dakota.

—Harold H. Schuler, Executive Secretary,
SDPhA and Board of Pharmacy, 1964-1986
Pierre, South Dakota

Benefactors

This book was made possible through the generous financial assistance of the following who contributed $100 or more to this project:

Steve & Robbie Aamot
Jeff Bertsch
Jim Bregel
Terry Casey
Yee-Lai Chiu
Marlyn Christensen
Shane Clarambeau
Robert Coolidge
Earle Crissman
Mark & Diane Dady
Sharon Dady
Philip J. Dohn
Roger Eastman
Robert & Mary Lou Ehrke
Galen Goeden
Robert Gregg
Russell Hatch
Bernard Hietbrink
Willis Hodson
Raymond Hopponen
Ronald Huether
The Hustead Family
Karla Overland-Janssen
Dennis M. Jones
James "Jack" Jones
Kenneth Jones
Lloyd Jones
Monica Jones
Pamela Jones
Galen & Ann Jordre
Brian Kaatz
Cheri Kraemer
Dave & Mary Kuper
Danny Lattin

Arvid Liebe
Dennis Ludwig
Pat Lynn
Earl McKinstry
Julie Meintsma
Duncan Murdy
John Nelson
Robert Overturf
Allen Pfeifle
Jo Prang & Wallace Arneson
Robert Reiswig
Ronald & Marilyn Schwans
Terry Setera
Dan L. Somsen
Steve Statz
Conley Stanage
Edward Staudenmier
Jim Stephens
Paula Stotz
Dale Stroschein
Renee Sutton
Ed Swanson
Cliff Thomas
Mary Thomas
Carv Thompson
Louis Van Roekel
Wiley Vogt
Murray Widdis Jr.
Robert Wik
Maris Williams
Margaret Zard
Albert Zarecky
Milo Zeeb

Thanks to these corporate sponsors:

Jewett Drug
McKesson Corp.

Amerisource Bergen
Pharmacists Mutual Ins. Co.

A History of Pharmacy in South Dakota

Table of Contents

South Dakota College of Pharmacy

South Dakota Society of Health-System Pharmacists (SDSHP)

South Dakota Association of Pharmacy Technicians (SDAPT)

Preface

Writing a history book that covers such a long span of time is a huge task. Harold Schuler has done an incredible job of sorting through dusty boxes containing photographs and documents and conducting interviews and turning these into a complete history of pharmacy in South Dakota. He has the unique qualities and experiences that have made him the perfect choice for such an undertaking.

Knowing where we have been and the path we have taken to get where we are is an important part of choosing our future direction. This is true in all areas. Harold has made it possible to know these important facts about pharmacy in South Dakota and has done it in an interesting and compelling way. He has personalized his book with the names and accomplishments of the leaders that have shaped our profession. I feel fortunate to have had even a small part in bringing this project to completion. On behalf of everyone involved with pharmacy in South Dakota, I sincerely thank Harold for giving us this wonderful documentation of the past.

I would also like to thank Cliff Thomas and Carveth Thompson for their extraordinary efforts in getting this book to publication. Their conviction in the need for the publication of this book carried the project forward to completion. They quickly raised the funds necessary for publication and associated costs so SDPhA could use the proceeds in its efforts to promote the profession of pharmacy.

I would also like to thank all of the individuals and organizations that donated money or purchased advertisements to pay for author and publication costs. These benefactors are listed in another section.

—Monica Jones
South Dakota Pharmacist Association
President, 2003-2004

Foreword

The pace of American life is undeniably speeding up, both at home and hearth, as well as in the marketplace. As we race along, it seems that almost every endeavor in which humans are involved can be characterized as undergoing enormous change, and often are said to be at "a crossroads".

Remarkably, these crossroads do not occur just once but usually over and over again. Professions seem to undergo a sea change and, within a generation or less, do it all over again.

As we strive to make sense of this, there is value in looking back in an effort to understand the trends and "trajectory" of the forces which influence the present. In a very real way, almost all of these forces can be traced to the past and can help explain the future.

Harold Schuler has done a great favor to the pharmacy profession in South Dakota by giving us a sweeping overview of the past, which in turn helps us understand the future. His *A History of Pharmacy in South Dakota* gives the reader a fascinating trip through the last 125 years or so of a great profession. Mr. Schuler is uniquely qualified to give us this perspective on pharmacy and history within South Dakota, having extensively participated, studied, and written about both.

It is remarkable to me that many of the "crossroads" that seem so unique today occurred in a previous version with circumstances not so very different from now. Mr. Schuler capably assists us in understanding these with this comprehensive journey through the state's pharmacy history.

The ideal educational preparation for pharmacists, the challenges of competitive forces, and discussions with other health professionals are just a few of the issues that seem to recur with regularity.

I applaud this addition to our history—it brings us nicely into the 21st century. Where will we go from here? I suspect many of the clues reside within *A History of Pharmacy in South Dakota*.

—Brian Kaatz
Dean, College of Pharmacy
South Dakota State University
April 2004

CHAPTER 1
Pharmacy in the Dakota Territory, 1861-1889

The story about *A History of Pharmacy in South Dakota* began in 1861. On March 2 of that year, the United States Congress created the Dakota Territory, consisting of present-day North and South Dakota. President Lincoln appointed William Jayne as governor. The first Legislature, meeting in Yankton on March 17, 1862, selected that city as the capital. Population of the Dakota Territory was 2,402.

Shortly after 1862, Charley Bramble, New York, opened the first drug store in the new territory at Yankton. F. A. Brecht, who later opened a drug store at Yankton in 1869, recalled that Bramble marketed "drugs, shot guns, hardware and everything else that was salable." Brecht and his family had traveled by train to Sioux City. From there they traveled by team and wagon to Yankton. Brecht said his "drug business was, of course, connected with groceries and everything salable. Two months later, there came L. M. Purdy from Wisconsin, he was sent out by Dr. Miltz, and the firm name was Miltz and Purdy until I bought them out."[1] [An 1869 prescription says Mills and Purdy] Purdy served as Territorial Auditor at the Yankton Capital, 1881-1882. In the 1898 list of pharmacists, F. A. Brecht holds a Ph.G. (Pharmacy Graduate) degree. E. M. Coates, Yankton, opened his drug store in 1870.

A provision of The Laramie Treaty of 1868 set aside all land west of the Missouri River, in a portion of the Dakota Territory that is now South Dakota, as the Great Sioux Reservation. Anyone using the land without permission from the Indians was trespassing. Following the discovery of gold near Custer in 1874, and near Deadwood in 1875, settlers began entering the Black Hills without permission. Doing business in Deadwood and the Black Hills was first legalized by an 1877 Act of Congress that opened the Black Hills for settlement.

Kirk G. Phillips, Maryland, was the earliest settler to open a drug store in Deadwood. He and his partner, Dr. A. M. McKinney opened their Main Street drug store in May 1876 in a log house without a floor. They sold great quantities of patent medicines, prescription drugs, paints, oils, window glass, etc. Phillips said, "J. B. Hickok, better known as Wild Bill, had a little to do with early pharmacy in Deadwood. He most graciously assisted me to unpack and place the first large invoice of goods I received. If he had lived, he might have become a member of this Association."[2] Phillips served as a delegate to the second Constitutional Convention at Sioux Falls, in 1885. He was elected South Dakota Treasurer and served 1895-1898. Phillips became the Republican candidate for Governor in the 1898 South Dakota general election, losing to incumbent Governor Andrew E. Lee by 325 votes. He died in 1913.

Julius Deetken opened his drug store in Deadwood on June 1, 1876. Deetken said, "I opened my store with a $1,200 stock...in one of the first log houses built in Deadwood. I occupied one-half of the building 20 x 30, the other half being occupied by a grocery store. We had no doors or windows—simply 'holes in the wall,' and at night we hung up a blanket to cover up the holes. The floor was mother earth covered with saw dust. My counter was two rough boards nailed across two tree stumps. My shelves were one-half dozen rough boards."[3]

Deetken described some of his business practices: "Prices were good then, freight [hauled by wagon trains] was high, about $.08 a pound from Cheyenne to Deadwood. Twenty-five cents or two bits was the smallest sale we made. One Seidlitz powder or one dose of pills, was $.25. There was little or no paper currency, gold dust was the universal money. A gold scale was on every counter and we took twenty-seven grains of gold dust for one dollar. No bank, no United States Mail, no express office during 1876. I use to hide my buckskin sack full of gold among the 'R' bottles where no one would ever look for money. No fire insurance company was doing business in Deadwood during those first two or three years. We constructed underground fire proof warehouses—a log house built underground, usually right back of our store, roof covered with dirt, just above ground, and sacks filled with sand near the trap door. In case of fire the sand was thrown on the trap door, making it perfectly fire proof."[4]

In a speech to the members of the 1901 SDPhA convention, Deetken related that on July 1, 1876, about sundown, he noticed an ox train moving along the street in front of his pharmacy. Walking along the side of the ox train, was "a slender 'beardless' youth with a Colt's Navy revolver strapped to his loins, a Remington rifle over his shoulder, his overalls tucked into his boots. The ox train stopped further up the street and soon began to unload." He later discovered it was another competitor, E. C. Bent from Cheyenne. Four months later, he and Bent formed a partnership. E. C. Bent later recalled that a clerk of his, C.D. Mattison [C.D. Matteson on 1898 list], started one of the first drug stores in Rapid City. In October 1878, E.C. Bent moved to Sioux Falls and then to Dell Rapids

A History of Pharmacy in South Dakota

in 1892, where he opened a pharmacy. Bent later served as Secretary to the Association and Board of Pharmacy, 1897-1923. He died in 1924.

There were no laws regulating the practice of pharmacy in the Territory between 1862 and early 1887. A person simply had to buy a stock of drugs and open a pharmacy. Presumably, that person had some apprentice training in a pharmacy. A few pharmacists had a little college training which had been obtained in other states. The Territorial Agricultural College at Brookings had opened in the fall of 1884. Pharmacy was first mentioned in the 1887-1888 catalog. In 1888, the catalog outlined a two-year course in pharmacy, "designed to fit young men and women for the business of druggists." In 1890, after South Dakota became a state, the first five students graduated and were awarded a certificate of completion for the two-year course.[5]

During the 1872 Legislative Session, a law was passed requiring a pharmacist to have a license to sell intoxicating liquor. Another law passed that same year gave authority to the town supervisors to act as a Board of Health, with power to control the sources of filth and causes of sickness. Although no laws regulated the practice of pharmacy, pharmacists were subject to territorial laws pertaining to the protection of public health.

In 1879, the Legislature authorized pharmacists to sell liquor for medicinal purposes, but only upon a doctor's prescription. However, a pharmacist could not sell wine for sacramental purposes. It was unlawful for any person to sell opium. The 1881 Legislature granted the control of public health to the Board of County Commissioners, who acting as a Board of Health, could pass rules to prevent the spread of contagious diseases.

Warren J. Page, Alpena, told the 1921 convention about his store of forty years ago [1881]. He reported that there was no Board of Pharmacy, no State Sheriff, no narcotic laws, and no special taxes. He stated:

"We were simply turned loose to do an unrestricted business. I remember with feelings of pride I placed a gold leaf mortar and pestle on a post in front of my store and how the glass show bottles filled with colored solution placed in the windows were in my mind things of beauty as well as necessary advertisements. The glass labeled shelf bottles were well placed to the front of the store so that a wayfaring man...need have no doubt as to the identity of the place. The cash register was represented by the money till with the bell, and a boy on horse back took the place of a telephone. One of my doctors made many of his calls with a high wheeled bicycle.

"We had no soda fountain, no luncheonette...no serum, no antitoxins with the exception of smallpox vaccines. Our line of perfumes consisted principally of Musk, Hoyts German Cologne, Imperial Cologne, and Florida Water. No talcum. In toilet soaps, Cuticura, Cashmere Bouquet and Castile practically covered the list. The only shaving soap being Williams Yankee. Very few face powders or lotions, no writing tablets or box stationery, no Kodak's or phonographs, no vacuum bottles, no manicure or toilet sets. Toilet articles consisted largely of hair brushes, tooth brushes and coarse and fine combs. Druggists manufactured most of their tinctures and pharmaceuticals, cold creams etc.

"They did not stock cottons, gauzes, bandages, and not many surgical requirements. Antiseptics either in solution, tablets or powders that are so plentiful now, were not much in evidence, the principle one then being carbolic acid. What is there in store for us in the future? Is the tendency toward separating technical pharmacy from its profitable commercial side lines? I hope not, for professional sentiment will not ring the bell on the cash register and drugs and medicines would have to necessarily sell at advanced prices. Will the time come when syndicates will control, own, and operate all the drug stores?"[6]

In 1885, the Legislature created a three-member Territorial Board of Health consisting of the Attorney General and two Governor appointees. One appointee needed to be a medical doctor, who served as Superintendent of Public Health, and was paid $500 per year. The board had power to pass rules for the prevention, cure, and spread of any contagious disease among persons and domestic animals. It also had authority to condemn and destroy any impure or diseased article of food offered for sale. The 1885 law also defined who could practice medicine and dentistry. However, no mention was made as to the practice of pharmacy. Interestingly, the 1885 Legislature defined how to mark and sell imitation butter by placing the word oleomargarine on the package in words not less than one inch in length.

Formation of Southern District Pharmaceutical Association, 1886

Between 1878 and 1886, railroad workers laid tracks into almost every part of the Dakota Territory east of the Missouri River. For example, in 1880, the Chicago and Northwestern Railway built a line from the Minnesota border through Brookings, Huron, and on to Pierre. The Chicago and Milwaukee Railroad completed a line from Canton to Chamberlain in 1881. Connecting lines were also completed to many towns east of the Missouri River. During that era, often called the

"Dakota Boom", many towns were formed along the new railroad lines. All types of businesses were undertaken in these new towns, including pharmacies. Therefore, many pharmacists believed that it was time to organize an association to promote the interests of the rapidly growing profession.

Thirty-eight young pharmacists, most of them in business for themselves and strangers to each other, met October 20, 1886 at the Alex Mitchell Hotel, Mitchell, Dakota Territory, to form an association. They represented twenty-six towns from the southern part of the Territory. Some of those towns included Yankton, Marion, Alexandria, Parker, Flandreau, Sioux Falls, Mitchell, Kimball, Chamberlain, Gettysburg, Mellette, Iroquois, Arlington, and Watertown. W. S. Branch, Parker, recalled, "I boarded the train at Parker on my way to Mitchell to assist in organizing the DPhA. I remember Captain D. S. White, then in business in Flandreau, being on the train, and at Alexandria W. J. Hull came aboard and went with us. F. M. Hammer and L. O. Gale of Mitchell, did all they could to make our stay a pleasant one. Our meeting was held in a room at the hotel, and when we finally adjourned an organization had been affected, duly officered, with a committee appointed on the work of drawing up a permanent Constitution."[7]

The purpose of the Association, as stated in its Constitution, was "to unite the educated pharmacists and druggists of the Territory, to improve the science and art of pharmacy, and to restrict the dispensing and the sale of medicines to educated druggists and apothecaries." Membership fee was set at $2.00. The group elected Daniel S. White, Flandreau, president and W. S. Branch, Parker, as secretary. White, born in Vermont in 1837, had served as a Captain in the Second Vermont Volunteers in the Civil War. He and his wife, Maria moved to Flandreau in the late 1870s where he opened a pharmacy. White died in 1912. In 1907, only seven of the original thirty-eight charter members were still practicing in the state.

The Code of Ethics for the new Association included these principles:
1. Accept the United States Pharmacopoeia (USP) as the standard for preparations
2. Condemn making alcohol a prominent feature of a pharmacy
3. No secret formulas between doctors and pharmacists
4. Decline to give medical advice
5. Encourage advancement of knowledge of pharmacy
6. Refrain from saying detrimental things about doctors and expecting the same from them.

Dakota Territory, 1887 Pharmacy Law

The pharmacists in the new Southern District Pharmaceutical Association began lobbying the 1887 Legislature to pass a pharmacy law. The Legislature, meeting in the new capital at Bismarck since 1885, passed a new pharmacy law March 11, 1887. For the first time in the Dakota Territory, it was unlawful for anyone other than a registered pharmacist to retail, compound, or dispense drugs, medicines, and poisons. Basically, all those persons practicing pharmacy before the new law were allowed to register as a pharmacist under the new Territorial law. All former pharmacists had ninety days to pay their $2.00 fee and register as a pharmacist. A person who met any one of the following standards could obtain a registered pharmacist certificate:

1. A graduate in pharmacy
2. Engaged in the pharmacy business on their own account in the Territory
3. Engaged in the dispensing of drugs for ten years
4. Licentiate in pharmacy.

A licentiate in pharmacy was required to have had two consecutive years of practical experience in a pharmacy and pass an examination administered by the Board of Pharmacy. The new statute also permitted persons not qualifying as a registered pharmacist to become "registered assistants." Such persons had to meet two standards: be at least eighteen years of age and have had two years of experience working in a drug store. After paying the $1.00 fee, they were granted a registered assistant certificate. Assistants could act as a clerk or assistant in a drug store, but they were not entitled to engage in business on their own account.

The 1887 statute created two association districts within the Territory. Dakota Pharmaceutical Association district lay north of the seventh standard parallel [present-day North Dakota]. Southern District Pharmaceutical Association lay south of the seventh standard parallel [present-day South Dakota]. Each district had a separate Board of Pharmacy. The executive committee of the Southern District met in Parker, March 30, 1877 and recommended five names for the Board of Pharmacy to Governor Louis K. Church. He appointed J. L. Kreychie, Iroquois, H. L. Warne, Mitchell, and D. S. White, Flandreau as the first Board of Pharmacy.

The new law required the board to meet and organize for business. Duties included granting certificates to practice pharmacy to those who qualified. W. S. Branch, Parker, was paid a small yearly salary as secretary to the Board of Pharmacy. Board members were paid $5.00 a day for attending meetings. Nothing in the new law could interfere with the business of physicians in their regular practice nor prevent them from supplying drugs to their patients. Every pharmacist proprietor of a drug store was held responsible for the quality of all drugs and medicines sold or dispensed, except those sold in the original packages known as patent or proprietary medicines. Any pharmacist knowingly selling adulterated drugs was subject to prosecution and a fine up to $500.

Territorial Pharmacists

There is no surviving record of the names of pharmacists who were practicing in the Territory between 1862 and up to the first pharmacy law in 1887. Many pharmacists had moved out of the territory, retired, or died before the first pharmacy law in 1887, which required registration of pharmacists.

No records of the Territorial Board of Pharmacy have survived. However, a list of all South Dakota pharmacists who were licensed between October 1, 1890 (effective date of new South Dakota pharmacy law) and June 3, 1943, was printed in the 1943 SDPhA Annual Proceedings. That list of 2,841 pharmacists, certificate No. 1 through certificate No. 2,841, showed their South Dakota certificate number as well as the number for those who had held a Territorial certificate. W. S. Branch, Parker, held Territorial certificate No. 1. He was also the first to register with the South Dakota Board of Pharmacy on October 1, 1890 and held South Dakota certificate No. 1. Certificate No. 2,841 was issued to Guilford C. Gross, Brookings, on June 3, 1943.

According to the 1943 list, the highest Territorial certificate number issued was 623 to Lora B. Clark, Lead. She also held South Dakota certificate No. 354 issued December 4, 1890. There were another 24 pharmacists who did not have a Territorial certificate number because they were pharmacists before the 1887 Territorial pharmacy law. The 1943 list carried them as DBpTBd—in the drug business prior to organization of the Territorial Board of Pharmacy. Therefore, according to that 1943 list, containing a record of pharmacists with territorial certificate numbers, 647 pharmacists were authorized to practice in the Southern District between March 17, 1887 and September 30, 1890, a period of three years and seven months. In 1891, 386 of the territorial pharmacists were still practicing. This was reduced to 263 in 1898. Their numbers dropped to 244 in 1901. There were 11 women registered to practice in 1890, 8 in 1898, and 8 in 1901.

A Polk Directory for Minnesota and Dakota Territory, 1882-1883, Volume 3, listed 75 drug stores located in 45 cities and towns within the South Dakota part of the Dakota Territory in 1882 (See Appendix J.). The number of drug stores in the South Dakota part of the Territory grew rapidly between 1882 and 1886. A Minnesota, Dakota, and Montana Gazetteer for 1886-1887, published by R. L. Polk & Co., showed there were 183 drug stores located in 97 towns in the South Dakota part of the Territory in 1886.

The 1943 list of 2,841 pharmacists with a South Dakota certificate, as well as those with a Territorial certificate, listed seventeen women. The list showed Jennie French, Beresford, and Mrs. Callie Miller, Kimball, were in practice before the Territorial Board of Pharmacy was organized on March 17, 1887. Therefore, they had no Territorial certificate number but were authorized to practice pharmacy. Ellen H. Coates, Yankton, who held South Dakota certificate No. 13, also held the lowest Territorial certificate No. 115. Those three women, according to available records, were the earliest practicing women pharmacists.

Mary G. McClain, Tripp, held registered assistant Territorial certificate No. 113, the first woman registered assistant. Mary assisted her husband, pharmacist John McClain in a drug store in Tripp, S.D., which they opened in 1882. John was president of SDPhA 1893-1894. Mary died in 1904 and John in 1909. [Note: the author, in the summer of 2002, while checking on the graves of his parents Herman and Frieda Schuler in the Tripp, S. D. Cemetery, saw the gravestones of both John and Mary McClain.]

The seventeen women who were authorized to practice pharmacy between March 17, 1887 and October 1, 1890, [between Territorial Law and South Dakota Law] according to surviving records, were: Jennie A. Chase, Artesian; Lora B. Clark, Lead; Ellen H. Coates, Yankton; Ida A. Estey, Cavour; Mrs. L. E. Ferris, Carthage; Jennie French, Beresford; June Gage, Parker; Rose L. Graham, Erwin; Nettie C. Hall, Wessington Springs; Mrs. Callie Miller, Kimball; Elizabeth Reid, Forest City; Viola K. Smith, Spearfish; May Delle Sturgeon, Chamberlain; Sarah Jane Sturgeon, Chamberlain; Mrs. H. A.Walker, Howard; Caroline Wettergreen, Bridgewater; and Julia M. Wheeler, Appomattox.

Southern District Pharmaceutical Association, 1887-1889

The second annual meeting of the Association was held in Sioux Falls on September 6, 1887. Secretary W.S. Branch reported that 127 pharmacists, all but six who were proprietors of drug stores, had paid their $2.00 membership fee and joined the Association. Papers read and discussed at the meeting included: "Our Pharmacy Law" by H. L. Warne of Mitchell; and "Weights and Measures Used in Pharmacy" by S. W. Cleave, Bridgewater. The following officers elected at the meeting included:

former Secretary W. S. Branch, Parker, president; A. A. Bartlett, Madison, and V.B. Diehl, Scotland, vice-presidents; I. A. Keith, Lake Preston, secretary; and L.T. Dunning, Sioux Falls, continued as treasurer. Sixteen members of the Commercial Travelers, salespersons serving the drug store business, challenged the pharmacists to an afternoon baseball game.

Huron pharmacists were the hosts for the third meeting held August 21, 1888. One of the officers remembered that the delegates participated in a moonlight ride in the boat *City of Huron* on the James River. Officers elected were: W. S. Branch, continued as president; C. Burtch, Huron, and N. G. St. Marie, Frankfort, vice-presidents; I. A. Keith, Lake Preston, continued as secretary as well as L.T. Dunning, Sioux Falls, as treasurer.

The year 1889 was a big year for the Dakota Territory as well as the Southern District Pharmaceutical Association. On March 2, 1889 the United States Congress, after setting aside land for five Indian Reservations, opened the remaining land between the Black Hills and the Missouri River for settlement. Settlers followed and more pharmacies were established in the newly opened lands, between Pierre and the Black Hills.

A statehood movement was brought to fruition when the United States Congress, on February 22, 1889, provided for the division and admission of North and South Dakota into the union. A South Dakota Constitution was adopted July 4, 1889 at a Sioux Falls Constitutional Convention. The delegates called for an October 1, 1889 election to approve the Constitution, select the temporary capital, and elect a slate of state officers. Pierre won the capital fight, defeating five other cities. Newly-elected Governor Arthur Mellette and the Legislature met in Pierre October 15, 1889 to be sworn in and form a government. The South Dakota Legislature agreed to hold its first session in Pierre January 7, 1890 in the new wooden capitol on the southwest corner of the present-day capitol grounds.[8]

The Opera House in Aberdeen was the headquarters for the fourth annual Southern District Association meeting August 20, 1889. President Branch proposed a reorganization of the Association. He asked that the Association be made statutory, each registered pharmacist becoming a member of the Association by reason of their registration with the Board of Pharmacy. He asked that the secretary and treasurer of the Association also be secretary and treasurer of the Board of Pharmacy. The convention approved the concept and agreed to support it before the 1890 Legislature in Pierre. Six papers were presented at the convention, one of which was by R. M. Cotton, Tyndall, "State Board of Pharmacy Examinations, What Should They Embrace?" The following officers were elected: R. A. Mills,

Aberdeen, president; H. A. Cadd, Dell Rapids, and R. T. Hill, Aberdeen, vice-presidents; I. A. Keith, Lake Preston, was reelected secretary and L. T. Dunning, Sioux Falls, was reelected treasurer. South Dakota's population in 1890 was 328, 808.

CHAPTER 2
1890-1899

SD Pharmaceutical Association (SDPhA), 1890-1899

On January 1, 1890, Governor Arthur Mellette and the newly elected South Dakota state officials moved into the new wooden capitol in Pierre. On January 7, the Legislature met. Association President R. A. Mills, Aberdeen, appointed a Legislative Committee to help carry the pharmacy bill through the Legislature. Evidently support for the bill was strong, because it passed on March 8, 1890 with an emergency clause that required a two-thirds vote of both the House and the Senate. With the emergency clause, and the Governor's signature, the law became effective March 8 rather than the usual day of July 1.

According to the law, only registered pharmacists could compound, dispense, and sell drugs and medicines. It also created the "South Dakota State Pharmaceutical Association." The purpose of the Association was "to improve the science and art of pharmacy, and restrict the sale of medicines to regularly educated and qualified persons as provided by this act." It was a broad purpose and used by the Association throughout the years to defend their position that only pharmacists could compound, dispense, and sell drugs and medicines. The secretary and the treasurer of the Association also held the same offices with the Board of Pharmacy. The secretary, the only paid officer, earned $500 per year.

Requirements for persons to register or reregister as pharmacists, as well as assistant pharmacists, were also outlined in the law. The annual $2.00 renewal fee was paid to the Secretary of the Board of Pharmacy, who then issued a renewal of the registration certificate [license]. Although pharmacists were automatically a member of the Association by reason of their registration as a pharmacist with the Board of Pharmacy, the renewal fee remained with the Board of Pharmacy according to the 1890 law. That feature was changed in an 1893 law which specifically stated that the renewal fee was paid to the Secretary of the Association, for which the pharmacist would then receive the renewal of the certificate of registration from the Board of Pharmacy. At first, the state appropriated $300 to the Board of Pharmacy to help with expenses. The annual $300 appropriation continued until 1914.

Apparently it made little difference whether the renewal fee was paid to the Board or to the Association. A close examination of the 1898, 1901, and 1905 financial reports shows that only one set of books was kept for the Association and Board. Secretary E.C. Bent's report to the 1905 convention listed total income of $2,082 from the following: $1,638 certificate renewals, $440 Board exam fees, and $4.00 for duplicate certificates. Expenses of $2,082 showed a mixture of Board and Association expenses. Some of these expenses were: $480 per diem for the Board; $38.75 for convention expenses and for a stenographer to record the Association's 1904 convention proceedings; and $5.60 to the Ladies' Auxiliary. Treasurer W. A. Nye, Salem, reported a similar mixture of expenses. In any event, the report was always turned over to an auditing committee, who reported their findings at a later convention meeting.

The Association held its first annual meeting at Watertown August 20, 1890, and met each year thereafter. One of the highlights at the first convention meeting was a spoof dethroning the old Territorial Board of Pharmacy and replacing it with the new South Dakota Board of Pharmacy. At the evening banquet, Governor Arthur Mellette spoke on "Our Commonwealth, Young in Years but Mighty in Resources." New officers elected included: W. A. Burnham, Groton, president; George C. Bradley, De Smet, first vice-president; Charles O. Hatch, Willow Lake, second vice-president; I. A. Keith, Lake Preston, secretary; and George W. Lowery, Sioux Falls, treasurer. A new Constitution and By-laws were adopted for the South Dakota Pharmaceutical Association.

Later that summer, Governor Mellette appointed A. H. Stites, Sioux Falls, O. H. Tarbell, Watertown, and D. K. Bryant, Huron, as the first South Dakota Board of Pharmacy. They organized and commenced business on October 1, 1890. A.H. Stites later served as a State Senator in the Legislature, 1898-1902. On August 18, 1891, there were 424 pharmacists registered to practice in South Dakota.

Pharmacies were not yet licensed, so it is not known how many existed in the state. Dr. R. M. Cotton, Tyndall, however, referred to "300 drug stores in South Dakota" in a speech to the 1898 convention. Forty counties were represented at the August 1898 Mitchell convention. Counties in western South Dakota with pharmacies included: Custer, Fall River, Lawrence, Mead, Pennington, Butte, Campbell, and Stanley. Twenty-eight pharmacists were practicing in Lawrence County compared to twenty-nine in Minnehaha. Other than a railroad running from Chadron, Nebraska into the Black Hills, there were no railroads crossing the

Missouri River in 1898. Consequently, it was difficult for West River pharmacists to attend conventions in eastern South Dakota. To handle Black Hills matters, there was a local "Black Hills Pharmaceutical Association." SDPhA President C. H. Lohr, Estelline, in naming his Legislative Committee, included L. P. Jenkins of Lead, because he had past experience with the Legislative Committee of the Black Hills Association. No records of the Black Hills group have survived.

Trade Interests

Several trade interests concerned pharmacists at the 1898 convention. Competition from manufacturers, department stores, and peddlers caused the greatest concern. President C. H. Lohr, Estelline, in a floor speech, expressed concern about "the competition of the department stores who buy their goods in large quantities, thereby securing extra rebates, enabling them to sell at a good profit for about what the druggists pay for [their goods]. For example, department stores advertise the sale of Hood's Sarsaparilla for $.58, while the druggist pays $.70."[1]

Another concern was the peddlers, who traveled house to house with team and wagon. President Lohr said the peddler "pays no taxes, trades worthless remedies for a living, and cuts into the druggist's business."[2] Pharmacist J. H. Ferris, Carthage, said "The past year the patent medicine peddlers, and the wall paper peddlers have come into competition with my trade a good deal. I find that in making my own preparations, there is...a good deal more money."[3] He recommended the Association start its own manufacturing plant to make patent medicines, similar to that performed by the Minnesota Association and the Minnesota Pharmaceutical Manufacturing Company.

Secretary E. C. Bent told the convention, "We are blind to our own interests, to work here in South Dakota trying to sell patent medicines for the eastern manufacturers, who have gotten rich off this country, when we can just as well put up superior preparations of our own and receive a larger profit on them."[4]

H. P. Pettigrew, Sioux Falls, in a prize paper presented at the 1898 convention said, "The preparation of medicine for the sick, is almost completely overshadowed by the patent medicines. The prescription business is now of little importance to the druggist. The only solution...is for the pharmacist to turn attention to manufacturing. Sell your own products and keep the manufacturers profit for yourself. In the year 1887 we put up several hundred $.05 packages; 520 $.20 articles; 1,793 $.25 articles; 403 $.50 articles; and 116 $1.00 articles. The sale amounted to $829 for that year. Total costs were $214 and the profit was $615."[5]

The convention agreed that President Lohr appoint a special committee of Secretary E. C. Bent, Dell Rapids; H. P. Pettigrew, Sioux Falls; I. M. Helmey, Canton; C. M. Serles, Salem; and A. H. Stites, Sioux Falls, to investigate and recommend some plan for a uniform line of home remedies and pharmaceuticals to be adopted by the retail pharmacists of the state. He asked them to make a report by November 1, 1898.

The study committee, reporting on that date, said that South Dakota was too young a state to organize a home plant to manufacture pharmaceuticals. They also said it was not feasible for pharmacists to each prepare their own remedies and sell them at a uniform price. While the preparations would be uniform in style, they would not be so in preparation nor would they possess the same degree of excellence. Lastly, they recommended that the Association work with the Minnesota Pharmaceutical Manufacturing Company to market their manufactured remedies in South Dakota.

Compounding vs. Manufacturing

John Wyeth and Brother, Philadelphia, paid for a one-page advertisement in the 1891 SDPhA Annual Proceedings announcing that they were manufacturers of elegant pharmaceutical preparations. The preparations included: compressed tablet triturates; sugar coated compressed pills; compressed hypodermic tablets; compressed lozenges of U.S.P.; compressed cocaine tablets and lozenges for hay fever; fluid extracts; elixirs; syrups; Peptonic pills; Menthol Pencils; and Marvins Pure Cod Liver Oil. They provided special price quotations for compressing pills in quantities.

Perhaps the advertisement was one of the sources John McClain, Tripp, 1893-1894 SDPhA president, used to prepare his award winning paper on compounding vs. manufacturing for the 1898 Mitchell convention. He said he was speaking about:

"The rank and file druggists who gain a living selling and dispensing medicines. I do not say compounding for that is almost a past art. In my younger days, I spent hours, yes, days at a time compounding and mixing, making pills, plasters, tinctures, elixirs, syrups, etc., but now alas, I hardly know how to roll up a pill mass.

"The physician in order to please his patient...began to seek how the obnoxious taste of the drug might be concealed. Thus the sugar coated pill was introduced, and the syrups and aromatic elixirs. Afterward came the wafer, then the capsule, and now we have the compressed tablet. Until recently these were made largely by the retail pharmacist. The work of the pharmacist ran along smoothly for some time, but as time passed the manufacturing chemists, those who had been formerly engaged in the manufacture of that branch of pharmaceuticals called chemicals, conceived the idea of enlarging their business and gathering unto themselves the emolument that was justly due the pharmacists.

"At first this was confined to the manufacture of pills, and the fluid and solid extracts, but gradually one after another of the original productions of the retail pharmacy have been gathered in by syndicates and centralized under the heading of pharmaceutical preparations, and sold to the trade in general, physicians and department stores not excepted. We must make our own remedies, not have them made."[6]

H. P. Pettigrew, Ph.G., Sioux Falls, in another paper at the same convention expressed strong support for preparing tinctures from fluid extracts rather than from crude drugs. He reminded the audience that in about 1888, pharmaceutical authorities were against the growing custom of preparing tinctures from fluid extracts. They preferred making a tincture from the crude drug by percolation. Pettigrew believed:

"there is no earthly reason why a fluid extract properly diluted, should not constitute a good tincture," [alluding to the fact that druggists were too busy working long hours each day to have time to be a manufacturing pharmacy.]

"Hence the growing custom of preparing tinctures from fluid extracts had been a growing one. This practice encouraged...the makers of fluid extracts who attach to their containers printed labels bearing directions for the preparation of tinctures and infusions.[7]"

Pettigrew presented statistical evidence from his pharmacy to back his argument. In October 1887, 42 out of 200 prescriptions called for one or two tinctures and by 1898, only 25 out of 200 prescriptions called for tinctures. He said:

"It seems...there is no good reason why two sets of fluid preparations of the crude drugs, to say nothing of elixirs, syrups, solid and powdered extracts, pills, and tablets should be kept in stock. The only fluid preparations needed in the practice of medicine are the fluid extracts, and the physician can more successfully prescribe the fluid extract, diluting it to suit the requirements of the case, than the tincture, expecting the druggist to always have in stock a lot of tinctures, many of which are seldom called for and to keep them always fresh. The use of tinctures should be abolished.

"Of the 70 tinctures of the pharmacopoeia, a few are in common and quite constant use, others being called for but at rare intervals. Fifty of the tinctures of the pharmacopoeia might as well be dropped, because...a fluid extract properly made, of official strength, and in the case of the powerful alkaloid drugs, assayed, is the only necessary and rational liquid preparation of the crude drug to use. Every pharmacist should have at least a moderate sized, clean, well-lighted laboratory furnished with the necessary apparatus, for carrying on this manufacturing process. It becomes then as easy to make and assay a fluid extract as a tincture."[8]

An example of the pharmaceutical industry of the late 1880s is described by Cowen and Helfand as, "The progress made by this new industry is demonstrated by the catalogue of the American firm, G.D. Searle, which by the late 1880s listed 400 fluid extracts, 150 elixirs, 100 syrups, 75 powdered extracts, and 25 tinctures and other drug forms. Searle, too, claimed uniformity of potency for its products."[9] They further report that "The 19th Century [1800-1900] did not see the end of the art of compounding, but the art did give way, however grudgingly, to new technology. It has been estimated that a 'broad knowledge of compounding' was still essential for 80% of the prescriptions dispensed in the 1920s."[10]

Conventions

Association annual meetings were held in Madison, 1891; Sioux Falls, 1892; Yankton, 1893; YMCA rooms Huron, 1894; a tent on the Chautauqua grounds at Lake Madison, 1895; Odd Fellows Hall, Madison, 1896; Germania Hall, Sioux Falls, 1897; Masonic Hall, Mitchell, 1898; and Watertown, 1899. Entertainment at Madison in 1891, included taking the conventioneers, via a motor line, to Lake Madison for a boat ride on the steamer *City of Madison*. The Ladies' Cornet Band of Madison furnished music for the boat ride. The Madison pharmacists must have been good hosts, because the annual meeting was held at Madison three times in eight years.

Papers were presented at each of the SDPhA conventions, including seven at the 1894 Huron gathering. One of those papers was "The Physicians" presented by Nettie C. Hall, Wessington Springs. Nettie C. Hall was elected second vice-president at the Huron meeting. The SDPhA Annual Proceedings for 1896, 1898, and 1915, all show that Nettie C. Hall was the first woman officer of SDPhA, serving in 1894-1895. Mrs. L. E. Ferris, Carthage, was elected second vice-president at the 1898 convention. Mrs. Ferris held Territorial certificate No. 620 and on October 1,

1890 she reregistered and was issued South Dakota certificate No. 279. E. C. Bent, Dell Rapids, was elected secretary at the 1897 Sioux Falls meeting. He served as secretary for twenty-six years, retiring in 1923. At the 1897 Sioux Falls convention, C. H. Lohr, Estelline, was elected president of the Association. Lohr had been elected to the S.D. House of Representatives in 1896 and served Deuel County in the Legislature, 1897-1898.

Pharmacists from forty counties attended the 1898 Association convention in Mitchell. The Association had five standing committees: Legislative, Education, Trade Interests, Finance and Auditing, and Pharmacy and Queries. Subjects for the Queries Committee were usually assigned by the president. The papers were read by the authors and then discussed on the convention floor. A prize committee judged who gave the best paper. First prize often paid as much as $15. Three members were assigned to each of the standing committees. However, five members were assigned to Legislative and Trade Interests. A delegate was selected to attend the APhA national convention. Pharmacists were selected to attend each of the nearby Association conventions in Minnesota, Iowa, North Dakota, and Nebraska. Travel expenses were paid by SDPhA. The National Association of Retail Druggists (NARD) was organized in 1899 to protect the interests of retail druggists.

Conventions in the 1890s included indoor and outdoor sports. Contestants participated in various kinds of events to be judged for one of three top prizes. Some of the indoor sports for the ladies, at the August 1898 meeting were: guessing the age of President Lohr, number of beans in a bottle, and most graceful lady waltzer. Some of the indoor sports for men were: guessing the number of wood toothpicks in a glass jar; over-stitch sewing contest, best work done in five minutes. Prizes included a Dickens Tobacco Jar, one-half pound White Rose extract, and one dozen Fuller and Fuller tooth brushes.

Outdoor sports at Mitchell consisted of seventeen different events. Some of them were: ladies' air-gun shooting contest, mens' bow and arrow contest, mens' thirty-yard foot race, ladies' thirty-yard hoop-rolling race, baseball throw for men and traveling men; tug-of-war with eight traveling men vs. eight men pharmacists, ladies' bicycle race, and ladies' twenty-yard teaspoon and egg race. Prizes for each event were awarded for first, second, and third. Some of the prizes included: one box Greenleaf Little Havanas, one-half dozen of Eli Lilly's Formaseptol, one dozen Euthymol Tooth Paste, six quarts Muscatel wine, box Violets, and a handsome fruit dish. One event for the gentlemen was to identify twenty-five specimens. First prize for the identification of specimens was awarded to H. P. Pettigrew, Sioux Falls, who was awarded six gallons of mixed paint donated by Heath and Milligan.

There were 40 different contributors of prizes and cash for the 1898 convention. Some of them were: Fuller and Fuller Co., Bartlett Cigar Co., Dr. Daniel's Medicine Co., Schlitz Brewing Co., Eli Lilly & Co., Merck Pharmacy, and Philadelphia College of Pharmacy.

A stenographer recorded the entire convention. The 1898 proceedings, consisting of 111 pages, were printed by State Publishing Co. of Pierre at a cost of $143 for 600 copies. On December 1, 1898, Secretary E. C. Bent mailed copies to all of the registered pharmacists and assistant pharmacists. The 1890 pharmacy law required that the Association provide an annual report to the Governor of South Dakota. A copy of the annual proceedings was provided to the Governor to meet that statutory requirement.

SD Board of Pharmacy, 1890-1899

Professional Titles

After a careful review of the pharmacy laws of 1887, 1890, 1893, and 1895, it is obvious that early lawmakers used a variety of words to describe pharmacists and pharmacies. Generally, bills in the Legislature affecting professions are carefully reviewed by the persons within those professions. Presumably, SDPhA legislative committees worked with Legislators to secure passage of the early pharmacy laws. A tabulation of the pharmacy laws shows that the following was used to describe the place of business: drug store 8; pharmacy or store 9; and retail drug store 2. The word pharmacy was used in a professional sense 25 times. The word pharmacist was used 62 times. The word druggist was not used in 1887, 1890, or 1893, however, it was used three times in an 1895 amendment.

Pharmacists used all of the above words in talking about their profession. For example, President C.H. Lohr speaking to the 1898 convention, used pharmacist 3 times, druggist 11 times, drug store 1 time, and quoted from the *Omaha Druggist*. He also mentioned the Druggists' Mutual Fire Insurance Co. (It wasn't until 1927 that the APhA House of Delegates favored the word "pharmacy" for drug store, and "pharmacist" for druggist, but the change was slow throughout the years. There was strong sentiment at the 1950 APhA convention to use pharmacist and pharmacy rather than druggist and drug store.)

1890 Pharmacy Law

With the advent of statehood, the South Dakota Legislature meeting in Pierre, was required to pass new laws. Much of the 1887 Territorial Law was carried over into the 1890 South Dakota Pharmacy Law.

The new pharmacy law regulated the practice of pharmacy in the state of South Dakota. It specifically stated that it shall be unlawful for any person, other than a registered pharmacist, to retail, compound or dispense drugs, medicines, or poisons. It was also unlawful for any person "to open or conduct any pharmacy or drug store" unless such person was a registered pharmacist.

Any person of good moral character and temperate habits, and paying the $2.00 registration fee, was entitled to register as a pharmacist if they met any one of these standards:

- licentiate in pharmacy or
- graduate from a reputable college of pharmacy or
- hold a certificate of registration from the South Dakota Board of Pharmacy at the time this act takes effect or
- engaged in practice of pharmacy in the Territory of Dakota, provided that they are now and have been, continuously engaged in said practice.

All of the above, except a licentiate, could register without a Board examination. A licentiate needed to be eighteen years of age, have had three years practical experience compounding drugs in a drug store, and pass a Board examination. Pharmacists from other states could register by producing proof that they had been registered by examination.

A person who was eighteen years of age, of good moral character, with two years service under a registered pharmacist, and who passed a Board examination was eligible to become a registered assistant pharmacist. Any registered assistant pharmacist had the right to compound medicines or sell poisons, under the direct supervision of a registered pharmacist, and take charge of a drug store or pharmacy during the temporary absence of the registered pharmacist. The 1887 law used the term "registered assistants" whereas the 1890 law used the term "assistant pharmacists."

Physicians were also affected by the new law. Firstly, nothing in the pharmacy act could interfere with the business of physicians or prevent them from supplying drugs to their patients. Secondly, no part of the law could be construed to give the right to a physician to furnish any intoxicating liquors to be used as a beverage, on prescription or otherwise.

The first South Dakota Board of Pharmacy organized for business on October 1, 1890. On August 18, 1891, the Board reported that 424 pharmacists were in good standing and registered to practice in the new state. The basis for their registration was as follows: 365 reregistered because they held a Territorial certificate (11 of whom were women); 21 reregistered because they were engaged in practice before May 17, 1887 when the Territorial Board was created; 18 were licentiates from other states and reciprocated into South Dakota; 9 were graduates of a college of pharmacy; and 11 registered by examination. Also practicing in the state were nineteen assistant pharmacists, six of whom were women.[11]

Of the 424 pharmacists, 51 held M.D. degrees and 16 held Ph.G. degrees. Of the 16 pharmacists with a Ph.G. degree, 9 showed the college of pharmacy from which they graduated: 6 from the Chicago College of Pharmacy; 1 from Massachusetts College of Pharmacy; 1 from Ontario College of Pharmacy; and 1 from the Philadelphia College of Pharmacy. Eleven of the pharmacists were women.

There were also thirty-one registered pharmacists who lived out-of-state.

An 1894 list of pharmacists showed 415 Territorial certificates and 26 had been engaged in practice before May 17, 1887 when the Territorial Board of Pharmacy was created. The increase over the 1891 list can be attributed to the fact it took longer for some pharmacists to reregister for the new 1890 South Dakota Law.

In 1898, there were 411 pharmacists practicing in 153 South Dakota towns in 52 counties. The college training of the 411 pharmacists was as follows: 19 with Ph.G. [Pharmacy Graduate], 37 with M.D. Most of the other 355 pharmacists were carry-over pharmacists with Territorial certificates; however, those with enough practical experience could qualify to take the Board examinations. Only a few would have had more than an eighth grade education. (It wasn't until 1906, that the Board of Pharmacy required at least one year of high school to take the Board examinations.) There were also 68 out-of-state pharmacists. Eight women were registered pharmacists, one of whom held an M.D. degree. Nettie C. Hall, Wessington Springs, was elected vice-president, 1894-1895. Fourteen registered assistants pharmacists also practiced in the state, two of whom were women. (The 1887 law referred to "registered assistants" whereas the 1890 law referred to "assistant pharmacists.")

Board Examinations 1890-1891

The first South Dakota Board of Pharmacy consisted of A. H. Stites, Sioux Falls; O.H. Tarbell, Watertown; and D. K. Bryant, Huron. The secretary was I. A. Keith, Lake Preston and the treasurer was G. W. Lowry, Sioux Falls. Board examinations in 1890-1891 were conducted in Sioux Falls, Pierre, Aberdeen, and Huron. Because of transportation problems to the Black Hills, the Board asked Julius Deetken, Deadwood, to conduct the exam in that city. The exams were mailed to Deetken who returned them to the Board for correction. At the five examination sites, 30 candidates appeared, of which 11 passed and were registered as pharmacists,

13 failed, and 6 were registered as assistant pharmacists. Candidates for the Board exams could purchase *Gray's Pharmaceutical Quiz Compendium*, to help prepare for the exams. The neatly-bound book cost $1.50 and contained 1,500 questions and answers on pharmacy, botany, and chemistry. According to the publisher, it was the only standard of its kind on the market.

Board member A.H. Stites gave the chemistry exam to the candidates. His chemistry exam consisted of twenty questions. Some of his questions were: What is the effect of dilute sulfuric acid on starch? Give the chemical names of the two official iodides of mercury. How is tannic acid prepared? How is citrine ointment prepared, what reaction occurs? Give the official name for lunar caustic and state its mode of preparation. How is boric acid prepared? Give the official chemical name for tartar emetic, calomel, white precipitate, alum, corrosive sublimate, and glauber salt.

Board member O. H. Tarbell presented nineteen questions on materia medica. Some of his questions were: What is an alkaloid? How and of what is saccharated pepsin made? Name two plants that contain strychnine. Name six coal tar products used as a medicine. What would be the effect of an overdose of antipyrine? How many grains of opium in ten grains of Dover powder? Give dose and medical use of chloral hydrate. What is the formula for U.S.P. compound cathartic pill?

Board member D. K. Bryant presented ten questions in pharmacy. Some of his two and four part questions were: What systems of weights based on the grain are used in pharmacy and state the denominations of each? What is specific gravity and how is it ascertained? Give formula for making paregoric and give its officinal name. How many grains of cocaine in seven drachms of a four percent solution? What are oleoresins? Is glycerite of tannin officinal?

The Board gave four examinations in 1890-1891, and it appears each board member had a different set of questions for each of the four examinations. Presumably, it was very difficult for candidates to pass on information about questions from one examination to the next.

Board examinations were conducted in one day. The exams given to six candidates in the Hotel Arcade, Watertown, October 4, 1893, started at noon and were over by 6:00 p.m. Board examinations given to sixteen candidates in the Kendall Opera House, Parker, January 10, 1894, started at 1:00 p.m. and lasted until 8:00 p.m. Of the 16 candidates, 6 were registered as pharmacists, 4 as assistant pharmacists, and 6 failed.

A. H. Stites, said this about the 1896 examinations: "At present the examinations consist of a written examination in pharmacy, which is partly theory; materia medica, and general chemistry; an oral examination, which consists of reading prescriptions, doses, toxicology; manipulation, which is filling prescriptions, making pills, powders, ointments, etc.; identification of specimens."[12] A list of twenty-five drugs was also given to the class for identification.

In 1896, the Board of Pharmacy consisted of A. H. Stites, Sioux Falls; C. F. Ayer, Sioux Falls; and N. J. Bleser, Milbank. They met four times in 1895-1896 and gave the examinations as follows: October 9, 1895, Sherman House, Aberdeen; January 8, 1896, City Hall, Sioux Falls; April 8, 1896, Depot Hotel, Huron; and June 24, 1896, Pierce Hotel, Yankton. Meeting times and locations were determined according to railroad transportation schedules. During the period, 46 candidates appeared; 28 were registered as pharmacists, 7 as assistant pharmacists, and 11 failed.

The Board always met the night before the exam day to organize the exam as well as conduct official Board business. The three Board members divided the exams among themselves, one chemistry, one materia medica, and one pharmacy, each containing twenty questions. At the end of the three exams, all three members united for the examination in manipulation, oral, and identification. Usually the one-day exam started at 9:00 a.m. and finished by 6:00 p.m. The Board took their exam papers and corrected them at home. Usually, it took six to eight days to send the results to Secretary I. A. Keith at Lake Preston. He notified the candidates of the results.[13]

At one 1896 business meeting, the Board reported they had received $1,476 in license renewals and fees. That same year they spent $1,279. Board Chairperson A. H. Stites, said "The Board has been handicapped in its efforts to enforce the pharmacy law by a lack of funds with which to conduct prosecutions."[14] The license renewal had been raised from $2.00 to $3.00 in 1894. Stites said "the majority of the druggists regard this as a burden. To increase the fees by statute would certainly cause a wholesale revolt."[15]

The board was required to keep a book containing information on each registrant. (These records are still in the possession of the South Dakota Board of Pharmacy.) The Board began regulating the practice of pharmacy according to law. The three-member Board of Pharmacy conducted examination for applicants and performed other duties. Such duties included reporting annually to the Governor and the South Dakota Pharmaceutical Association upon the condition of pharmacy in the state. The board enforced the provision of the law which made it illegal for any pharmacist to adulterate drugs or substitute one material for another. Any person violating any part of the law, was subject to prosecution by the state's attorney in the county where the violation occurred.

1893 Pharmacy Law

In the 1893 Legislative Session, H. B. 104 was introduced to create a new pharmacy law. It is not clear as to the reasons for this act however, there are a few changes. Almost all of the 1890 law was included in H. B. 104. Some significant additions included:

- Name changed to South Dakota Pharmaceutical Association

- To register as a pharmacist, one needed to be a licentiate in pharmacy, or a graduate from a reputable college of pharmacy

- Licentiates in pharmacy needed to be eighteen years of age, (1) have had three years experience in the practice of pharmacy, or (2) hold diploma from a medical college, and (3) pass board examinations. A graduate from a college of pharmacy and a graduate from a medical college needed to pass a board examination.

- Unlawful for anyone to use the title of registered pharmacist if not registered as a pharmacist

- The $3.00 renewable fee for a certificate of registration was payable to the secretary of SDPhA, however, the renewal certificate was issued by the secretary of the Board of Pharmacy

- Salary of SDPhA secretary set at $500 per year

- Pharmacist selling poisons must keep a poison register and record the name and address of the purchaser

- Board given power to revoke a pharmacist's certificate of registration, should that person become incompetent or disqualified. That person had the right of a hearing before the Board and could appeal its decision to the Circuit Court.

1895 Pharmacy Law Amendment

Chapter 149, Session Laws of the 1895 Legislature, provided a clear directive to the pharmacy school at South Dakota Agricultural College. The law provided two more ways for pharmacy students over eighteen years of age to register as licensed pharmacists:

Section 1. Persons holding diplomas entitled to license. Any person who has received a diploma for the pharmacy course at South Dakota Agricultural College, and who has, before or after graduation, practiced pharmacy for one year under a licensed druggist in South Dakota, in a drug store where prescriptions are compounded, shall, upon passing a Board of Pharmacy examination, receive a license from the Board to practice pharmacy in any county in South Dakota. Said Board shall grant said license to said applicant without unnecessary delay.

Section 2. Examination. Any person who has made the following preparations shall be entitled to a druggist's license upon passing a satisfactory examination before the Board of Pharmacy; one year's work in college of pharmacy course and two year's work in an accredited drug store.

Required Board Examination Grades

Board of Pharmacy Regulations approved in October 1897 stated that applicants for registration by examination are required to obtain an average grade of 65%, and not less than 50% in any of the following branches: Pharmacy, Materia Medica, Chemistry, Manipulation, Oral Examination, and Identification of Drugs. For an assistant pharmacist certificate, an applicant must have an average of 60% and not less than 40% in any of the above named branches. New regulations approved in October 1899 required an average grade of 70% and not less than 55% in any of the branches to register as a pharmacist. Registered assistant pharmacists needed an average grade of 55% and not less than 45%. Candidates registering by reciprocity needed to have an average of 80% passing grade in their board examinations from their home state.

The Board of Pharmacy gave the same examination to candidates for registered pharmacists and for assistant pharmacists. Those with lower grades at least had a chance to qualify as a registered assistant pharmacist. However, a SDPhA Committee on Board of Pharmacy, chaired by R. M. Cotton, Tyndall, presented a resolution to the 1898 SDPhA convention urging the Board to give separate examinations for those seeking registration as a registered pharmacist and for those seeking to be registered as an assistant pharmacist. The resolution was adopted. It was some time before the Board acted upon the resolution.

Educational Requirements for Board Examinations

The Board of Pharmacy apparently had great latitude as to the educational requirements needed for an applicant to take the board examinations who had three years of practical experience in a drug store. In some cases, applicants had less than graduation from the eighth grade. The Committee on Board of Pharmacy at the 1898 convention presented this resolution which was adopted: Before an applicant for either a registered pharmacist or registered assistant pharmacist can take the Board examinations, they must show proof they have an education equivalent to the common school requirement of the state [eighth grade], either by examination or certificate from such school.

In 1898, the Board of Pharmacy, consisting of N. J. Bleser, Milbank; James Lewis, Canton; I. A. Keith, Lake Preston, and Secretary E. C. Bent, Dell Rapids, met four times—Redfield, Parker, Watertown, and Mitchell. During the year, thirty-eight candidates took the one-day board examinations, 8:00 a.m. to 9:00 p.m. Twenty-eight were registered as pharmacists, five were registered as assistant pharmacists; and five failed.

Four of the thirty-eight had a Ph.G. degree from a College of Pharmacy. All four of the Ph.G. applicants passed the examinations and became registered pharmacists. Board Secretary E. C. Bent earlier had purchased needed chemicals and supplies for the practical work in the examinations. The Board that year had a total income, including renewal fees, of $1,561. Their total expenditures were $1,263.

Some of the complaints before the 1898 Board of Pharmacy were:
- A pharmacist at Hazel was violating the pharmacy law and Secretary Bent was asked to investigate
- A pharmacy operating at Mound City without a pharmacist in charge was ordered to comply
- A complaint that the pharmacy law was violated at Blunt was handled by the Board when the pharmacist agreed to comply
- A registered assistant pharmacist was conducting a drug store at Marion without a registered pharmacist. The Board agreed to prosecute the assistant pharmacist, however, the owner secured a registered pharmacist immediately
- A delinquent pharmacist who had not renewed his license was dropped from the roles.

SD College of Pharmacy, 1890-1899

The Territorial Legislature, meeting in Yankton, passed an Act to establish an Agricultural College at Brookings. Governor N. G. Ordway signed the Act on February 21, 1881. The citizens of Brookings had donated an eighty-acre tract of land northeast of the city for college purposes. It wasn't until 1883, however, that the Legislature approved the sale of $25,000 in bonds to finance the construction of a college building.[16]

Dr. George Lilley, Corning, Iowa, was selected as president in June 1884, at a salary of $1,500 per year. The building, known as Old Central, was partially opened for classes on September 24, 1884. The staff consisted of two paid instructors and two volunteers. That year's catalog stated that a candidate for admission must be at least fourteen years of age, and pass examinations in Arithmetic, Geography, Reading, Spelling,

Penmanship, History of the United States, Hygiene, and English Grammar. Tuition, room, fires, and lights were free for residents. Nonresidents paid $5.00 a term. Board was $2.50 per week.

A pharmacy school was established at State College, Brookings, by an act of the Board of Regents, June 19, 1888. Pharmacy was first mentioned in the 1887-1888 catalog. It read "A couple of terms of elective work are offered in the senior year of both courses [Agriculture and Domestic Economy] to students who may desire to enter upon a preparation for the business of druggist. This new course requires considerable work in weighing, measuring, making decoctions, distilling, and filtering."[17] The pharmacy laboratory and classroom space were located on the third floor of Old Central.

The 1888-1889 catalog listed the courses for a two-year course in pharmacy.

First Year
  Fall Term; Physics, English Composition, Bookkeeping,
      Elementary Algebra
  Spring Term; Physics, Physiology, Rhetoric, Elementary Algebra
  Summer Term; Chemistry, Materia Medica, Botany, Geometry.

Second Year
  Fall term; Chemistry, Materia Medica and Toxicology,
      Geometry, Botany
  Spring Term; Chemistry, Pharmacy, General History, Latin
  Summer Term; Pharmacy, English History, Physiology and
      Hygiene, Latin.

The course was "designed to fit young men and women for the business of druggists." Ten students enrolled in the course, under the direction of Professor James H. Shepard who taught the first course in pharmacy. Shepard Hall was named after him. The faculty, in August 1890, recommended that five of the students be awarded certificates of completion of the two-year course in pharmacy.

The five graduates and their theses were: Irwin D. Aldrich, Elmira, SD, *Some Unsolved Problems for Pharmacists*; William S. Bentley, Detroit, Michigan, *Why not the Metric System?*; Grant Houston, Virgil, SD, *Symptoms and Physiological Action of Poisons*; Farley D. McLouth, Brookings, SD, *The Birth of Chemistry*; Hugh H. West, White, SD, *A Few Facts About Homeopathy*. There was a public reading of the theses in the College Chapel at 10:00 a.m. Tuesday August 19, 1890.

Cyril G. Hopkins was Acting Professor of Pharmacy 1893-1894. It wasn't until 1895, however, that five students were awarded a Ph.G.

[Pharmacy Graduate] degree. That 1895 class was recognized as the first class graduating in pharmacy. Class members included: Elmer E. Briggs, William H. Knox, Elmer A. Lents, William Murphy, and Bower T. Whitehead.

In 1895, David F. Jones, Ph.G. Northwestern University, was named to lead the new Department of Pharmacy. He stayed one year and then purchased a retail drug store in Watertown. In August 1896, Professor Bower T. Whitehead, Ph.C. (Pharmaceutical Chemist) Northwestern University, was named Head, Department of Pharmacy. Whitehead earned his B.S. degree in 1897 and his M.S. Degree in 1901, both from the Agricultural College in Brookings. In 1898, the Department of Pharmacy announced that Ph.G. graduates could obtain a B.S. in Pharmacy with two more years of study. However, most of the pharmacy students were satisfied with the Ph.G. degree and few pursued the four-year course for a B.S. degree.

SDSU College of Pharmacy Professor Clark T. Eidsmoe, in 1974, praised Professor Bower T. Whitehead, "It is conceded moreover that the burden of the development of the Department of Pharmacy was borne by Professor Whitehead, who almost single-handedly brought pharmacy to a standard where it commanded respect second to no other department of the college."[18]

SDSU College of Pharmacy Professor Dr. Kenneth Redman said in 1983, "the College of Pharmacy has a long and illustrious existence. With its start in 1887, it is the second oldest school still in existence in the states bordering South Dakota and it is the eighth oldest College of Pharmacy in the United States."[19]

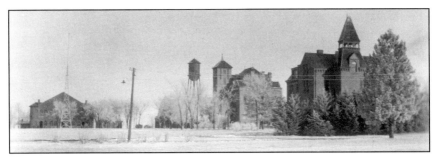

Early view SD State College. Old Central right, next Old North.

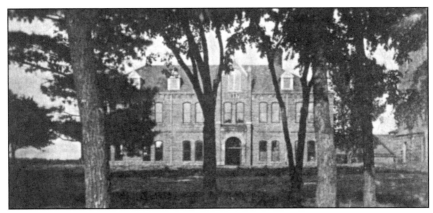

Old Chemistry Building.

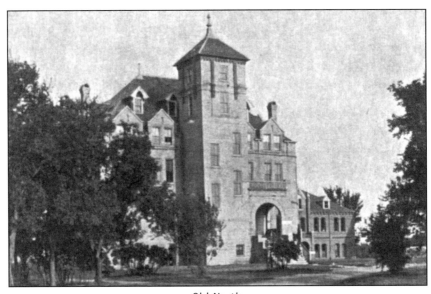

Old North

A History of Pharmacy in South Dakota

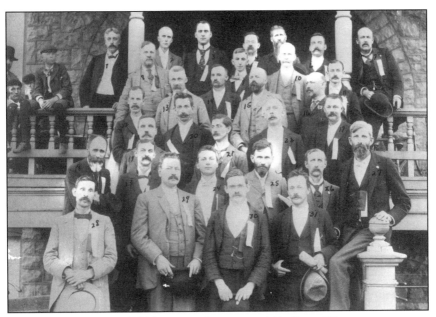

1896 SDPhA convention group at Madison, SD.

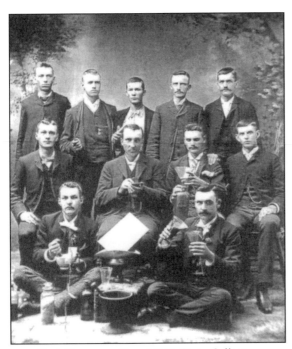

First Pharmacy Class 1889, State College.
Professor Shepard, second on left middle row.

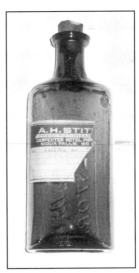

A.H. Stites prescription
bottle from his pharma-
cy in Carpenter Hotel,
Sioux Falls, 1890.
Member of first SD
Board of Pharmacy.
*(Photo courtesy of Bill
Juffernbruch)*

CHAPTER 3
1900-1909

SD Pharmaceutical Association (SDPhA), 1900-1909

Board of Pharmacy members were appointed by the Governor, one from each of three districts according to the 1890 law. Governor Charles N. Herried, in a 1903 meeting with the SDPhA Legislative Committee, said he was satisfied with the combined statutory relationship of the Board and the Association. However, he felt that Board members should be selected at large from throughout the state, rather than by districts. The pharmacists agreed and the law was changed. Each year, the Association needed to recommend the names of three practicing pharmacists, doing a retail drug business in this state, to the Governor. The Governor appointed one of them to the three-member Board of Pharmacy, who had staggered three-year terms.

A resolution adopted at the 1901 convention, designated *Northwestern Druggist* as the official news organ of the Association. Secretary E. C. Bent later reported that his office received complimentary copies of *Merck's Report*, *American Druggist*, *Pharmaceutical Era*, *Northwestern Druggist*, *Meyer Brothers' Druggist*, *Druggists' Circular*, *Wisconsin Pharmaceutical Review*, and *Retail Druggist*. Bent, who owned and operated a pharmacy in Dell Rapids, was paid $50 a month for being secretary to the Association and to the Board.

There were 445 in-state pharmacists, sixty out-state pharmacists, and twenty-seven assistant pharmacists on the membership roles in 1901. Drug stores were located in fifty South Dakota counties. Drug stores were not yet licensed so no record was kept as to the number of stores throughout the state. However, as an example, the drug store owners in the City of Yankton in 1901 included: F. A. Brecht, E. M. Coates, and George Tammen. A drug store was also located in each of the towns of Gayville, Lesterville, and Volin. The population of Yankton County in 1900 was 12,649.

Conventions

The highlight of the year for many pharmacists was the business and social gathering at the annual SDPhA convention. Mrs. Abbie Jarvis,

M.D. and pharmacist, Faulkton, served as vice-president in 1899. Forty-two pharmacists and twenty-four spouses and commercial travelers met in the Opera House at Redfield August 1901. Guessing contests, games of chance, and foot races, totaling twenty-seven events, kept the pharmacists, commercial travelers, and ladies entertained. A dance sponsored by the Commercial Travelers at the Opera House was well attended.

Similar events occurred at Flandreau in 1902. Fifty dollars in prizes, divided between first, second, and third, were awarded for the best papers presented at the convention. Papers needed to be typewritten and on scientific subjects. A $5.00 gold piece was also available to unregistered drug clerks for writing the best paper on "The Ideal Pharmacist." The Ladies' Auxiliary was organized in the parlors of the Woodmen Hall at Flandreau, August 5, 1902. Twelve charter members elected Mrs. W. A. Simpson as the first president. A constitution and by-laws were approved in 1903. Eighty-two pharmacists gathered for the 1904 convention. Forty-five of them attended the opening session at the Mitchell Courthouse to hear President F.G.Stickles, Mellette, greet the members and report that the Association was in a good financial condition. Forty-six ladies and nineteen commercial travelers also joined in convention events. There were sixty-four donors of prizes and cash to the convention. Dr. Oscar Oldberg, Dean Northwestern College of Pharmacy, Chicago, spoke to the delegates.

At Aberdeen in 1905, 146 people, of which fifty-seven were pharmacists, all from east of the river, joined the festivities. The group went as a body to visit Jewett Wholesale Drug House. On Friday, all went by special train car to Tacoma Park along the river, about ten miles away, where they participated in foot races, ball games, rooster catching, and guessing games. But were good times coming to an end? Delegates approved the following resolution at the Aberdeen meeting: "Although we favor the social features at our [conventions], we are of the opinion that they should be so limited and arranged as not to interfere with the regular business sessions, which should always be regarded of first importance."[1] The Commercial Travelers' Auxiliary was organized August 1, 1905 at the Aberdeen convention.

At the Association gathering at Sioux Falls in August 1906, automobiles were loaded with people at the Cataract Hotel, and driven to all parts of the city before returning for a Wednesday evening banquet. The Brown Drug Company had provided transportation for those wanting to visit the State Penitentiary. On Friday morning, at 9 a.m., the delegates boarded a train at the Great Northern Depot to be taken to a picnic in the Sioux Falls area. Conventioneers were reminded that the train would return to the city at 7:45 p.m. that day. At Huron the next year, thirty-seven pharmacists and seventeen ladies toured Huron College before going to the State Fairgrounds for contests, sports, and a picnic, after which Governor Coe Crawford spoke.

In 1908, 264 badges were issued at the Watertown convention. Entertainment that first evening at the Courthouse was a concert played by the Fourth Regiment, South Dakota National Guard Band. The Ladies' Auxiliary offered a $5.00 gold piece for the best typewritten paper on any subject. That same year, there were 518 registered pharmacists and twenty registered assistant pharmacists practicing in the state. Lead was selected for the August 1909 convention.

Very few west river pharmacists were able to attend east river conventions until 1908. In 1907, the Chicago Northwestern Railway built a bridge across the Missouri River at Pierre and then finished a line of track to Rapid City. The Chicago, Milwaukee, & St. Paul Railway built a line from Chamberlain to Murdo in 1906, from Murdo to Rapid City in 1907, and from Mobridge to Lemmon in 1909. Not only did this permit statewide travel, it also resulted in many new pharmacies being started in newly formed towns. Automobiles were also chugging along on county dirt roads. By 1912, there were 30,000 automobiles in South Dakota. That year, South Dakota State College, to meet the demand for auto mechanics, began offering a three-week course on gas engines, ignitions, electrical and cooling systems, and car repairs. Tuition was $1.00.

The three-day August convention at Lead was well attended. A reception, followed with readings and musical numbers, provided entertainment the first evening. There was a grand ball at the City Park the next evening. On the last day, conventioneers boarded a special train at 8:00 a.m., traveled through Spearfish Canyon and stopped at Spearfish Falls. A stop at Spearfish for a clay-pigeon shooting contest was included in the round-trip. Those riding on the engine's 'cow-catcher' had a spectacular view of the scenery.

SDPhA President H. A. Sasse, Henry, reminded the delegates at Lead that this was the first convention ever held in the Black Hills. He also had special praise for "Our late brother, pharmacist John C. McClain, Tripp, who so nobly stood in the forefront of battle for sixty long days [lobbying for the Association at the Legislature in Pierre for the state's first Pure Food and Drug Act approved in 1909]. Much credit is also due Senator L.E. Highley, Hot Springs, for his untiring efforts. The Pure Food and Drug Act of this state is in conformity with the national law."[2] H. A. Sasse, a State Representative, also served in the South Dakota Legislature, 1909-1913. Representative Sasse and Senator Highley had both worked for passage of the Pure Food and Drug Act in the 1909 Legislative Session.

Kirk G. Phillips, the first pharmacist in business in Deadwood in 1876, was still active during the 1909 convention. Julius Deetken, the second pharmacist in business in Deadwood in 1876, was elected president of the SDPhA for 1909-1910. E. C. Bent, the third pharmacist to open a drug store in Deadwood in 1876, was reelected as secretary. A. A. Woodward, Aberdeen, was reelected as treasurer. L. E. Highley, Ph.G., Hot Springs, and George G. Nelson, Ph.G., Volga, were elected as vice-presidents. F. W. Brown, Lead, served as the local secretary for the 1909 convention. South Dakota Congressman Eben W. Martin, 1901-1907, 1909-1915, from Deadwood, told the convention that the 1900 Census showed that the average wealth of each man, woman, and child was $1,250. He expected it to grow to $1,500 per person by 1910.

Changing Pharmacy Practice

Between 1900 and 1909 the growing practice of eastern drug companies manufacturing prescription drugs, which pharmacists had compounded themselves, was of concern to some pharmacists. Isaac M. Helmey, Canton, in presentation of a paper at the 1901 convention, reported that prescriptions prescribed for proprietary medicines or special manufacture were growing in his pharmacy. In 1891, it was 12% which grew to 25% in 1900. He expected the ratio of manufactured proprietary medicines and special manufactured prescriptions to increase. Helmey served as SDPhA president, 1904-1905.

S. H. Scallin, Mitchell, won a $10 third prize for his paper "Phases of Commercial Pharmacy" at the 1904 convention in Mitchell. He forewarned pharmacists that "in order to make a financial success in the average South Dakota city, it is necessary to supplement the [prescription business] with other lines of goods."[3] Some lines he sold in his store along with a prescription drug stock included: books and stationery, jewelry and silverware, eyeglasses, China, wall paper (one of his best paying departments), paints and oils, cigars, candy, magazines, and Kodak's. He also operated a soda fountain, and recommended "honest goods and honest dealings" throughout the drug store.

Dr. Ratte, a pharmacist and Rapid City doctor, speaking at the 1909 Lead convention, remembered his days as a pharmacist when "we rolled our pills, it was in the days of making our own plasters. Today, we receive these products in a neatly wrapped package. Every druggist that knows his business can put up any prescription that I am able to write. I plead with the doctors and the druggists to go back to the old times."[4] In response, SDPhA President Julius Deetken, Deadwood, agreed saying "the majority of prescriptions...used, are manufactured in the east and sent out here, largely...in the form of pills and tablets."[5] A longing to return to the old days when pharmacists performed most of the compounding was contrary to ever changing business and professional practices.

Dr. F. E. Walker, Hot Springs, addressed the same convention and said "I cannot help but feel that outside of the thousands of different pharmaceuticals manufactured purposely for the doctor, as patent medicine is manufactured for the layman, the difference and the breach between the professions is due largely if not entirely, to the doctors themselves. While I am especially favorable to several standard manufactured preparations, yet I am convinced that your profession has greater cause for alarm because of manufactured products, than you have from a lack of prescription writing."[6] Pharmacist James Lewis, Canton, thanked the presentations by the doctors and said "We as druggists would like to see the physicians confine themselves more closely to the U.S.P. and N.F. and write their own prescriptions instead of allowing the houses to manufacture the goods for them. They are in harmony with the view of druggists."[7]

Some pharmacists believed that a well-equipped laboratory where chemical, microscopical, and bacteriological examinations were performed, was the best way to maintain a good prescription business. Leo M. Baughman, Ph.G., Watertown, chairman of the Education Committee, reported at the 1909 meeting that "A well-equipped laboratory in the drug store is not only necessary for manufacturing pharmaceutical products, but we should be able to do work superior and more technical than this. A microscope, centrifuge, incubator, and a small assortment of chemicals and apparatus is all that is necessary for testing and examination of milk, water, blood, etc. The examination of sputum, urine, and blood will be almost a daily requirement."[8]

NARD and SDPhA

National Association of Retail Druggists (NARD) was organized in 1899 to promote the advancement of commercial pharmacy. Secretary Thos. V. Wooten in a speech to SDPhA pharmacists in 1901, indicated that price cutting on proprietaries was a large problem for the average druggist. However, there is "certain improvement in prices on these goods as the result of the cooperation between manufacturers, jobbers, and retailers, which our organization has brought about."[9] He reported that thirty-five states belonged by 1901 and urged SDPhA to join. The membership fee was $.50 per member.

SDPhA did not belong, but contributed $50 each year to the national association. In 1904, the South Dakota Pharmaceutical Association voted to send I. A. Keith as a delegate to NARD and pay his train fare and hotel expense. At the 1907 gathering of SDPhA at Huron, a motion was presented not to pay the $50 to NARD, and let pharmacists join individually. After a lengthy floor fight, the pharmacists voted 21 against paying the contribution, and 10 in favor. However, they did vote to send Fred G. Stickles, Mellette, to the Atlanta NARD convention. Stickles later reported that he had traveled by train to Chicago where he boarded a special train of delegates going to Atlanta. After a three-hour stop at the Chickamauga, Tennessee, famous Civil War battlefield, they arrived at Atlanta the next day. Over 1,700 delegates attended the meeting, the largest in its history. His expenses for the trip totaled $93.00.

Pure Food and Drug Act

The United States Congress in 1906, passed a Pure Food and Drug Act, effective January 1, 1907. The Act pertained to drugs in interstate and foreign commerce. It prohibited the sale of adulterated drugs, false or misleading labeling, and improper packaging. The label had to show the presence and amount of dangerous drugs, including any narcotic drugs. If a drug differed from the standard of test or purity laid down in U.S.P. or N. F., it was considered misbranded.

It was necessary to pass a similar law in South Dakota. The Association believed that the administration of a law relative to the purity of medicines should be placed in the hands of the Board of Pharmacy, or some competent pharmacist. The 1907 Legislature passed a South Dakota Food and Drug Law along the lines of the federal law. Fred G. Stickles, Mellette, explained the new law to pharmacists at the 1907 convention: "As I understand the law the manufacturers and wholesalers are supposed to furnish the retail druggist with pure drugs and are charging us accordingly, and we should be prepared to verify the purity of the article and not depend wholly on the imprint or the rubber stamp in the corner of the invoice stating that these goods are guaranteed under the Pure Food and Drug Act."[10]

However in 1908, the South Dakota Supreme Court declared that a section of the 1907 South Dakota Act was unconstitutional. It was detrimental to South Dakota druggists and of no value to the public. Pharmacy leaders in the Association worked to obtain a new law to include the provision that the South Dakota Board of Pharmacy have a voice in administering the law.

A new South Dakota Pure Food and Drug Act was enacted at the 1909 Legislative Session. The law warned pharmacists not to buy any drugs that were not guaranteed. Dr. Alfred N. Cook, Vermillion, was appointed as the Pure Food and Drug Commissioner to administer and enforce the law in the state. James Lewis, Canton, of the Board of Pharmacy reminded pharmacists: "For your own protection insist upon every package bearing a guarantee, not with a rubber stamp...but a plainly printed guarantee attached to each bottle, package, or container...by the manufacturer, jobber, or wholesaler."[11]

SDPhA and APhA

The American Pharmaceutical Association (APhA) was established at Philadelphia in 1852 to promote the profession of pharmacy. Henry A. Cadd, Dell Rapids, after serving as an Association delegate to APhA in 1887 and 1888, served as acting president of APhA at its 1890 convention. He died in 1892, after which E. C. Bent purchased Cadd's pharmacy. APhA membership in 1894 was 1,600. The SDPhA annual proceedings for the 1898 convention shows that a delegate was sent to the 1899 APhA annual meeting. D. F. Jones, Ph.G., Watertown, a delegate to the 1901 convention, indicated that only he and two other South Dakota pharmacists belonged to APhA. He urged pharmacists to pay the $5.00 annual fee and join the national group. According to Jones, the APhA printed annual proceedings on the progress of pharmacy, "is worth the membership fee." The delegates voted to send Jones to the 1902 APhA convention in Philadelphia.

Jones not only attended the 1902 Philadelphia meeting, but also the 1903 meeting at Mackinac Island, and reported on both meetings at the 1903 state convention. Membership in APhA at the time, included retail pharmacists, scientific pharmacists, and those teaching in colleges of pharmacy. Over 1,000 people attended the Philadelphia meeting to celebrate the 50th birthday of APhA. Annual meetings were divided into three sections: commercial, scientific, and education and legislation. Jones, as a member of the section on education and legislation, said a motion was made and passed to establish "a conference of states boards of pharmacy...to create uniformity among the different state boards and bring about an exchange of certificates throughout the United States."[12]

Jones also referred to the Conference of American College Faculties, connected with APhA, whose objective was to equalize the requirements and regulations governing the Colleges of Pharmacy. The concept was that a conference of state Boards of Pharmacy and a Conference of Faculties could work to develop uniformity of pharmacy education and Board of Pharmacy testing to enable pharmacists to reciprocate between states. The National Boards of Pharmacy was organized at the 1904 APhA Kansas City convention, with only two state boards present. However, it was not perfected until the 1905 APhA Atlanta meeting which I. A. Keith, Lake Preston, attended as SDPhA's delegate. R. M. Cotton, Tyndall, attended the 1908 meeting in Hot Springs, Arkansas.

State Price Mark

Pharmacists not only faced competition from peddlers, mail order houses, and manufacturers, but they also faced a wide variance of prescription charges by competing pharmacists. To help develop some uniformity in price, the pharmacists at their 1903 annual meeting in Canton approved a state Price Mark. The Price Mark consisted of alphabetical letters C O P Y R I G H T S Z and numerical letters 1 2 3 4 5 6 7 8 9 0. After checking with a number of drug stores around the state, the secretary made up the Price Mark listing, which was a fair price for mixtures; capsules, pills (freshly made), and powders; ointments; and suppositories (freshly made). Mixtures were as follows: 1 oz. mixture $.25; 2 oz. mixture $.35; etc. up to $1.00 for an 8 oz. mixture. One dozen pills $.25; 2 dozen $.40; 3 dozen $.50; 75 to 100 $1.00 to $1.50. Similar prices were shown for ointments and suppositories. If the prescription called for one dozen pills for which the pharmacist charged $.25, the pharmacist would mark on the container the letters OR. The letter O (for 2) and R (for 5).[13]

When the Price Mark was discussed, pharmacists were more concerned that some pharmacists were charging too high a price. This system would avoid that and create some uniformity. The notice on the Price Mark stated that the prices were not "arbitrary in any locality, but simply a guide that prices may be uniform as far as possible."[14] One pharmacist said that we can recommend but we can't enforce. The Price Mark was carried in the annual proceedings for 1903 through 1907. Apparently the policy did not exist after 1908.

Peddlers

President C. W. Peaslee, Redfield, in a 1903 convention speech expressed a concern about traveling vendors. He also noticed "a few jobbers [wholesalers] were selling to department stores certain drugs in their original packages as glycerin, carbolic acid, castor oil, etc. This hardly seems right, and [we should] show our displeasure to the houses that are practicing this."[15] Peaslee was guided by the South Dakota law which stated that only registered pharmacists had the right to dispense and sell drugs, medicines, and poisons. The Board of Pharmacy had no drug inspectors at the time and the law was difficult to enforce. However, the Legislature in 1903 passed a law requiring that peddlers be licensed to sell their products. License fees were determined by how the peddler traveled. For example, a peddler traveling with a bicycle, on foot, or by railroad, paid $30 for the license. If using a single horse and wagon to carry goods, the fee was $60. A fee of $100 was charged if the peddler used an automobile or two horses and wagon. Each peddler had to display the license number on the wagon or automobile. The South Dakota Attorney General later ruled that it was constitutional to license peddlers.

Ladies' Auxiliary

A Ladies' Auxiliary was formed in the parlors of the Woodmen Hall at Flandreau August 5, 1902. Twelve charter members elected Mrs. W. A. Simpson, Flandreau, president; Mrs. D. F. Jones, Watertown, vice-president; Mrs. W. A. Nye, Salem, secretary; and Mrs. E. C. Bent, Dell Rapids, treasurer. Mrs. E. C. Bent and Mrs. F. C. Smith, Madison, were asked to prepare a Constitution and By-laws and present them at the next meeting. Twenty-five ladies met in the parlors of the Rudolph Hotel in Canton in August 1903 and adopted the Constitution and By-laws. The main purpose of the Auxiliary was to promote an acquaintance among the spouses, sisters, and daughters of pharmacists and advance the social interests of the Association. Annual dues were set at $.50 a person. After participating in the various convention activities, the ladies stopped at the home of Mrs. O. S. Gifford [Oscar S. Gifford served as a Delegate to Congress, 1885-1889] for refreshments. An evening ride was taken on the *Sioux Queen* on the Big Sioux River. Mrs. W. A. Simpson was reelected president.

The 1904 August meeting was in the Masonic Hall at Mitchell with thirty ladies present. After a Corn Palace visit, the delegates elected Mrs. George C. Bradley, De Smet, president. At the time, Mitchell and Pierre were competing for the state's capital. It had been at Pierre since 1889, but the Legislature asked the people to decide if it should be moved to Mitchell. Consequently, the pharmacists and spouses were entertained by the Mitchell Band, which was ready to play anywhere to promote Mitchell for state capital. Pierre won the November 8, 1904 election, and construction of a new stone capitol began in 1905.

A highlight of the thirty-five ladies at the Aberdeen 1905 meeting was a tour through the Jewett Wholesale Drug House. Thursday morning, the ladies assembled on the courthouse steps for their annual photograph. Dinner was at the Commercial Club dining hall, followed by ice cream at Woodward's Drug Store. Mrs. George Sabin, Clark, was elected president. Later, Mrs. E. M. Jones, Clark, at the 1917 convention, reviewed the history of the Ladies' Auxiliary. She told about her train trip to Aberdeen in 1905: "To attend a state meeting was a much greater event in the early years than at the present time of fast-moving automobiles. I believe it required a night and almost a day to reach Mitchell, [from Clark] spending most of the time at an eating house at some junction. On this trip to Aberdeen in 1905, I remember waiting several hours at Elrod for such accommodation which finally appeared in the form of a red caboose hitched behind several freight cars. I had a large lunch box. We started for Aberdeen early in the morning; we arrived late at night."[16]

A gala time was held in Sioux Falls at the August 1906 SDPhA convention. On Wednesday afternoon, Brown Drug Company provided transportation for an auto ride around the city. That night, delegates and spouses attended a banquet at the Cataract Hotel. The next day the women visited Brown Drug House, where they ate lunch. Friday's events at the Palisades were rained out. At the business meeting, the thirty-one ladies elected Mrs. Fred G. Stickles, Mellette, president.

Thirty-three ladies participated in many Auxiliary events at the Royal Hotel for the 1907 Huron convention. Thursday afternoon they were entertained at a lawn party where Miss Wheeler played her gramophone [early record player] during the event. On Friday, the women toured the State Fairgrounds. Mrs. John E. Heisler, Centerville, was elected president. At Watertown in 1908, Mrs. E. M. Jones, Clark, was named historian for the Auxiliary. Later, the women were invited to Mrs. D. F. Jones' home for a reception to meet the spouses of the Watertown doctors and dentists. Mrs. W. F. Michel, Willow Lake, was elected president. The group of thirty-five ladies met in Lead in 1909, and elected Mrs. D.F. Jones, Watertown, president. After touring Spearfish Canyon by train, the ladies visited the fish hatchery.

Commercial Travelers' Auxiliary

A resolution was passed at the 1903 convention authorizing the Association president to appoint a five-person committee to encourage the organization of a Commercial Travelers' Auxiliary. Twenty-one travelers, sales persons, at that convention believed it was a good idea. An organization was not perfected until the Association convention in Aberdeen, August 1, 1905. Thirty-two charter members met and formed the Commercial Travelers' Auxiliary. The aim of the Auxiliary, according to its Constitution, was to "unite the druggists and traveling men, promote good fellowship, and assist in the entertainment at the annual meetings of the South Dakota State Pharmaceutical Association."[17]

Elected officers included a president, three vice-presidents, secretary, treasurer, and a five-member executive committee. Every commercial traveler calling upon the drug trade was eligible for membership. Dues were set at $2.00 a year. New officers were: President, A. H. Rogers, Noyes Bros. & Cutler; First Vice-President, C. H. Coleman; Second Vice-President, C. A. Robinson, Park Davis; Third Vice-President, Sam H. Lewis; Secretary, R. T. Wincott; and Treasurer, C. A. Haley.[18]

Carl Mueller was elected president in 1906 by the fifty-seven members. The Auxiliary's total expense was $19.75 which included $9.00 for convention badges. During the Association convention that year, a specific time was set aside for pharmacists to inspect the various lines of goods displayed by the travelers. R.T. Wincott was elected president at the 1907 meeting in Huron. Fifty-one members were present at the Watertown meeting in 1908. Money on hand totaled $202.45, of which $102 came from dues. Expenses at Watertown included: printing $8.25, badges $7.00, transportation to Lake Kampeska $25.00, and cafeteria lunch at Lake Kampeska $101. J. H. Brown, Minneapolis, was elected president for 1908-1909.

South Dakota's population had grown from 401,500 in 1900 to 583,888 in 1910. The state consisted of 304 incorporated towns and cities in 1910, and about 300 drug stores. In 1900, wheat was $.58 a bushel, corn $.29, and oats $.24. In 1910, wheat was $.89 a bushel, corn $.40, and oats $.30. There were about 70,000 farms. South Dakota's new stone capitol was dedicated in Pierre on June 30, 1910. It easily accommodated the state's 110 employees.

SD Board of Pharmacy, 1900-1909

The Board of Pharmacy was charged with regulating the profession of pharmacy in the state. Its duties included examining and licensing pharmacists, passing regulations, and enforcing such regulations and laws. Pharmacists violating laws and regulations could be punished by verbal warnings, fines, or revocation of license. In 1901, a doctor and pharmacist, after a trial, were convicted and fined $50 each. A person in Meckling was convicted in a Clay County trial for conducting a drug store without a registered pharmacist in charge. In a 1904 annual report to Governor Charles N. Herreid, Board President D. F. Jones, Watertown, said, "Very few cases of open violation have been reported and there seems to be a growing disposition to respect and comply with the pharmacy act. Most of our trouble arises from the general and department stores who are being supplied with patents and many drugs that should be handled only by registered pharmacists, and by the wholesalers. In many cases this operates in direct opposition to the interest of the real drug trade and public welfare who ought, instead, to be protected by the jobbers and wholesalers."[19]

Board Examinations

One of the primary functions of the Board of Pharmacy was to conduct examinations for applicants seeking to register as pharmacists. Candidates needed to meet certain educational standards to take the examinations. Those standards were frequently discussed at Association,

Board, and College of Pharmacy meetings, mostly to upgrade the profession. According to the 1903 South Dakota law, candidates who were at least eighteen years of age, and who could meet any one of the following standards were eligible to take the board examinations:

    a. Three years experience in the practice of pharmacy in a drug store, or

    b. Hold a diploma from a medical college, or

    c. Hold a diploma from the pharmacy course of South Dakota Agricultural College, plus one year of practical pharmacy in a drug store, before or after graduation, or

    d. One years work in a college of pharmacy course and two year's practical pharmacy work in a drug store.

To pass the examination, a candidate for registered pharmacist needed an average grade of 70%, and not less than 55% in any one of the following branches: Pharmacy, Materia Medica, Chemistry, Manipulation, Oral Examination, and Identification of Drugs. Assistant pharmacists needed grades of 55% and not less than 45%. The same test was given to all candidates. The grade received determined whether candidates would be registered as pharmacists or as assistant pharmacists.

The Board of Pharmacy had a rule that a candidate must have at least a common school education (eighth grade) if they used (a) above. Sometimes that rule was not enforced. At the 1901 Association convention, there was considerable floor discussion on a motion that the Board require at least one year of high school. I. H. Keith, Lake Preston, noting that South Dakota Law had no requirement relative to preliminary education, supported the motion. The motion passed. Keith also recommended the Board enforce their present rule requiring an eighth grade diploma, until a change was made.

In 1903, 123 candidates appeared for the Board examinations. The educational training of the eighty-five who passed was: 27 had a Ph.G. degree; 14 had a M.D. degree, and 44 had three years of experience. Some, with the three years of experience, may also have had some high school work or partial course work from some college or institute of pharmacy. Twelve passed as assistant pharmacists. Of 123 candidates, 26 failed, 5 of whom had their Ph.G. degrees. However, three of the Ph.G.'s had a grade high enough to be registered as assistant pharmacists. Records did not show the name of the college from which the candidates graduated. In 1909, Professor Whitehead, Department of Pharmacy, State College, reported to the convention that all but one of sixty-five of their graduates who took the examinations were registered pharmacists. He was referring to those who graduated between 1894 and 1909. Some of the Department's graduates may well have gone to other states to take their board examinations.

A high school requirement was decided at the 1903 Association meeting. After much debate, the pharmacists approved a motion asking the Board to gradually raise the high school requirement in four stages: one year of high school by 1907, two years by 1908, three years by 1909, and four years by 1910. Later, the Board agreed to the new standards, but moved them up a year requiring one year high school in 1906, two years in 1907, three years in 1908 and a diploma in 1909. They also added a provision that if a candidate could not produce a diploma, that person had to pass a preliminary examination with a grade of 60%. A lower grade barred that person from taking the regular Board examination. They also required an apprentice, gaining practical experience in a drug store, to register that practical experience with the Board of Pharmacy.

In 1906, the Board gave the examinations at Watertown, Canton, Aberdeen, and Mitchell, where 102 candidates appeared. Their training included 27 with a Ph.G. degree, 2 with a M.D. degree, and 73 with the three years of experience and the necessary one year of high school. Forty-five were registered as pharmacists and 20 as assistant pharmacists. Three women took the examinations and two passed. Of the 27 with a Ph.G. degree, 17 were licensed as pharmacists, 6 as assistant pharmacists, and 4 failed. Overall, 65 candidates passed and 37 failed the examinations. Later that year, the Board raised the examination passing grade from 70% to 75% for those seeking to be registered as a pharmacist. In 1906, there were 580 registered in-state pharmacists, 72 out-state pharmacists, and 47 assistant pharmacists.

The Board of Pharmacy gave four Board examinations in 1907-1908. A total of 97 took the exams: 10 had Ph.G. degrees and 87 met the three years experience in a drug store requirement, plus three years high school. Nine appeared for reciprocity license, 43 were licensed as pharmacists, 20 were licensed as assistant pharmacists, and 25 failed. Two women, one of whom was Carrie M. Sacker with a Ph.G. degree, passed and were licensed as pharmacists. The Board favored a change in the law raising the age requirement to take Board examinations from 18 to 21. The age for assistant pharmacists to take the exams remained at eighteen. SDPhA president H. A. Sasse, Henry, in 1909, recommended to the Board of Pharmacy they hire an inspector to check compliance of drug stores, grocery stores, etc. The Board took no action on the recommendation.

National Association of Board of Pharmacy (NABP)

For years, the South Dakota Board of Pharmacy accepted reciprocity candidates provided the candidates produced evidence that they had passed the Board examinations in other states with a grade of 80%. For several years, the APhA and the American Conference of Pharmaceutical Faculties had been working for a uniform national system to permit the exchange of pharmacists between states. NABP was organized in Kansas City in 1904, with two Boards of Pharmacy present. It was perfected at Atlanta in September 1905, with twenty Boards of Pharmacy present. The purpose of NABP was to "provide for interstate reciprocity in pharmaceutical licensure based upon a uniform minimum standard of pharmaceutical education and uniform legislation."[20]

I. A. Keith, Lake Preston, member of the South Dakota Board of Pharmacy, 1897-1906, had a leading role in forming NABP. He was elected president of NABP in 1905 at the Atlanta meeting. SDPhA President Issac M. Helmey, Canton, praised I. A. Keith and D.F. Jones, Watertown for their untiring efforts in organizing NABP. South Dakota was the second state to join the organization.

At the 1908 NABP meeting, the delegates did not approve a National Examining Board. They believed that the examination of candidates to practice pharmacy was a state function. However, there was a NABP Committee on Questions and Methods, who believed that the foundation of all questions given by any Board should be the United States Pharmacopoeia and National Formulary, and that the written examinations should be part of the examination. The Committee surveyed thirty-one states in 1908 and reported this information on examinations: [Numbers do not add up because some did not respond to all questions.]

- 31 states had a written examination,
- 17 states had oral examination, 13 did not,
- 26 states had identification of specimens, 4 did not,
- 15 states had practical work in dispensing, 12 did not,
- 20 states required 4 years practical experience, 10 required 3 years,
- 22 states issued an assistant certificate, 8 did not,
- 24 states used reciprocity, 7 did not, and
- 16 states required 75% grade to pass, 4 states 70%, and 1 state 67%.

Some of the Board examination questions provided to the Questions Committee were:

Definitions
- Define levigation, lixivation, trituration.
- Define terms as to crystals: acicular, clinometric, holohedral.

- Define terms as applied to botany and Materia Medica: gladiate, glucosides, alkaloids.

Physics Pharmaceutical
- Define specific volume as applied to pharmacy.
- If one fluid ounce of liquid weighs 569.63 grains, what is its specific volume?
- For what uses are hydrometers intended in pharmacy?
- Describe the principal uses of heat in pharmacy.
- Explain the theory of freezing mixtures.

Chemistry
- How would you distinguish tannic acid from gallic acid by a chemical test?
- How would you purify zinc chloride or zinc sulphate from iron salts?
- What action has iodide of potassium upon the insoluble mercurous salts?

Meteria Medica—Botany
- What is styrax, and from what is it obtained?
- Name six medicinal plants belonging to the natural order compositae (sunflower family) and describe the chief characteristics of this order.
- Cardamomum: state origin, habitat, description, constituents, names of pharmaceutical preparations in which it is used.

Pharmaceutical Arithmetic
- How many fl.ounces will 10 av.ounces of glycerin measure? Sp.grav. 1.246.
- A doctor requests a 4-ounce solution of Nitrate of Silver in distilled water, so made that he can use a teaspoonful in a pint of water and obtain a solution 1 to 10,000. How much silver nitrate would you use? Show figures.
- How many grams of oxygen are contained in one liter distilled water? (H_2O, 17.88)[21]

SD College of Pharmacy, 1900-1909

Dean Frederick Wulling, College of Pharmacy, University of Minnesota in speaking to the pharmacists at the 1901 convention, suggested "that you request the schools of pharmacy to have an entrance requirement of at least one year of high school work, and establish a research scholarship."[22] Dean Wulling addressed the delegates again in

1903. He believed the Board of Pharmacy should be the first to set the educational requirement of one year high school before taking the Board examinations. If so, the Department of Pharmacy [Officially called Department of Pharmacy between 1895 and 1924 when it became the Division of Pharmacy] at Brookings would be sure to follow. At that same meeting, R. M. Cotton, Tyndall, agreed with Professor Wulling, "Any one can readily see that there is no inducement for a young man to go to college if he can spend a few months studying privately and pass an examination. If the Board of Pharmacy requires this, of course the School of Pharmacy naturally must follow."[23] It was at that 1903 meeting where the Association recommended that the Board of Pharmacy require four years of high school credit, graduated over a four-year period.

At the 1905 Association convention, D. F. Jones, Watertown, asked what support may be expected from the Department of Pharmacy on these matters. He stated, "I have attended, I guess ten of these meetings, and, as I said yesterday, in one instance only did we find the School of Pharmacy represented. I guess it was two."[24] In 1906, President Robert Slagle, State College, was scheduled to appear at the convention, but an unexpected problem arose and he was unable to make it. E. M. Jones, Clark, of the Association Education Committee read a statement from President Slagle, "As to Query No. 4, my position is that our College should be closely identified with the work of the Association—we should always have representatives there to take part in the discussions. Please state that as my view."[25]

Dr. Robert L. Slagle, President of State College, did appear at the 1907 convention held in Huron. He said, "I understand that for a number of years the institution has not been represented and that you have the idea that we take no interest in the proceedings of the Pharmaceutical Association. Now I hope that in the future this idea will not prevail. Requirements for admission to the first year class has been a preliminary or equivalent of two year's high school training."[26] [Dr. Slagle had served as Professor of Chemistry at State College 1895-1897 and at the School of Mines 1897-1899. He served as President School of Mines 1899-1905, President State College 1906-1913, and began as President University of South Dakota in 1914.]

It was clear that the Department of Pharmacy was moving along with the same high school entrance requirements as the Board of Pharmacy. Professor Bower T. Whitehead, Brookings, talked after Dr. Slagle and told the delegates, "We require more than most schools require. Most of them require one year of high school work, and we are pushing it up just as fast as we dare to. I am very glad that the Board made the requirement of high school work before they could take the examination."[27]

In 1908, the Department of Pharmacy, State College, Brookings, was approved for membership in the American Association of Colleges of Pharmacy. That same year Professor and Department Head, B. T. Whitehead, assured the pharmacists that any student seeking admission for the pharmacy course, "has to have the same preparation [as those taking] the regular college work."[28] In 1908, the Board of Pharmacy required three years of high school before an applicant was eligible to take the Board examinations.

Department Head and Professor B.T. Whitehead again addressed the Association convention in 1909. He presented statistical information about the ninety Schools of Pharmacy in the nation. Ten of them required over two years of high school, but a large majority of the Schools of Pharmacy only required one year of high school, and some not any. At the time, the Department of Pharmacy at Brookings required three years of high school in order to be eligible to take the pharmacy course. He also said "we stand ready to make any change in the course of study that you wish to recommend and of the sixty-five of our graduates who have tried the state examinations sixty-four are registered. (Applause)"[29] Following Whitehead's talk, the Association delegates passed a special resolution: "The Association highly commends the course of study in pharmacy pursued by the Brookings Agricultural College."[30]

The Growing Numbers of Ph.G. [Pharmacy Graduate] Degrees

The number of practicing pharmacists with Ph.G. degrees grew dramatically between 1898 and 1908. Five earned their Ph.G. degree from the Pharmacy Department, State College at Brookings in 1895, the first graduating class.

In 1898, there were 411 pharmacists practicing in South Dakota: 19 with a Ph.G. degree, 37 with a M.D. degree, and 355 had passed the examinations with the practical experience requirement. Some of the 355 may have had some pharmacy course work from a college of pharmacy or institute of pharmacy.

In 1904, there were 481 registered pharmacists in the state: 86 with a Ph.G. degree, 49 with a M.D. degree, 2 with a P.C. degree, 1 with both a M.D. and Ph.G., and 341 had passed the examinations with the practical experience requirement.

In 1908, there were 518 registered pharmacists practicing in South Dakota: 123 with a Ph.G. degree, 50 with a M.D. degree, 2 with a P.C. degree, 1 with a M.B.S. degree, 1 with a D.D.S. degree, 1 with both an M.D. and a Ph.G. degree, and 340 had passed the examinations with the practical experience requirement. There were also 39 assistant pharmacist certificates in force, with 19 practicing in the state.

Annual proceedings of the Association did not show where pharmacists received their Ph.G. degrees. Not all of them were graduates from State College Department of Pharmacy. State Historian Lawrence Fox, published a *Who's Who Among South Dakotans* in 1924. Seventeen pharmacists were included in the 238 page publication, nine of whom held a Ph.G. degree. They are listed as follows:

- University of Illinois:
    - Ph.G. Lincoln L. Eves, Meckling
- Northwestern U, College of Pharmacy, Chicago:
    - Ph.G. David F. Jones, Watertown
    - Ph.G. Frank D. Kriebs, Beresford
- Highland Park, College of Pharmacy, Des Moines:
    - Ph.G. Chris Hansen, Woonsocket
    - Ph.G. Henry A. Perriton, Huron
    - Ph.G. Louis F. Chladek, Tyndall
    - Ph.G. Lawrence G.France, Canistota
- State College, Brookings:
    - Ph.G. Ernest J. Quiggle, Groton
    - Ph.G. Guy Abbot, Yale.

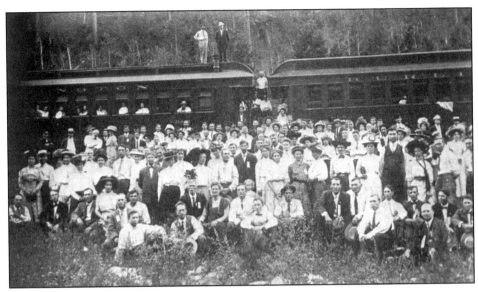
SDPhA 1909 Lead conventioneers ready to take the train to Spearfish Falls.

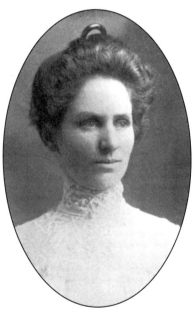
Mrs. W. A. Simpson, Flandreau,
was first president of Ladies'
Auxiliary 1902-03.

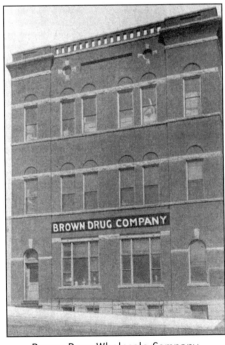
Brown Drug Wholesale Company,
Sioux Falls SD, 1906.

A History of Pharmacy in South Dakota

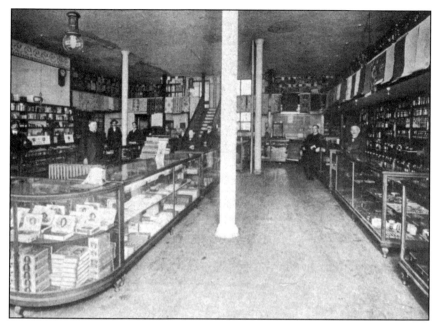

Pharmacy of Kirk G. Phillips, Deadwood, SD, 1909

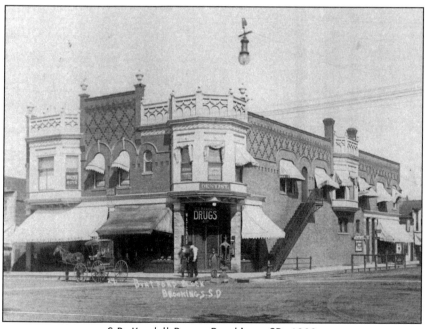

C.D. Kendall Drugs, Brookings, SD, 1909
(Photo courtesy of Robert Kolbe Collections, Sioux Falls, SD)

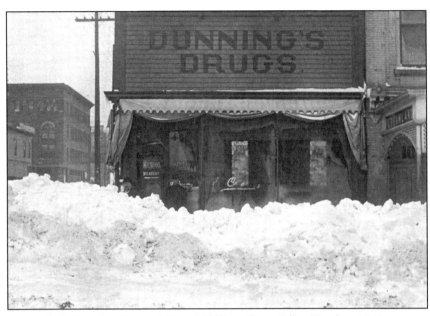

L. T. Dunning Drugs, 8th and Philips, Sioux Falls, SD, circa 1909.
(Photo courtesy of Robert Kolbe Collections, Sioux Falls, SD)

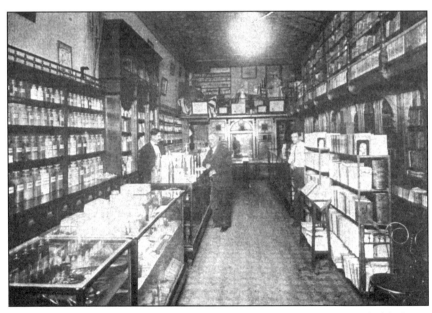

David F. Jones Pharmacy, Watertown, SD, 1908. Jones, left side behind
counter, was a past president of SDPhA and APhA.

A History of Pharmacy in South Dakota

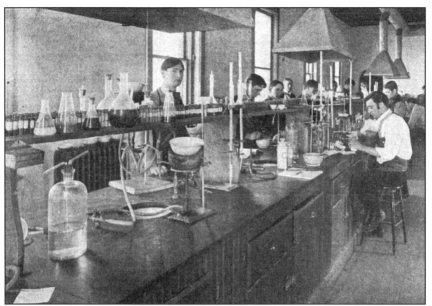

Pharmaceutical Laboratory, State College, Brookings, SD, 1908.

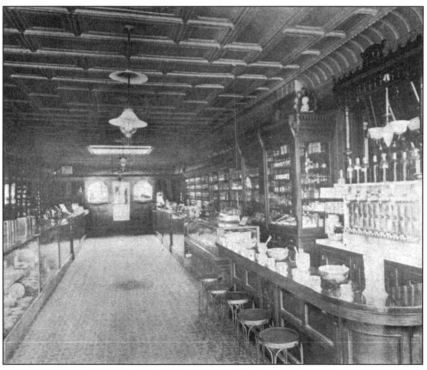

A.A. Woodward Pharmacy, Aberdeen, SD, 1905

CHAPTER 4
1910-1919

SD Pharmaceutical Association (SDPhA), 1910-1919

Attendance at conventions continued to increase. At Yankton in 1910, United States Senator Robert J. Gamble, Yankton, congratulated the Association for its rapid growth during its first twenty-five years of existence. Dr. Alfred Cook, Commissioner of the S.D. Pure Food and Drug Act, with his office in Vermillion, explained the provisions of the law. At one of the meetings, the Commercial Drug Travelers presented a chest of silverware to Mr. and Mrs. I. A. Keith, Lake Preston, for years of service rendered to the Association and Board of Pharmacy. He had served as secretary 1887-1897. Also honored were Mr. and Mrs. E. M. Coates, Yankton, who had operated a drug store in that city since 1870. A first prize of $10 in silver was offered by the Association for the best exhibit of a National Formulary preparation made by a registered pharmacist. The Ladies' Auxiliary offered a $5.00 prize to a lady for the best paper, *Reasons Why Women Excel as Pharmacists*. In November 1910, J. W. Brackett, Sturgis, was elected to the South Dakota House of Representatives and served one term. He was a part of the 1911 Legislature which held the first session in South Dakota's new stone capitol, opened in June 1910.

At the 1911 gathering in Huron, United States Senator Coe I. Crawford, Pierre and Huron, greeted the delegates. Fifty-three ladies attended the meetings of the Auxiliary and enjoyed a picnic dinner sponsored by the Commercial Travelers' Auxiliary. The following year in 1912, the Association met at the Evans Hotel, Hot Springs. One of the excursions included a trip through Wind Cave. Bower T. Whitehead, Head of the Department of Pharmacy at Brookings, reported on the status of the Department of Pharmacy. Ph.G. L. E. Highley, Hot Springs, was elected Association president. Magdeline Gernon, Westport, was elected vice-president.

Mr. and Mrs. C. A. Smith, Mobridge, won first prize for the longest distance traveled by auto at the 1913 Sioux Falls convention. Delegates heard from Governor Frank M. Byrne and Professor Remington of the

Philadelphia College of Pharmacy. The fifty-two ladies from the Auxiliary were entertained at the home of former State Senator and Mrs. Albert H. Stites. The group posed on the balcony of the Stites' home for their annual picture. Stites had graduated from the Philadelphia College of Pharmacy in 1879. He opened a pharmacy at Sioux Falls in June 1881, at the corner of Tenth Street and Phillips Avenue. Stites, holder of South Dakota Board of Pharmacy Certificate No. 2, continued in the drug store business at various locations on Phillips Avenue for forty-four years. He served as mayor of Sioux Falls in 1896 and in November was elected to the State Senate where he served two terms. Ph.G. H. G. Schnaidt, Parkston, was elected Association president, Mrs. Jean M. Kenaston, Bonesteel, and Laura May Carroll, Aberdeen, were elected vice-presidents.

Pharmacists met in Aberdeen in 1914. Convention headquarters was at the Grand View Hotel at Lake Madison in 1915. Business meetings were held on Wednesday and Thursday afternoons. Conventioneers were entertained one night at the hotel by a band concert followed by a performance of the Broadway Players. Herbert A. Keith, Lake Preston, was elected Association president. Mrs. Austin Mankey, Webster, was elected vice-president. A baseball game was played between the pharmacists and Commercial Travelers. A ball was held that night at the Huntimer Hotel.

Chairpersons of eight Association committees gave reports at the convention: Legislative, Education, Auditing, Botany and New Medicinal Plants, Queries for 1916, Trade Interests, National Legislation, and College of Pharmacy. Votes cast for the 1916 convention site were as follows: Mitchell 25, Sioux Falls 14, Redfield 13, and Forestburg 0. Almost everyone attended the Mitchell convention by automobile in 1916.

During World War I, the organization met in the Lincoln Hotel at Watertown, August 1917. It was the Association's largest gathering, up to that time. Two hundred ninety-four pharmacists and auxiliary members jammed the city to take part in the presentation of a new Motor Army Ambulance to the State of South Dakota. The opening session was held in the Metropolitan Theatre. Festivities included an auto ride throughout the city, picnicking and boating at Lake Kampeska, and a National Guard band concert. The Commercial Travelers' expenses included: Lincoln Hotel lunch, 280 plates at $.60 each; rent for dance hall and fee for musicians $38; and free movies at the Lyric Theatre $20. The Commercial Travelers' Auxiliary elected I. A. Helmey, (Hornick, More, and Porterfield), Sioux Falls, president. Forty-eight members of the Ladies' Auxiliary elected Mrs. E. M. Jones, Clark, president. Members of the Association elected Fred L. Vilas, Pierre, president. E. C. Bent, Dell

Rapids, was reelected secretary for the 21st time. Sixty-three business units advertised in the convention program and there were 103 cash donors to help defray convention expenses. The memorial program included a remembrance for Professor Bower T. Whitehead, Head Department of Pharmacy, State College, Brookings, who had died April 1, 1917.

The major activity of the convention was the presentation of the Motor Army Ambulance to the State of South Dakota. During the early part of 1917, D. F. Jones, Watertown, led a statewide fund drive to buy a Motor Army Ambulance for the South Dakota National Guard. Three hundred and eleven individuals, mostly from the pharmaceutical business within the state, contributed $1,700 to pay for the ambulance, built to Army specifications. Pharmacists, spouses, two marching bands, members of the Grand Army of the Republic, members of the South Dakota National Guard, Red Cross workers and nurses, Boy Scouts, and citizens paraded to the City Park in Courthouse Square for the presentation ceremony. President J. A. Pool, Redfield, greeted the crowd, estimated at 5,000, and introduced Governor Peter Norbeck. The Governor thanked the pharmacists and others for helping with the war effort, and accepted the ambulance for the South Dakota National Guard and the State of South Dakota.

Because of World War I, the Association did not hold a convention in 1918. The next meeting was at Lead in 1919.

Peddler Medicine Wagons

Traveling vendor wagons had been operating in South Dakota since statehood. C. R. Noyes, St. Paul, told the pharmacists at the 1915 convention, "You cannot legislate these peddlers out of business. It has been tried, and it is impossible."[1] However, the South Dakota Legislature in 1903, required that all peddler medicine wagons be licensed. Raleigh, Watkins, Ward, and Baker were the principal out-of-state companies operating medicine wagons in the state. It was the general feeling of most operators of drug stores that they had lost business to the wagons. R. O. Grover, Huron, decided to do something about it. He presented an excellent paper at the 1915 convention pertaining to his experience of operating a peddler medicine wagon as a part of his pharmacy business.

Grover found that out-of-state companies take few chances. "When they make a contract with a man to take a territory, they require him to put up a bond for all the medicines...and this bond must be signed by two responsible parties. They in turn sell him their [patent] medicines, extracts, spices, etc., at a very reasonable price. In many instances far less than we pay for our...lines. The agent, I am told, buys his own wagon,

A History of Pharmacy in South Dakota

furnishes his own team or auto, pays his own expenses and really owns the line. He sends them a certain percentage of all monies received for which they credit his account."[2] A Mr. Alley of the Webster Line reported from the convention floor, that a man must sell at least $100 a week in order to hold the agency for his wagon.

Grover further reported, "I decided in March 1914, to put out a wagon and go after the same business that they were getting. I purchased an up-to-date [roof covered] medicine wagon with shelves, drawers, etc. [It cost Grover about $500 to start a medicine wagon business.] Made a contract with a man, I to furnish the stock and wagon and pay one-half of the expenses on the road. He to furnish the team, do the selling, pay one-half the expenses and then divide the profits equally. We have an advantage over the foreign medicine houses in being able to handle more lines than they. In my case carrying four lines, namely a remedy line of about 100 different items, a sundry line of goods in common use, a list of common household drugs, and a veterinary line. We aim to make the territory about every three months. A man would [earn about] $60 to $75 a month. [Grover's share was from $600 to $900 a year.]"[3]

"I think the real purpose for the wagon is not the money you can make on the wagon itself, but it is the means of getting business into the drug store. I think the patent medicine wagons have taken a vast amount of business out of the drug store. You can work every department of your store with a wagon. Take for instance, in the way of a Victrola. A great many of these wagons the druggists are running take a Victrola with them. When they stop over night they take out the Victrola and give them a concert. They get the people out in the neighborhood to listen to the concert."[4] It was generally agreed that making from six to nine hundred dollars a year on a five hundred dollar investment was a good profit.

Early Narcotic Laws

Secretary E. C. Bent in 1904, surveyed 100 leading South Dakota pharmacies as to their procedures for selling cocaine. At the time, only pharmacists had authority to sell narcotics, such as morphine, opium, and cocaine. Twenty-nine pharmacists replied they only sold cocaine by prescription, except to doctors and dentists. Twenty said they sold cocaine without a prescription to a 'limited extent' when they know their customers. One pharmacist from Bonesteel, where people were waiting for a land drawing reported, "We have several hundred calls a day by as many cocaine fiends, who are in town [for the drawing]." Some stated that if they didn't sell it to patients, someone else would. Other pharmacists responded they favored a law limiting the sale of narcotics by a doctor's prescription only.[5]

In 1914, Congress passed the Harrison Narcotic Act that regulated the puchase and sale of morphine, codeine, herion, cocaine, and opium or any of their derivatives. The law was placed under the administration of the Internal Revenue Department. Under the Act, narcotics could only be dispensed by registered pharmacists upon a doctor's prescription. Only medical doctors with a federal license could prescribe narcotics. South Dakota Legislators passed a similar law effective March 1915. Dr. G. G. Frary, South Dakota Commissioner of Food and Drug Law, informed pharmacists that records kept for the Harrison Act were sufficient for the South Dakota Act. One feature of the law was the requirement that a person receiving a narcotic prescription from a pharmacist, must sign for it on the back of the prescription.

Ph.G. F. W. Halbkat, Webster, reviewed the new South Dakota law at the 1915 convention. He considered it "a good law to control the sale of narcotics in the drug stores of South Dakota. Let the good work go on. If, under our law and the Harrison Act it is unlawful to sell medicines containing more than two grains to the ounce of gum opium or extract, that it is an outrage to all patent medicines like Chamberlain's Colic, containing 1.99 grains of opium to the ounce to be dealt out without restriction, or Ward's Liniment containing 1 grain of opium to the ounce or any cough medicine or other mixtures containing such drugs."[6]

Ph.G. D. F. Jones, Watertown, reported that since the new law, he would not take any phone prescriptions because there were too many chances for mistakes. Jim Lewis, Canton, reviewed the procedure he used to take a telephone prescription for a narcotic. First, the doctor read the prescription to him. Then he repeated it back to the doctor, and then he read the whole thing again to the doctor. After filling the prescription, he wrote on the original written order, that it was a phone prescription and that he had verbally rechecked it with the prescribing doctor. S. H. Scallin, Mitchell, followed the same procedure but still believed it wasn't wise to take a narcotic prescription by telephone.[7]

Impact of World War I

World War I affected South Dakota pharmacies as early as 1915. That year Ph.G. F. W. Halbkat, Webster, chairperson of the Association's National Legislation Committee said, "The prolonging of the European War has effected the drug markets to an astonishing degree; in fact we do not think any retailer, broker or wholesaler could have seen or comprehended such a demoralized epoch. Increased prices of goods due to lack of importation and facilities for manufacture in this country, abnormal demands for certain classes of disinfectants due mostly to the war, epidemic diseases among cattle, also chemicals for manufacturing explosives

A History of Pharmacy in South Dakota

have brought about conditions which only the ending of the European conflict can right."[8]

During 1916, prices of all goods rose dramatically. In South Dakota, the price of gasoline rose from $.12 a gallon to $.22 a gallon. Hogs were selling for $11 a hundred, the highest since the Civil War. The price for a pair of shoes increased 40%. Fred Vilas Sr., Blackhawk Drug, Pierre, reminded his customers that during 1916, 75% of the drugs had doubled in price. On April 6, 1917, the United States declared war on Germany. Between that date and the end of the war on November 11, 1918, 32,791 South Dakotans either enlisted or were drafted to serve their country. Included in the group were over forty pharmacists. The South Dakota Legislature created a State Council of Defense. Governor Peter Norbeck appointed its executive committee, which included State College President, E. C. Perisho.

A. A. Woodward, Aberdeen, at the 1917 Watertown convention told about shortages and increased prices of pharmaceutical products. He said, "Figured in percentages, drugs and chemicals have advanced [in price] far more than other classes of merchandise, amounting in some instances to 500 or 600 percent. Articles like castor oil have advanced two and one-half times its normal value; glycerin about four times...; saltpeter four times...; and potassium permanganate, twenty times its normal value. One should keep thoroughly in touch with market changes. When advances [increase in prices] are noted, your stock [prices] should be made to conform whether it be a drug, chemical, proprietary or patented articles. We are entitled to the market advances the moment we get notice of such advance, you must replace your stock as fast as sold and you will have to pay market prices. Do not wait until you have sold your present stock and have to pay the higher price before you raise your price. We have good reason to suppose that [prices] will increase again, when the pending War Revenue Tax [on medicines] becomes a law."[9]

There was also a shortage of bottles, paper, and twine. B. H. Neumayr, Vermillion, urged pharmacists to conserve on these items because of their scarcity and increased price. He told them, "The supply of bottles is so short that we are justified in requesting customers to bring in their bottles to be refilled. Take care of every bottle which comes into the store, and washing all emptied stock bottles promptly...and not overlooking the important precaution not to use any of those second hand bottles for prescriptions. Another item...is wrapping paper, this increased expense can also be offset...by saving all the paper from incoming packages. While considering the saving of bottles and paper, the small item of twine should not be lost sight of, since the price of that article has advanced almost fifty percent. Save the twine from packages. If the war should continue for any length of time it will not be a matter of choice, but an actual necessity."[10] D. F. Jones, Watertown, installed a Stokes' Tablet Machine which he used to compound aspirin tablets. The machine cost him $40, but he made thousands of aspirin tablets.

Medicines were taxed during the Spanish-American War, and also during World War I when the tax on medicine was 2%. Freighting of goods was slow and uncertain, and in some cases taking twenty days to deliver goods instead of the normal five days. The Board of Pharmacy accepted candidates to take Board examinations with only fifteen months of practical training, rather than two years. The Board would not cancel a license while a pharmacist was on military duty. However, pharmacists entering the service didn't always end up practicing their profession or were not awarded an advance rank for their skills. A special 1917 convention resolution urged the South Dakota Congressional Delegation to ask the military to give a higher rank to pharmacists in the United States Service and also place them upon an equal footing and pay with other branches of the service.

No information was found as to the number of South Dakota pharmacists killed or wounded during World War I. However, a total of 995 South Dakotans died during the war: 441 died in American camps, 205 killed in action, 83 wounded in action, 233 died from disease, and 33 died from other causes.

Drug Store Laboratory vs. Manufacturers Laboratory

Dr. J. H. Beal, Urbana, Illinois, former APhA secretary, presented a paper at the 1917 Watertown convention. He spoke about the practice of compounding medicines in the drug store laboratory being replaced by making medicines in the manufacturers laboratory. He referred to a time fifty years earlier when most towns had individual craftsmen like the shoemaker, harness maker, pottery maker, etc. These craftsmen were replaced by large factories in centers of population. A similar change had occurred in the field of pharmacy.

Dr. Beal said, "One very influential factor in lessening the importance of the drug store laboratory, as the source of pharmaceutical preparations, has been the constantly increasing complexity in manufacturing processes and the refinements introduced into the methods of testing medicinal products. When tinctures made by maceration and other galenicals of simple character were the staple articles of the drug stock, they could be readily manufactured by the apothecary. When fluid extracts were introduced, with their theoretical relation of grain of crude drug to minum of liquid, a more complicated process of manufacture became necessary, and the first step was taken toward the elimination of the drug store laboratory.

"The next refinement was the development of elaborated processes for the assay of galencial preparations and for the testing and grading of chemical compounds other than galenicals, which all require a higher degree of technical skill. A second important factor in the transfer of the manufacturing operations from the small to the large laboratory has been the rapid introduction of entirely new classes of medicinal products which can be prepared only in establishments much more extensive than any retail dealer can hope to maintain. From the very nature of these products it is impossible that the dispensing pharmacist should seriously undertake their manufacture, and he must content himself therefore to act mainly as their distributor to the medical profession and the public.

"Pharmacy is gradually going through an evolution, which will result in there being two distinct classes of pharmacists, the professional and the commercial pharmacists. In this connection I must protest against the limitation of the title 'ethical pharmacy' to a business consisting exclusively of the compounding and dispensing of drugs and medicines to distinguish it from a business in which many other things are dealt in besides drugs and medicines. The selling of the mixed merchandise of a modern drug store is just as truly ethical in substance and fact as the manufacture of a fluid-extract or the compounding of a prescription.

"But someone will say: what becomes of pharmaceutical education and what is the use of our colleges of pharmacy if we once admit that the principal function of the pharmacist is to act as the distributor of preparations manufactured by other people instead of his own manufacture. The answer is that the pharmacist's education will be just as valuable. The frank acknowledgement of the fact that the majority of pharmacists must be commercial pharmacists rather than compounding and prescription pharmacists will not make the college curriculum useless. Let us for once and all get rid of the fantastic and snobbish notion that the so-called 'professional pharmacy' is the only kind of pharmacy worth cultivating. Let us frankly acknowledge that commercial pharmacy has a legitimate place and purpose in the social economy, and then let us devote the best that is in us to making it ethical, respectable, and profitable."[11]

That same day at the 1917 convention, D. F. Dexter, Canton, talked to the pharmacists about *Drug Store Side Lines*. Dexter said, "Side lines in a drug store include all the articles handled which are not drugs...and the handling of side lines is the part of the business which we do not learn in colleges of pharmacy nor...in textbooks. I believe the time is not far distant when commercial pharmacy will be added to the pharmacy course.

The druggist who can look at his books at the close of a month's business and see in detail the conditions of each department of his store and ascertain whether he has made or lost money is in a better position...than one...better qualified in chemistry and Materia Medica, yet lacks good business instincts and training.

"Every druggist, [should have] a clean and modern drug department...partitioned from the general store by transparent partitions, so that customers entering the store can see that the prescription and drug department are the principal business and not a side line. There are certain things that custom has settled which druggists should handle that are not strictly a part of a pharmacy. The principal ones and most profitable ones are toilet articles, surgical dressings, rubber goods, and stationery. These lines sell 365 days a year. My idea is to make a complete department of each of these four lines.

"In connection with toilet articles, carry a face powder, hair tonic, cold cream, lotion, and perfume. What the druggist needs is gross profits. Some goods give 10% others 15%, and still others 33%, some 50%, and some 100%. With reference to rubber goods...I select one hot water bottle, one combination outfit, one atomizer, and several other items and mark them 20% above the ordinary profit. Treating of stationery, visiting cards, social cards, blank account books, and fountain pens...can be made to pay at least 40% actual profits on gross sales.

"Cigars, candy and the soda fountain lines...give a splendid profit. Kodak's require little room...and while they are sold at a fixed profit (33 1/3%) their accessories (films etc.) are quick sellers and bring customers to the store. Gift goods such as French and Persian lines, hand painted China, leather, manicure sets, all go to make up a splendid assortment that will sell during the year. Stock tonics and veterinarian preparations...are good sellers, especially the preparations of one's own making. I have a barb wire liniment and hog worm remedy that I make and sell with a guarantee. Stock condition powder, dips, and poultry remedies are very profitable side lines. Side lines actively pushed will make good returns and are perfectly legitimate."[12]

SD Board of Pharmacy, 1910-1919

The Board met in the Carpenter Hotel, Sioux Falls; Woodmen Hall, Pierre; Department of Pharmacy, Brookings; and High School, Lead in 1915. Fifty-nine candidates were licensed: 21 as pharmacists, 26 as assistant pharmacists, and 12 by reciprocity. Those from other states included 6 from Nebraska, 5 from Iowa, and 1 from Kansas. The Board passed a special regulation requiring all reciprocity candidates to meet in person with the Board of Pharmacy at any of its meetings. A resolution was also approved stating that all candidates appearing for Board Examinations holding a Ph.G. degree from State College have shown commendable proficiency. Ph.G. Wm. P. Loesch, Oldham, with the spring class, received 92%, the highest exam grade. SDPhA awarded Loesch a year's membership in APhA. A complaint was presented to the Board at the Lead meeting. It pertained to a pharmacist from Lily who, by reason of excessive use of intoxicants, became incompetent to dispense drugs. After a regular hearing in court, the Board cancelled the pharmacist's registration certificate for conduct unbecoming to the profession and drunkenness.

Board member F. W. Halbkat, Webster, reported that after examinations in five places in 1917, 30 were licensed as pharmacists, 30 as assistant pharmacists, 6 by reciprocity, and 4 failed. At the April examination in the Chemistry Building, Brookings, 16 with Ph.G. degrees appeared, 14 with a South Dakota address and 2 with a Minnesota address. Those holding Ph.G. degrees passed the examinations: 10 were licensed as pharmacists, and 6 were licensed as assistant pharmacists. Disciplinary matters before the Board included two hearings, after which two pharmacist licenses were revoked because of a violation of the state's liquor laws. They were advised that they could be reinstated later, if they proved their fitness.

There were 853 registered pharmacists in South Dakota in 1915: 661 in-state, and 192 out-state. The educational status of the 661 in-state pharmacists was as follows: Ph. G. degree, 181 men and 5 women; M. D. degree, 38; M.D. and Ph.G. degree, 6 men and 1 woman; and 1 dentist; for a total of 232 with degrees. Those who were registered by passing the examinations with the practical experience requirement included 9 women and 420 men.

The 1916 Legislature asked South Dakotans to vote, at the fall general election, on the question of prohibiting the sale of liquor in the state. The vote was 65,334 Yes to stop the sale of liquor, and 53,380 No to continue the sale. In 1917, the Legislature passed a prohibition law, or as some called it the "Bone Dry Law." Pharmacists could sell liquor upon a doctor's prescription or upon a signed affidavit that the liquor was for legitimate purposes. Not many pharmacies sold liquor upon signed affidavits because if the purchaser got drunk or into trouble, both the seller and the buyer were liable for fines. The State Sheriff was charged with administering the law. Pharmacies selling liquor by either of the above methods had to conform with strict record keeping procedures. They needed to show amounts on hand at the beginning of the month, amounts purchased during the month and from whom, amounts of liquor sold, and the amounts used in compounding medicines, extract and other preparations. The monthly report was sent to the Commissioner of Prohibition. It was estimated that from 60% to 70% of patent medicines contained alcohol. In regard to the sale of patent medicines, pharmacists needed to make a judgment whether or not the buyer would be using the patent medicines as a beverage. The prohibition law was repealed in 1934, both in the nation and in South Dakota. SDPhA President James Lewis, Canton, reported that the ninth edition of U.S.P. did not have whiskey or brandy mentioned, because they had no medical value.

A lively discussion occurred at the 1915 convention at Lake Madison. Chairman of the Board of Pharmacy, F. W. Halbkat, Webster, made these remarks as to the four-year high school needed to take the Board examinations: "As the Board [understood the direction from the Association] it did not mean specifically that a person have four years in a high school, but should have educational requirements that would be necessary for [that person] to take the examination. We have passed upon individuals and permitted them to take the examination when we felt that they were qualified as though they had a diploma from a high school."[13] David Jones, Watertown, thought the instruction to the Board was to require a full four-year course, or its equivalent, which would be determined by a preliminary examination. Professor B.T. Whitehead added that the Department of Pharmacy requires a full four years of high school to enroll for pharmacy courses. After more discussion, no further action was taken.

Secretary E. C. Bent, who had been a delegate to the NABP 1914 meeting in Detroit, reported that the organization had hired a full-time secretary, H. C. Christensen, Chicago, at $1,800 a year. There were thirty-six active state Boards of Pharmacy who had paid the $15 annual dues for membership in NABP. Secretary Bent kept one set of books for both the South Dakota Board and Association. Receipts included pharmacist renewal fees $2,507, examination fees $547, other fees $47 for a total of $3,101. The $300 appropriation provided by the state had ended in 1914. Disbursements were $3,889, the shortage was made up from the previous year's balance on hand. Some of the disbursements included: executive secretary's salary of $1,200 a year; expense for delegate to APhA, $81; legislative expense in Pierre, $364; expense for delegate to NABP, $76; per diem for Board, $440; rent for tables in Chemistry Building for Board exams, $1.00; printing 1,250 copies of annual proceedings, $328. After a reconciliation with the treasurer's books, the account was submitted to the auditing committee. Later in the convention, the committee reported that the books were correct. Their report was adopted by the convention.

SD College of Pharmacy, 1910-1919

The Department of Pharmacy originally had its laboratories on the third floor of Old Central. From there it moved to the basement of the North Building, and then to the old Chemistry Building. In 1919, it moved again, this time to the first floor of the Administration Building where it remained for sixty years. State College President E. C. Perisho, in a 1915 letter to the Association convention, announced that the College would establish a garden of medicinal plants upon the college grounds. It would be administered in conjunction with the Department of Botany. Their instructors would give a specialized course in the knowledge of plants. It lapsed after a couple of years, but was rejuvenated in 1917 by Professor Anton Hogstad Jr. The garden was located just north of the Old College Stores Building.

Professor Bower T. Whitehead reported that the 1915 graduating class included ten graduates with a Ph.G. degree and three graduates with a B. S. degree. The Board of Pharmacy required four years of high school to take the Board examinations. Professor Whitehead said, "Our requirements are four years in high school...and that is much higher than most of the schools. Both Minnesota and Wisconsin, for the first time, during this coming year will require four years of high school. Candidates write and want to come to our school, and their qualifications are not what they should be to meet our requirements, and we refuse to admit them, and then they go to some other school...and in some way get around the requirements, and then they take the examination."[14]

James Lewis, Canton, wondered if South Dakota's four-year high school requirement might be too severe. It had been required since 1909. He understood from Professor Whitehead's remarks that the requirements caused some students to go to different schools with a lessor requirement or take a 'plugging course' and then take the Board examinations.

Professor Bower T. Whitehead, Head of the Department of Pharmacy, State College, died Sunday morning, April 1, 1917 at Brookings. He was born on a farm in Hand County. Whitehead earned a Ph.G. from State College in 1895, a Ph.C. from Northwestern in 1896, and a M.S. from State College at Brookings in 1901. He was named Head of the Department of Pharmacy in 1896 and served until his death. James Lewis, Canton, knew him from the time he was appointed and said in remembrance, "The School of Pharmacy was then a struggling infant and Professor Whitehead was very anxious to get into close relationship with the pharmacists of the state and build up and develop such a school as would be a credit to the state and of benefit to the students. He grew into the lives of the students and while stern when occasion demanded, yet they all loved him as they knew he was just."[15]

Earl R. Serles, a native of Unityville, S.D., had been a graduate assistant under Whitehead. After Whitehead's death, Serles was named as Head of the Department of Pharmacy. Serles, at the August 1917 convention, provided information about the pharmacy school: "We have a two-year and a four-year course. The two-year course comprises such subjects as have a direct bearing upon the State Board examinations. Since its foundation twenty-three years ago, [State College's] Department of Pharmacy has graduated from the two-year course and the four-year course combined about 160 persons, of which 18 have become physicians, 2 dentists, 7 chemists, and 7 are with colleges of pharmacy...and I am proud to say that 110 out of the 160 are actively engaged in practice in the State of South Dakota today. We have made some changes...for instance we are teaching business law and accounting. In placing of the pharmacy laboratory, which includes the making of tinctures that are made from crude drugs. We have substituted that, and we have installed a prescription case, not quite as modern as some, but it has the same purpose to serve. We expect as soon as possible to increase the drug garden."[16]

Professor Serles continued in that position until he entered the military in 1918. While Serles was in the military, Charles A. Locke, Ph.G. 1906, assisted by Anton Hogstad, Jr. ran the department. In the fall of 1918, a Ph.C. [Pharmaceutical Chemist] degree, which was a three-year course, was offered along with the Ph.G. two-year pharmacy course. In early 1919, shortly after the war, Serles returned to his old job.

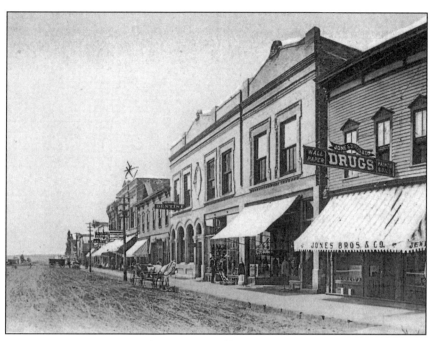

Jones Brothers Drug, Madison, SD, circa 1910.
(Photo courtesy of Robert Kolbe Collections, Sioux Falls, SD.)

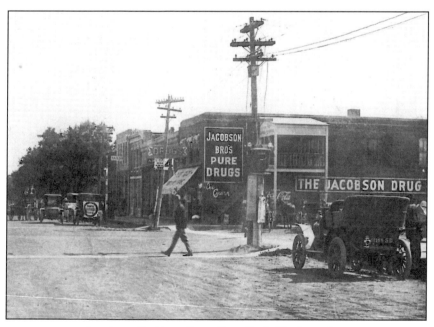

Jacobson Brothers Drug, Beresford, SD circa 1915
(Photo courtesy of Robert Kolbe Collections, Sioux Falls, SD.)

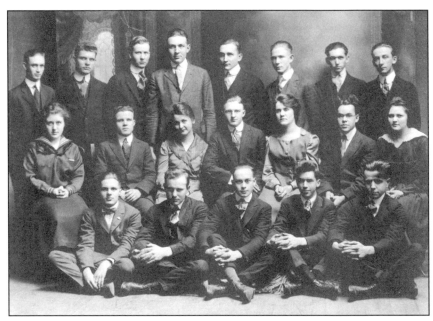

Department of Pharmacy Head Earl Serles, left third row, with Class of 1918.
Bliss Wilson, second from left second row, became NABP president in 1963.

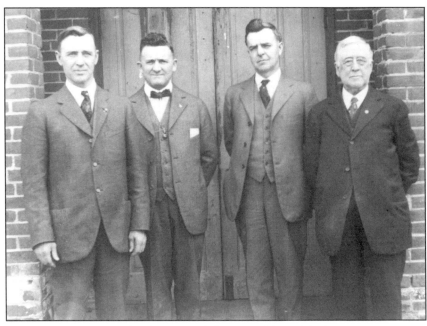

Executive Secretary E. C. Bent, right, with the
1919 South Dakota Board of Pharmacy.

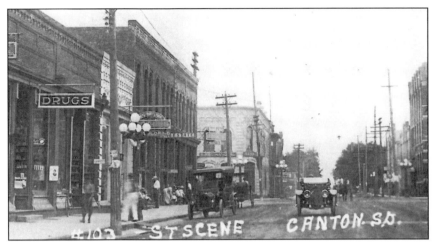

I. M. Helmey Drug store, center; A.G. Noid Drug store, corner, Canton, SD, circa 1910. *(Photo courtesy of Robert Kolbe Collections, Sioux Falls, SD.)*

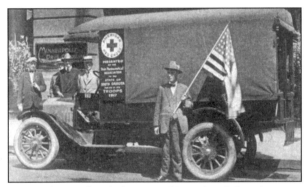

SDPhA donated ambulance to SD National Guard, 1917.

J. F.Casey Drug Store, Vivian, SD, circa 1912.
(Photo courtesy of Terry Casey)

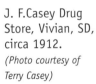

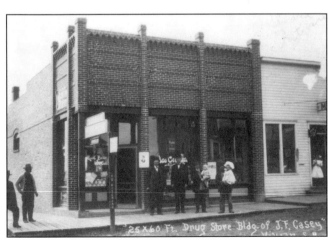

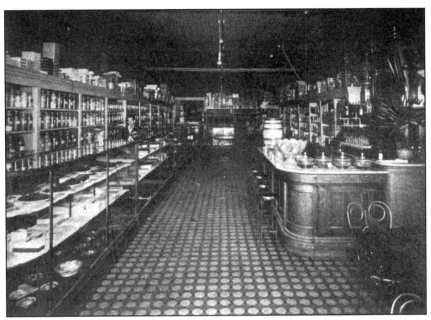

Pharmacy of Perriton & Son, Huron, circa 1910.

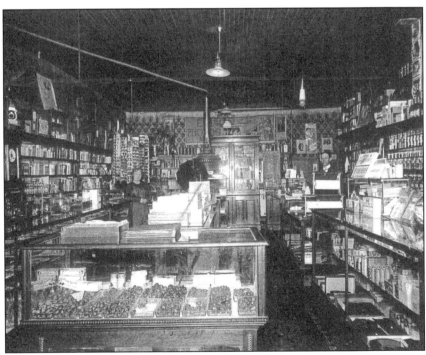

Weisflock Brothers Drug Store, Frankfort, 1914. *(Photo courtesy of Jim Weisflock)*

A History of Pharmacy in South Dakota

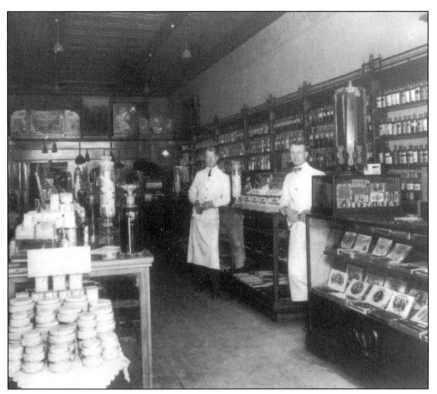

Joseph H. Statz Drug Store, Parkston, circa 1915.
(Photo courtesy of Stephen R. Statz)

CHAPTER 5
1920-1929

SD Pharmaceutical Association (SDPhA), 1920-1929

Association Business

The Commercial Travelers approved a new constitution at the pharmacists' August 1921 convention in Sioux Falls. Sixty travelers reaffirmed their prior objectives which were to unite and promote fellowship between the traveling salesmen and druggists of South Dakota, to urge better attendance at annual meetings and to provide entertainment for the same. The group sponsored a dance in the Cataract Hotel which cost them $40 for hall rent, $63 for music, $22 for hats and decorations, and $34 for punch. A raffle for an Edison phonograph was conducted during the dance. Proceeds were donated to a new scholarship fund for the Department of Pharmacy, State College. Three hundred and sixty-four registered at the Cataract Hotel convention headquarters. The 200 page 1922 convention proceedings cost $115 for a stenographer, $457 for printing 1,200 copies, and $179 postage to mail them to 931 in-state and out-state pharmacists.

J. Chris Schutz, Madison, was elected Association president and Mrs. Clara Conkey, Brookings, vice-president at the 1923 gathering. E. C. Bent, Dell Rapids, who had served as secretary since 1897, retired in 1923. D.F. Dexter, Canton, was elected secretary that same year and served until 1925. At the 1924 convention in Rapid City, the Ladies' Auxiliary, chaired by President Mrs. H. A. Perriton, Huron, promoted their scholarship fund that provided $20 tuition for some sophomore girl in the Department of Pharmacy. Each of the ladies paid $.50 toward the fund. The thirty-five members of the Commercial Travelers' Auxiliary, meeting in the Elks Lodge, elected George McCullum, Fargo, ND, president and Carl H. Dailey, Sioux Falls, secretary. Later in the day, the pharmacists defeated the Travelers in a baseball game. Pharmacists' activities included a clay-pigeon shoot, fish fry, and various business meetings. At one of the business meetings, a $500 contribution was approved to help with the building of an all Pharmacy Headquarters Building in Washington, D.C. Only 178 registered for the Black Hills convention, including Dean and Mrs. Earl Serles, Brookings. At the time, there were 644 in-state-pharmacists.

Association Secretary D. F. Dexter, Canton, in 1924, mailed out a supply of five bulletins to pharmacies as part of a publicity program. These bulletins were mailed thirty days apart: Beware of the Peddler, Do you Realize, Public Notice, The Public to Think About, and Pharmacist Today. The free bulletins were placed as part of an official SDPhA Bulletin Board for use by the public. Few orders were received from pharmacies to replace the original supply. Some replacement orders were made for the one bulletin, Beware of the Peddler. Because of few requests, no other bulletins were mailed. Dexter however, recommended that one carefully selected bulletin be sent out each month during the coming year. The meeting in 1925 was at the Grand View Hotel at Lake Madison. The hotel was located four miles from the city on a graveled road. It had forty rooms, a large lobby, and ample porches. Good fishing, bathing, rowing, dancing in the largest pavilion in South Dakota, and all electric-lighted grounds were featured. President W. L. Buttz, Aberdeen, at one of the business meetings recommended that the Executive Committee be trimmed from ten to five members. W. P. Loesch, Oldham, was elected secretary of the Association and the Board at the 1925 meeting.

Three hundred and forty-three registered for the 1926 convention at Watertown. A Veteran Druggists Association was formed for the first time, at one of the business meetings. Pharmacists who had been in the retail drug business for twenty-five years were eligible for membership. Members elected C. C. Maxwell, Arlington, president. Twenty-five veteran druggists were recognized as members at the 1927 convention.

The Association's first Memorial Hour was conducted at the 1927 convention in Mobridge. As Secretary W. P. Loesch, Oldham, read the names of each of the deceased, pharmacists spoke some kind words or read a biographical sketch about them. Four past Association presidents died that year: J. A. Lewis, Canton, 1894-1895; C. M. Serles, Salem, 1901-1902; F.G. Stickles, Mellette, 1903-1904; and Perry Clute, Murdo, 1919-1920. B. H. Neumayr, Vermillion, president of the Board of Pharmacy was also memorialized. It was agreed by resolution to include a Memorial Hour in future conventions. Pharmacist and State Senator William L. Buttz, Aberdeen, was the toastmaster at the banquet in the Masonic Temple. Buttz had been elected State Senator in November 1926 and served during the 1927 and 1929 Legislative Sessions in Pierre. One hundred thirty-four men and fifty-six women registered for the convention.

A part of the 1928 Huron convention business was the approval of an official invitation to the American Pharmaceutical Association (APhA) to hold its 1929 national meeting in the Black Hills. The invitation called the Black Hills 'The Switzerland of America.' Included in the invitation was the reminder that Rapid City's 3,000 seat convention hall and exhibit center would be finished by the fall of 1928. David F. Jones, Watertown, formerly SDPhA president 1899-1900, had been elected president of APhA at its 1928 meeting. Early in 1929, APhA officials advised SDPhA president F. W. Brown, Lead, that APhA had accepted the invitation and would hold its meeting in Rapid City, SD during August. Many pharmacists from around the nation traveled by train to the Black Hills. President David F. Jones, Watertown, welcomed the pharmacists as a part of his presidential address at the opening session in the convention hall at Rapid City. APhA membership in 1937 was 3,400. It grew to 15,707 members by 1947, of which 63 were from South Dakota.

Earlier in 1929, the State Association convention had been held in Mitchell. The printed proceedings for that state convention contained advertisements for Brown Drug, Sioux Falls; Jewett Drug, Aberdeen; Northwestern Drug, Minneapolis; and McKesson Drug, Sioux City. J.J. McKay, Pierre, was elected president. Rowland G. Jones, Jr., Gettysburg, was elected executive secretary, replacing W.P. Loesch, Oldham, who had served 1925-1929.

Commercial Section

Allen R. Fellows, Sioux Falls, Chairman of the Trade Interests Committee, told the pharmacists at their 1923 meeting that on average only two percent of the people in any given community are taking medicine at any one time. Therefore, pharmacists must sell to the other 98 percent such items as: perfumes, soaps, electrical supplies, sporting goods, stationary, cigars, proprietary medicines, and items from the soda fountain, to name a few. At the same meeting, another pharmacy owner said that after expenses from $40,000 in gross sales, he had about six percent or $2,400 left. Another pharmacist report listed the percentage of total sales from some of the departments in his drug store included: proprietary medicines 22%; prescriptions 10%; soda fountain 14%; toilet articles 10%; cigars 8%; and candy 5%. Some pharmacies reported that gross profit for the average drug store was 33%, which left a net percentage margin on gross sales of about 5%. Gross sales of $40,000 netted about $2,000 a year. Some Board of Pharmacy members complained that they can make $10 a day in their pharmacy but are only paid $5.00 per diem when on official Board business. Obviously, net profits varied from pharmacy to pharmacy.

Department stores and chain stores provided the most competition to community pharmacies. Some manufacturers gave a twenty-two percent

A History of Pharmacy in South Dakota

discount to chain stores when buying in gross lots. Pharmacists maintained that manufacturers should sell products to pharmacies for the same price they sold to chain stores. The pharmacists believed that the commercial side of SDPhA must be expanded. At the 1924 convention, they amended the constitution to create two new committees: Commercial Section and an Educational and Legislative Section. They also changed their name to South Dakota State Pharmaceutical Association. The Commercial Section was designed to secure better prices from manufacturers and promote cooperation between pharmacies, retailers, jobbers, and manufacturers. Generally, it was supposed to further the interests of drug stores from a commercial standpoint.

The new program got underway in 1925 when C. L. "Roy" Doherty, Rapid City, was named chairperson of the new Commercial Committee. Doherty, a three-term mayor of Rapid City, was later elected and served on the State Public Utilities Commission, 1936-1965. D. F. Jones, Watertown, was named chairperson of the new Education and Legislative Committee. Remaining committees included Board of Pharmacy, Business Ethics, College of Pharmacy, Publicity, and Finance. Ph.G. W. F. Michel, Watertown, was hired as manager of the Commercial Section. Association and Board Secretary Ph.G. W. P. Loesch, Oldham, would continue his job. Michel's first task was to raise money from participating pharmacies. Dues were recommended in the range of $10 to $40 a store. In 1925, he sold 223 memberships.

In 1927, Michel collected $2,562. That year the Committee edited and printed a bulletin, *The Optimist*, and mailed it to the members. Michel had to drive around the state to collect the dues. He estimated it cost him $.40 to collect $1.00. In 1928, Michel collected $2,788 and spent $2,684. It was obvious that the program was not going to work. Later that year, the delegates at the convention voted to end the program. Secretary Loesch would continue handling the work of the Association and Board of Pharmacy. The name which had been changed to South Dakota State Pharmaceutical Association remained.

Druggists' Mutual Fire Insurance Co.

Druggists' Mutual Fire Insurance Co. was organized by South Dakota pharmacists and managed by them since its origin in 1895. Secretary S. H. Scallin, Mitchell, generally made a report at each of the Association conventions. In 1917, he told delegates that the company returned thirty-four percent of the premiums in the form of dividends. The company has $13.75 of actual assets for every thousand dollars of insurance in force. Scallin said the company is "The child of the Association. Your stock is worth twenty-five percent more today that five years ago."[1]

About seventy-five percent of the pharmacies did business with the company. However, a number of other businesses in the state were also insured by Druggists' Mutual. Insurance was only sold on property in the city, such as houses, business buildings, business inventory, etc. In 1921, the company had $3.4 million dollars of insurance in force. All of their policies were reinsured. If the company had a $20,000 loss, the company would pay $1,000 and the reinsurance paid the remainder. Of the approximate 325 pharmacies in the state, 268 did business with the company. In 1933, the company had 3,300 policy holders. Secretary S. F. Scallin, Mitchell, reported in 1942, that on December 31, 1941 the company had $2,516,435 net amount of insurance in force. (The corporation was dissolved and its charter surrendered to the South Dakota Commissioner of Insurance in 1951.)

Changing United States Pharmacopoeia (U.S.P.)

Dean Earl Serles, a member of the U.S.P. Revision Committee, reported that a new U.S.P. was being compiled and would be issued in 1930. Two-thirds of the committee working on the project consisted of pharmacists, chemists, and allied workers; one-third were physicians. David F. Jones, Watertown, president of APhA, presented an interesting treatise on the U.S.P. at the 1929 SDPhA convention in Mitchell. Ph.G. Jones had led the Department of Pharmacy at State College in 1895-1896.

Jones maintained that the Pharmacopoeia "over a period of years seems to have grown of less practical value to the retail and dispensing pharmacists and the physician. With each revision, it seems to have become more and more a book for the manufacturing pharmacists, the teacher, and those employed in law enforcement, and of less use to the pharmacist who desires to make and standardize his own preparations.

"The working formulas which made the old revisions books of value, have largely disappeared. Years ago, referring to my own experience, in a [ten year period] I was accustomed to use four or five copies of the Pharmacopoeia. They were literally worn out from use. Now, one or two copies seem to suffice for the entire ten-year period. Is it not possible, however, that this is due to the fact that it is of less practical value as a reference book in every-day work? The present revisions, I fear, are becoming of more value to the manufacturer and of less value to the dispensing pharmacist.

"Today, one will find that the average prescription pharmacy is becoming more and more dependent on the store's private books of working formulas, and less concerned with the official books, aside from their presence as a legal obligation. And, at the same time, the practicing physician is experiencing the same difficulty, and is working more closely with

A History of Pharmacy in South Dakota

his nearby pharmacist, and the U.S.P. and N. F. are not now frequently found in his library. These working tools must be restored."[2]

Perhaps the use of the U.S.P. had decreased for the compounding of prescriptions, however, it was required for many years as an official publication in a licensed South Dakota pharmacy. In fact, a licensed pharmacy was required to have both the U.S.P. and the N. F. on file. The law was changed in 1987 requiring a licensed pharmacy to have only one of the following on file: United States Pharmacopoeia; National Formulary; USPDI drug information for the health care provider; Facts and Comparisons; or American Hospital Formulary Service. The U.S.P. is still listed as one of the five choices, in 36-11-41, October 2000 South Dakota Pharmacy Law and Information. Drugs are defined in 36-11-2.1 with four definitions, one of which is; articles recognized in the official U.S.P. or the official N.F. as adopted by the Board of Pharmacy.

Dean Earl R. Serles, a member of the 1931 U.S.P. Revision Committee, said, "There are more than 600 monographs of items in the U.S.P. In the committee on the Standards of Cod Liver Oil, more than fifty men...have been invited to express their opinions. The pharmacopoeia is the standard, which must be authorized by an Act of Congress and is the backbone of the Pure Food and Drug Acts."[3] Serles was the first member of SDPhA to be appointed to the U.S.P. Revision Committee.

SD Board of Pharmacy, 1920-1929

Examinations

Forty-nine candidates appeared for the Board examinations in 1921. All were high school graduates. Twenty-one held a Ph.G. degree from State College, and five from other Colleges of Pharmacy. Seven of those with Ph.G. degrees were women. After examinations, 30 were registered as pharmacists by examination, 5 registered by reciprocity, 5 registered as assistant pharmacists, and 9 passed the exams, but were short the required one year of practical experience or were under twenty-one years of age.

Regulations required those candidates holding a Ph.G. [Pharmacy Graduate] degree from State College to have one year of practical experience in a pharmacy, either before or after graduation. Those who passed the exams but were short the practical experience or who were not of age, were registered as assistant pharmacists until the full requirements were met. Twenty questions were asked in each of the following exam subjects: Materia Medica, Pharmacy, Chemistry, Orals, and Identification of Drugs. The number of questions asked in Manipulation was up to the individual

Board member. Norma Robbins, Redfield, obtained a 90% grade average in the Board exam and was awarded a one year membership in APhA.

The same exam was given to those seeking registration as pharmacists or as assistant pharmacists. A grade average of 75% and not less than 60% in any one subject was needed to register as a pharmacist. To be registered as an assistant pharmacist, a candidate needed a grade average of 65% and not less than 55% in any one subject. One addition to the 1924 exams required the compounding of five prescriptions. That year, 46 candidates completed the examinations, of which 22 held Ph.G. degrees from State College.

Candidates who had no college diploma were required to show evidence that they had three years of practical experience in a pharmacy, before taking the exams. C. B. Baldwin, Rapid City, and president of the Board of Pharmacy, believed the time had come for all candidates to have a two-year Ph.G. degree before taking the exams. President William E. Bissell, Plankinton, was concerned that too many out-of-state candidates took the South Dakota exams because of the less stringent educational requirements. NABP and twenty other states, as of 1924, required graduation from a reputable College of Pharmacy in order to take the Board examinations. Forty-four states belonged to NABP, whose office handled over 1,200 reciprocity transfers each year.[4]

In 1927, the Board required that all apprentice time be registered with the Board of Pharmacy office. In 1928, the Board of Pharmacy began to give separate exams for registered pharmacists and for registered assistant pharmacists. However, a candidate for a registered pharmacist needed to be 21 years old, whereas a candidate for registered assistant pharmacist only needed to be 18 years old. The Board in 1929, because of excellent facilities at the Division of Pharmacy, State College, voted to give all examinations at the College.

Poison License Law

South Dakota law stated that only registered pharmacists could sell poisons. When making a sale, the pharmacist was required to keep a register showing the name of the poison and the purchaser. Some farmers maintained that pharmacists were charging too much for Paris green, lead arsenate, and formaldehyde. A bill was introduced in the 1924 Legislature to permit lay persons to also sell certain designated poisons under a poison license. Association President J. C. Schutz, Madison, and the Association lobbyist argued against the proposal at the Legislature. However, the Legislature passed a Poison Law permitting lay persons, for the first time, to also sell certain poisons under a $1.00 license. The administration of the law was placed under Commissioner Guy Frary,

South Dakota Food and Drug Department. In 1925, the Legislature transferred the Food and Drug Department to the Department of Agriculture.

The new law also transferred administration of the Poison Law to the Board of Pharmacy. Lay persons could sell such poisons as Paris green, arsenate of lead, insect powders, and formaldehyde in the original packages under the $1.00 license. J. C. Schutz, Madison complained at the 1926 Association convention that whoever obtains the state license thinks it is a license to practice pharmacy and sells products they have no authority to sell. He recommended that the license read Poison Permit, issued by State Board of Pharmacy. The change was made and in 1927, 223 Poison Permits were sold to lay persons throughout the state.

South Dakota Pharmacy Law still restricted the sale of drugs, medicines, and patent medicines to registered pharmacists. Pharmacists could also sell poisons. South Dakota's Attorney General Byron S. Payne ruled in 1923 that it was illegal for anyone other than a registered pharmacist to sell aspirin. The 1903 Pharmacy Act, still in force in 1928, stated that only a registered pharmacist could own and operate a pharmacy.

Records and Record Keeping

A pet project of Governor W. H. McMaster was to consolidate all State Boards and have one secretary. A bill was introduced in the 1923 Legislature to make the consolidation. It was killed in committee. Association and Board finances, however, were always reviewed and discussed by the secretary and the treasurer at the state convention. After their presentation, a motion was made and approved to refer their report to an auditing committee of pharmacists appointed by the president. Later, at a convention business meeting, the auditing committee reported their findings. Association and Board finance reports, as well as the findings of the audit committee, were always published in the annual proceedings of the convention. The 1927 financial records show that only one set of books had been kept. Obviously, it was commingling of state funds and Association funds.

W. P. Loesch, Oldham, was named secretary to the Board and Association in 1925. There was no central office, the secretary kept the records where he lived. Before Loesch, the records were carried between secretaries in tied bundles. One of Loesch's first tasks was to order file cabinets. He spent a year reorganizing the records. CPA F. L. Pollard, Watertown, was asked to audit the records. He reported at the 1929 convention:

> "Although no mishandling of records or money took place,"
> Auditor Pollard reported that the "accounting records of the
> Association are practically nil. Even minute books only cover the

past two years. Although the records of previous years appear to have been lost or misplaced, the statement on page 1 [of his report] is at least a starting point for good future records and I would advise officers to require efficient records at all times. A more appropriate record should be provided for keeping the minutes. It appears Secretary Loesch has maintained a good account of finances. The balance on hand is $1,261."[5] Rowland G. Jones, Gettysburg, was elected as the new secretary of the Association and Board of Pharmacy in 1929. An inventory of his office equipment at Gettysburg, included 1 office desk, 1 office table, 1 wood filing cabinet, 1 steel filing cabinet, 1 Board of Pharmacy seal, for a total value of $325. Presumably he used his own typewriter.

In 1930, Association and Board funds were no longer commingled. Secretary Jones began keeping separate financial accounts for the Association and for the Board of Pharmacy.

Registered Women Pharmacists 1890-1929

Between October 1, 1890, when registered certificate No. 1 was issued under the new South Dakota Pharmacy Law, and the end of 1929, the Board of Pharmacy issued 2,543 registered pharmacist certificates. During the period, 2,413 registered pharmacist certificates were issued to men, and 130 to women.

Registered Assistant Pharmacists 1890-1929

The Territorial Pharmacy Law of 1887 referred to "Registered Assistants" who could assist registered pharmacists in a pharmacy. The new 1890 South Dakota Law referred to "Registered Assistant Pharmacists." A registered assistant pharmacist could only dispense drugs and medicines under the immediate supervision of a registered pharmacist. The first registered assistant pharmacist license issued by the Board of Pharmacy was to Jennie A. Chase, Artesian, on October 1, 1890. The last registered assistant pharmacist license issued was to Cedric J. Sowne, Lead, on May 26, 1926. During the thirty-six year period, the Board of Pharmacy issued 575 registered assistant pharmacist licenses.

In 1924, 52 were licensed as registered assistant pharmacists, of which 33 practiced in South Dakota. In 1927, there were 70 registered assistant pharmacists, of which 45 were practicing in the state. Five of the 45 were women. In 1932, there were still ten registered assistant pharmacists practicing in the state, three of whom were women. Two registered assistant pharmacists were still practicing in 1940, 2 in 1949, 1 in 1969, and none in 1970. The annual renewal fee was $1.00.

A History of Pharmacy in South Dakota

SD College of Pharmacy, 1920-1929

Dean Earl R. Serles noted in his 1921 report that enrollment for 1920-1921 included 28 freshmen, 20 sophomores, 1 junior, and 1 senior, for a total of 50. Sixteen graduated, 14 with Ph.G. degree, 1 with Ph.C. degree, and 1 with B.S. degree. The Department of Pharmacy received a $5,000 appropriation for the purchase of desks, wall storage cases, and drug and laboratory supplies.

Serles also reported that the following courses were being taught in the Department of Pharmacy: Inorganic Chemistry, Organic Chemistry, Pharmaceutical Problems, Business Law and Accounting, Physiology and Hygiene, Bacteriology, Materia Medica, Pharmacognosy, Pharmacy Botany, Pharmacy Latin, Pharmacy, Dispensing, Drug Assaying, Urine Analyses, Toxicology, and Pharmacy Laboratory. A new proposal included a college dispensary which would give practical training to pharmacy students. The dispensary would be for college students only and not be a money maker. In 1926, it was an adjunct to Student Health Service with a pharmacist in charge.

The Department of Pharmacy graduated 21 with Ph.G. degrees in 1923. Tuition per student was $20 and $25 for fees. The number of pharmacists practicing in the state with degrees continued to grow. In 1924, there were 644 in-state pharmacists practicing. Their degree status was as follows: 204 Ph.G.; 21 M.D.; 1 M.D. Ph.G.; 1 Dentist; 1 Ph.G. B.S.; and 2 M.S. for a total of 230 with degrees. The other 414 pharmacists were registered after meeting practical experience requirements and passing Board exams.

On January 22, 1924, the Board of Regents approved a reorganization that included changing the name of Department of Pharmacy to Division of Pharmacy. Earl R. Serles was named Dean of the Division of Pharmacy. Actually, Serles had been running the Department of Pharmacy since Whitehead's death in 1917. Dean Serles later earned his Ph.D. from University of Minnesota in 1934.

The Secretary of National Association of Boards of Pharmacy (NABP) spoke at the 1924 Association gathering in Rapid City. He urged that South Dakota change its pharmacy law to require graduation from a school or college of pharmacy in order to take the Board examinations. Twenty-four states, at the time, required graduation from a College of Pharmacy including North Dakota in 1915, Iowa in 1917, and Minnesota in 1919.

Improvements for the Division of Pharmacy in 1924 included hiring of Floyd Le Blanc as an instructor in pharmacy, providing an extra room and research laboratory, adding of the Schwartz Sectional System in the dispensing laboratory, and enlarging the drug garden. The three faculty and one employee were paid $8,530 in salaries. A faculty member was paid about $2,100 per year. The 1925 budget permitted the purchase of an electric centrifuge, balances, refractometer, microtone, embedding ovens, still for distillation of oils, and an electric still for distilled water. Needs for the next year's budget included a new mill for grinding drugs in the drug milling room in the basement. Total enrollment in the Division of Pharmacy was 68 in 1924, 75 in 1928, and 65 in 1929.

The last two-year class for the Ph.G. degree was in the fall of 1923. The two-year Ph.G. course had been eliminated with the last class graduating in the spring of 1925. This action conformed with the American Conference of Pharmaceutical Faculties, of which State College had been a member since 1908. The two-year course would be replaced with a three-year course wherein a student would earn a Pharmaceutical Chemist (Ph.C.) degree. In 1925, 24 graduated with Ph.G., 4 with a Ph.C., 2 with B.S., and 1 with a M.S. In 1926, only one graduated with a Ph.G. degree, 2 with Ph.C. degree, and 3 with a B.S. degree.

The graduating class in 1927 consisted of 8 with a Ph.C., 2 with B.S., and 1 with a M.S. to Floyd Le Blanc. The Division of Pharmacy in 1927, consisted of four well- equipped laboratories, however, they still were in need of one more laboratory and an extra faculty member. The graduating class in the spring of 1929 consisted of 16 with a Ph.C. degree, and 5 with a B.S. degree.

Whitehead Chapter of SDPhA for pharmacy students was organized in 1923. The first year, 100 percent of the membership paid their $1.00 per quarter dues. The purpose of the student organization, a branch of SDPhA, was to encourage the advancement of pharmacy as a science and a profession. Their meetings were held once a week and consisted of "a regular program planned by the students and consisted of the discussion of current topics dealing with all phases of the drug [profession]. In addition to their regular meetings they found time to make a float for the Hobo Day parade which took first prize. Their six-page edition of the *Industrial Collegian* was mailed to all pharmacists. They were the first student organization in America to pledge money to the APhA headquarters building fund."[6]

In 1928, the American Association of Colleges of Pharmacy asked Dean Frederick J. Wulling, College of Pharmacy, University of Minnesota, to inspect the Division of Pharmacy, South Dakota State College, to determine the quality of its educational program. He gave a favorable rating as to the accreditation of the Division of Pharmacy.

That same year, Professor Floyd LeBlanc spoke at the Huron convention on the subject *Gleanings From Our Garden*. He was referring to the drug garden maintained by the Division of Pharmacy, Brookings. The garden consisted of one-fourth acre with 3,000 plants. They had several plots of belladonna and also grew chenopodium which is used for the treatment of worms in animals. The plants under cultivation furnished much of the material used in the crude drug laboratories. The Division of Pharmacy obtained the oil from the seed and leaves. Dr. Carl Rang, director of the garden, later reported they planted 250 ephedra seeds from China in their garden. Ten plants were germinated in the green house and were transplanted.

A. A. Woodward, Aberdeen, Chairman of SDPhA's Division of Pharmacy Committee presented a good talk explaining the relationship between the Association, Board of Pharmacy, and Division of Pharmacy. He said:

"The work of the Division of Pharmacy, the State Board, and the Association are in a sense the same, inasmuch as each is charged with the safeguarding of the public against unprofessional service.

"It would seem proper to say that the Division of Pharmacy should develop the major portion of the training of young men and women for the profession, that the State Board should, in the best manner possible, determine the fitness of the applicant for the practice of pharmacy, and the State Association should foster these principles which may insure the pharmacist both public and private esteem. The pharmacist reflects his professional training in the conduct of his business.

"During the past five years more than 60% of all the pharmacists registered in the state received their training in our own Division of Pharmacy, and the number is rapidly on the increase."[7]

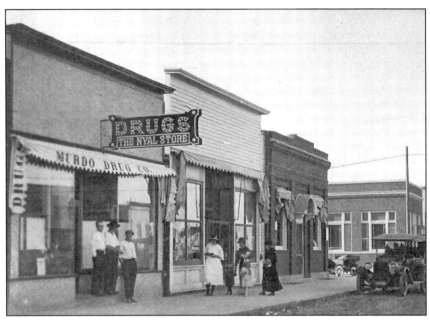

Chas. E. Clute, Murdo Drug Co. circa 1922.

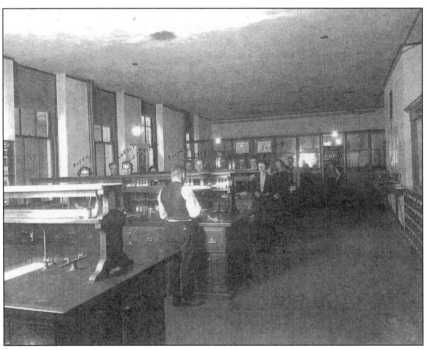

Department of Pharmacy Laboratory, circa 1922, Brookings, SD.

A History of Pharmacy in South Dakota

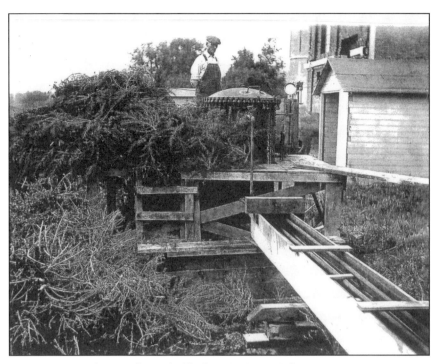

Chenopodium Distillation, SD State College, 1924.

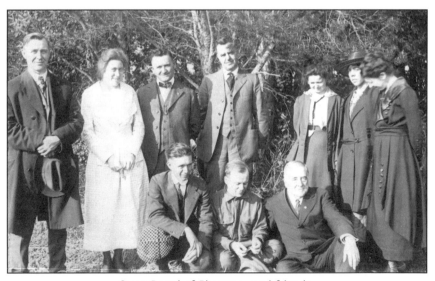

State Board of Pharmacy and friends,
seated left Earl Serles, seated right E. C. Bent, 1919.

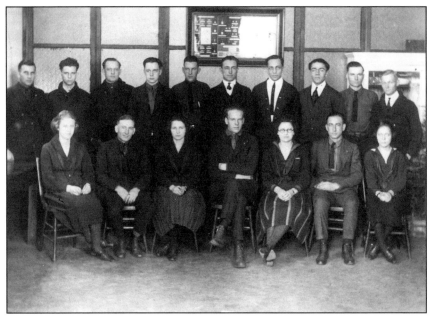

Division of Pharmacy, Class of 1924, Floyd LeBlanc top left.

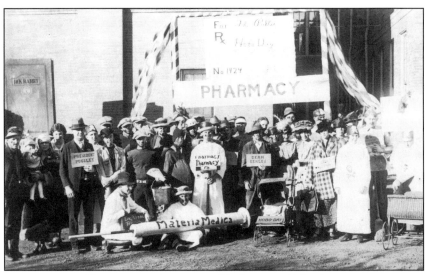

Pharmacy students assemble for 1924 Hobo Day.

A History of Pharmacy in South Dakota

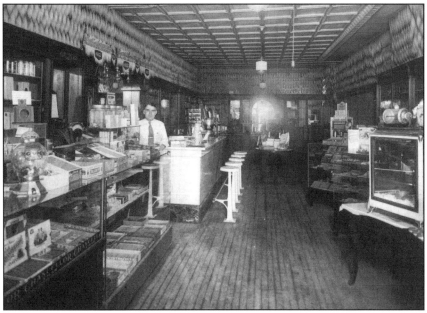

Herbert S. Crissman, standing left, in Crissman Drug, Ipswich, SD, 1925.
(Photo courtesy of Earle T. Crissman)

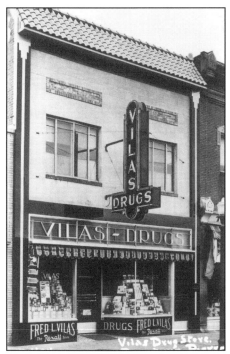

Vilas Drug, Pierre, SD, circa 1930s

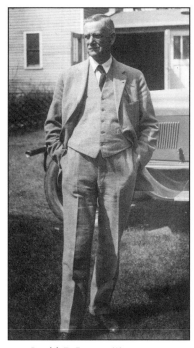

David F. Jones, Watertown,
Pres. APhA, 1929

Chapter Five, 1920-1929

CHAPTER 6
1930-1939

SD Pharmaceutical Association (SDPhA), 1930-1939

Association Events

Secretary Rowland Jones, Jr., Gettysburg, elected at the 1929 convention, informed the members of the 1930 Sioux Falls convention that the new bookkeeping system, recommended by CPA Auditor F. L. Pollard, was working well. Rowland said that Pollard's recommendations had been carried out and that full and complete records were now being kept of all business of the Association and of the Board of Pharmacy. The commingling of the records of the Board and the Association had been replaced with separate records for each entity. Jones also reported that his joint salary from the Board and the Association was $1,500 a year, and that he had spent $254 for a fireproof safe. Jones continued operating his pharmacy in Gettysburg while serving as secretary. He also favored hiring a drug inspector. Membership of out-state and in-state pharmacists in 1930 totaled 691. The $5 renewal fee produced $3,455 for the Association account. A $1.00 renewal fee was also collected from each of the fifteen practicing assistant pharmacists. In 1939, there were 673 in-state and out-state registered pharmacists and two registered assistant pharmacists.

Cyrus B. Warne, Redfield, conducted the Memorial Hour in the ballroom of the Cataract Hotel, for three deceased pharmacists. Warne, who had been one of the organizers of the first Memorial Hour in 1927, had been in Rapid City and said it took him eight hours to drive to Sioux Falls. He averaged about forty miles per hour. The Commercial Drug Travelers who had reorganized in 1921, reorganized again and changed their name to Allied Drug Travelers. They elected W. F. Ottman president. Association President J. J. McKay, Pierre, recommended the Association form statewide districts similar to the Minnehaha County Druggists' Association. The Sioux Falls group had from twenty-five to thirty members attend their business and social meetings.

The following year at the Madison convention, a pharmacist round-table discussion was held pertaining to the business impact of lay persons selling poisons. Lay persons had been authorized to sell certain poisons by the 1924 Legislature. Ralph Williams, Wakonda, said he tried to make a thirty-three percent gross profit on the poison products he sells. J. C. Schutz, Madison, remarked that a licensee in Madison sells Paris green for $.05 a pound less than for what he can buy it. D. F. Jones, Watertown, believed that there was no profit left for pharmacists to sell poisons. H. L. Lewis, Hartford, told the group that he had a registered pharmacist in his drug store at all times who can sell poisons, but there are also five lay persons, in his town of 640 people, with the $1.00 poison license doing the same thing. Karl E. Mundt, professor at the college in Madison, was speaker at the banquet in St. Thomas School.

In 1931, there was a growing practice among pharmaceutical manufacturers to compound various well-known formulas and then introduce them to physicians under proprietary names. Nina Lund, Oldham, Chairperson of the Association's 1931 Resolution Committee introduced a resolution wherein the following was maintained:

- that the ingredients of such formulas are found in the prescription departments of all drug stores
- that pharmacists are able to compound these preparations
- that the identifiable packages leads to self-medication
- that a prescription for the patent medicines creates an unqualified endorsement of the preparation

therefore the South Dakota Pharmaceutical Association deprecates the practice of prescribing and fostering the use of such preparations under proprietary names.[1]

A Prescription Department Sales Analysis, dealing with the professional side of pharmacy, was reviewed at the 1932 convention by J. W. Vander Laan, Minneapolis. The survey study included 70,000 prescriptions. The average prescription department stock, it was found, comprised 29% (1,500 items) of the total number of items stocked by the store, but only 17% ($1,140) of the average store inventory of $6,800. Analysis of the prescription stock inventory showed it to be divided into 30% to 40% specialties, 20% to 30% galenicals [medicines], and 11% to 14% chemicals. Official U. S. P. and N. F. chemicals and galenicals were found to account for about 80% of the total ingredients used, and manufacturing specialties for the remaining 20%. Some 61% of the prescriptions in the study were liquids, 17.5% were capsules, 10% tablets, 3.8% ointments and 3.3% divided powders. Sixty-five percent of all prescriptions studied called for more than one ingredient.[2]

Secretary Rowland Jones, Jr. and President C. L. "Roy" Doherty, Rapid City, had attended the 1931 NARD convention in Detroit. The total attendance at the gathering was 2,800. Expenses totaled $160 for Doherty and $156 for Jones. Henry J. Schnaidt, Parkston, delegate to the 1931 APhA convention in Miami, reported that the $800,000 American Institute of Pharmacy Building, in Washington, D.C. would be completed soon. A half-day discussion was held pertaining to the Army's practice of using privates to dispense drugs. However, the Army Medical Department planned to establish an Army Pharmacy Corps in the future. In 1934, Secretary Rowland Jones was invited to the dedication of the new marble building called The American Institute of Pharmacy. It was located on the west end of Constitution Avenue, not too far from the Lincoln Memorial. At the time, fifty South Dakota pharmacists were members of APhA.

One resolution approved at the 1934 convention in Brookings pertained to grocery stores: "Considering we expect grocers to refrain from carrying drug store items in stock for sale, we hereby go on record as opposed to drug stores handling for sale any grocery store items."[3] That year the total Association finances included income of $3,996, including pharmacy renewal fees, and $4,553 expense. A loss of $557 was made up from the prior year balances. The Association Constitution was amended in 1935 giving the Executive Committee the power to employ the Association secretary and set the salary. The final vote was 40 Yes and 1 No. Prior to this time the secretary was elected by ballot at the convention.

The Executive Committee, appointed Kenneth Jones, Gettysburg, a brother of Rowland Jones, Jr., as Association secretary, in 1935. The prior year, Secretary Rowland Jones, Jr., Gettysburg, was called to Washington, D. C. to serve as the Washington Representative for NARD. About a third of the nation's pharmacies belonged to NARD. Also in 1935, President George W. Lloyd, Spencer, reported that eighteen districts had been formed within the Association. The district in the northeast corner was chaired by F. M. Cornwell, Webster. At one of their meetings, area doctors and dentists had been invited to hear speaker Earl Serles, Dean of the Division of Pharmacy, State College. That same year, an Allied Council had been formed including representatives from the dental, nursing, veterinary, hospital, pharmacy, and medical associations. The purpose of the Council was to promote the science and art of practice of the member professions, in so far as they affect...the practice of the healing arts in South Dakota.

In 1935, the Legislature approved a three percent sales tax to replace the gross income tax. A $.50 license fee was charged by the Department of Taxation to collect the tax for the state. The collection formula was as follows: $.01 for sales between $.15 to $.64; $.02 for sales between $.65 and $1.25; and $.03 for sales between $1.26 and $1.74. Pharmacists were informed to collect the tax as they rang up the sale.

William G. France, Canistota, a student from the Division of Pharmacy, presented a paper at the 1937 meeting of pharmacists. He said his research indicated that in 1917, 90% of a pharmacies income was from these prescription items: pills, powders, mustard plasters, tonics, nerve remedies, cough medicines, etc. However, in 1937, only 10% of the pharmacies income was from those prescription items, and 90% of the income was from other departments within the pharmacy. In 1937, there were 165,000,000 prescriptions dispensed in the nation, costing an average of $.85 each.[4]

"Merchandising in the Modern Drug Store" was the theme at the April 1938 convention in the Sioux Falls Coliseum. Seventy-five manufacturers' and wholesalers' exhibits were on display at the drug show. Secretary Kenneth Jones, Gettysburg, announced at a business meeting, that he was sending a new monthly bulletin to each of the pharmacies in the state. It had been the practice to send the current Association president to the APhA convention. President Tom Haggar, Sioux Falls, recommended a resolution requiring the incoming president to attend that meeting so that person could institute what he had learned. It passed. Over 450 people jammed the Coliseum for the evening banquet and to hear a speech by Governor Harlan Bushfield. C.A. Locke, Brookings, was elected president for the year 1938-1939.

Congressman Karl E. Mundt was the speaker at the 1939 Association banquet in the Brown Palace Motel, Mobridge. The printed annual proceedings of the 1939 convention cost $2.05 a page to print. Included in the proceedings was the salary of $25 a month for the office secretary who was also paid $25 by the Board. Yearly Association salaries included treasurer, $100; president, $50; and a grant to the Ladies' Auxiliary, $25. The Executive Committee members were paid $.05 a mile for driving their cars. Herb Crissman, Ipswich, was elected president for the 1939-1940 year.

Northwestern Druggist

In 1901, the Association had adopted *Northwestern Druggist*, Minneapolis, as its official publication. News, information, and convention meeting notices were provided to the magazine by the secretary or a member of the Publicity Committee. News items were printed in a special South Dakota Section. George A. Bender, Watertown, frequently wrote articles for the magazine. Bender, who spent his early years in Webster, graduated from Division of Pharmacy, State College, Brookings in 1923. He practiced six years in Watertown before going to Minneapolis in 1929 to join the staff of *Northwestern Druggist*.

In 1933, Bender became editor of the *NARD Journal* where he served twelve years. After a period with *American Druggist*, he joined Parke-Davis & Company in Detroit as editor of *Modern Pharmacy* in 1947. By 1958, he had become Director of Institutional Advertising and the company's historian. Also in 1958, Bender was awarded an honorary degree from South Dakota State University. In 1966, with the cooperation of Artist Robert A. Thom, Bender developed and published two series of historical articles and the original oil paintings that comprised *Great Moments in Pharmacy and Great Moments in Medicine*. Those articles and paintings have encircled the world. Later, he joined the faculty of the College of Pharmacy, University of Arizona. In 1985, he wrote *A History of Arizona Pharmacy*.

Northwestern Druggist continued carrying South Dakota pharmacy news until 1947. That year, SDPhA and SDMA agreed to jointly publish the *South Dakota Journal of Medicine and Pharmacy*.

Drought, Dust, and Hard Times

During the 1920s and the 1930s, thousands of South Dakotans lost money in failed state banks and the stock market crash, while thousands more lost their farms by mortgage foreclosure. Drought, grasshoppers, and dust storms were next in line. Main Street South Dakota was barely surviving. The Civil Works Administration, Public Works Administration, Work Progress Administration (WPA), and other relief programs helped the unemployed, needy farmers, and businesses in South Dakota. WPA work programs, such as building roads, dams, schools, auditoriums etc., helped people earn from $32 to $45 a month. In 1936, there were 39,350 rural persons and 10,082 city persons working on WPA in South Dakota.

One of the private programs to help farmers was the Farmer's Aid Corporation. Farmers, who were clients of the Farm Security Administration, paid $2.00 a month for which they were promised payment of their doctor, drug, and dental bills. In 1934, SDPhA worked out a program with the Farmer's Aid Corporation whereby pharmacists would sell drugs to their clients at a ten percent discount. The program continued until 1939. A final tabulation showed that pharmacies were only paid for about twenty percent of their bills, even after giving a discount of ten percent. It wasn't until 1947 that Farmer's Aid Corporation was liquidated in Circuit Court. Only enough funds were left to pay five percent of the original unpaid bills.

Because of the depression, a motion was made at the 1932 Association convention to cut the meeting from three to two days. The motion lost. After a call for a standing vote, the motion still lost. Generally, the conventioneers favored business sessions in the morning and sports events in the afternoon. The convention in Rapid City in 1933, however, lost money due to a small attendance.

In 1932, there were 342 licensed drug stores compared to 315 in 1939. President Charles Locke, Brookings, reported to the 1939 convention that the United States Department of Commerce statistics show that the retail drug business suffered less in 1938 than any other business.

Fair Trade

The depression was not the only business problem facing drug stores during the 1930s. President A. C. Thompson, Colton, in his convention address at the Alex Johnson Hotel in Rapid City in 1933 tells about other problems. He said, "Things are happening too fast today to safely permit any druggist to go to sleep on the job. Today one hears of cut prices, pine board stores, pharma-groceries, super markets, and every kind of competitive inroads on the drug store. Our old-time competitors: the peddlers, mail order houses, department stores, are still in the running and must be dealt with. A druggist must give full attention to business. Keep alert, with your finger on the community pulse. Endeavor to make your drug store the center of drug purchases in your community, and to make people want to trade with you."[5]

The larger problem facing the average drug store and other main street businesses, was price cutting by chain stores. Chain stores and others sold products for less than the price shown on the package, sometimes almost at cost. Some chain stores were thinking of adding a drug department, presumably staffed by a registered pharmacist. Chain stores cutting prices was of concern to main street businesses, both in small towns and large cities. A movement began in the country to approve legislation, called Fair Trade Laws, making it illegal to sell products for less than the minimum price printed on the package. Some people argued there was a precedent for Fair Trade Laws. At one time, railroads were prohibited from giving service for less than the regular price. Laws compelled telephone companies to maintain a uniform schedule of rates for their customers. Insurance companies were not allowed to collect different premiums for policies carrying the same risk. Public warehouses were required to charge the same price for storing grain and other commodities.

Fair Trade Laws were being passed by a number of states. The reason, as explained by Secretary Kenneth Jones, Gettysburg, was to allow a retailer to "sell merchandise at a price marked on the package at a reasonable profit to retailer."[6] Rowland Jones, with the NARD in Washington, described the Fair Trade Law as an "act of a State Legislature aimed at the elimination of loss leader selling. Generally, these acts make lawful contracts between the manufacturers, and distributors [retailers] whereby minimum resale prices are set up for trade marked merchandise, which is in free and open competition with other merchandise of the same general class."[7]

In 1937, The South Dakota Legislature passed a Fair Trade Act. The bill passed unanimously in the Senate and 90 Yes to 6 No in the House. State Representative George T. Mickelson, Selby, told the legislators that "The chain stores have forced themselves into our communities to such an extent we must protect the small town merchant. I believe this bill is a step in the right direction."[8] In general, the Fair Trade Act, according to the South Dakota law, was a contract between a wholesaler and a retailer, wherein the retailer would not resell the same except to consumers for use and at not less than the stipulated minimum price. The Act only pertained to trade-marked and brand name products. When Governor Leslie Jensen signed the Fair Trace Act into law, the following witnessed the event: W. C. Botkin, Secretary SD Retail Merchants Association; Kenneth Jones, Secretary SDPhA; and Representative George T. Mickelson.

The South Dakota Legislature, to help protect retail merchants, passed a Chain Store Tax on March 7, 1939. The bill passed the House 64 Yes, 9 No. In the Senate the vote was 29 Yes and 6 No. The tax amounted to $150 per store, upon a chain of fifty or more stores, whether or not all of the stores were located inside South Dakota.

In 1940, the Fair Tract Act was challenged in the South Dakota Supreme Court. The Court upheld the Fair Trade Act because it did not violate the anti-trust and anti-monopoly clauses of the South Dakota Constitution. The United States Supreme Court had upheld the California and Illinois Fair Trade Laws. However, there were other legislative and court hurdles ahead.

During the era of Fair Trade Laws, the South Dakota Pharmaceutical Association took another step to limit price cutting. In the 1936 convention, a resolution was passed approving a uniform price schedule to correct a wide variation in prices charged for prescriptions. The schedule was mailed to all pharmacies for a one-year trial period. The schedule was reaffirmed in later conventions up to 1940. A prescription price schedule was discussed again at the 1951 convention. Secretary Bliss Wilson reminded delegates, "While we cannot adopt it as an Association, we can send it out to all members as a recommendation." Secretary Wilson was instructed to mail a copy to all the members. (The uniform price schedule was disbanded in 1961, because of anti-trust concerns.)

Pharmacists were guided by the statutory phrase in the South Dakota Pharmacy Act wherein the purpose of the South Dakota Pharmaceutical

Association was defined: "The purpose of which shall be to improve the science and art of pharmacy and to restrict the sale of medicines to regularly educated and qualified persons." Pharmacists believed that it would be difficult to improve the science and art of pharmacy, if pharmacies were driven out of business by price cutters and other monopolistic practices. They also believed the Legislature created their profession to protect public health, by restricting the practice to educated and qualified persons.

In time, Fair Trade Laws ran their course in American business. The South Dakota Supreme Court in 1970, ruled that the non-signer provision of the Fair Trade Act was constitutionally invalid as an unlawful delegation of legislative power to private parties.

Ladies' Auxiliary of SDPhA

The Ladies' Auxiliary, organized at Flandreau in 1902, continued its annual meetings during the conventions of the Association. At the 1932 convention in Aberdeen, June 14, 15, 16, they met in the ballroom of the Alonzo Ward Hotel for their opening session. After a business meeting, the group attended a bridge luncheon at the Aberdeen Country Club. That evening, they joined other convention members at a dancing party in Wylie Park Pavilion, hosted by the SDPhA.

On Wednesday, the Ladies' Auxiliary joined with Association members at the Memorial Hour, conducted by A. C. Thompson, Colton. At the Auxiliary business meeting, chaired by President Mrs. O. C. Nicolls, Mitchell, the group voted to convert their scholarship fund into a student loan fund. Principal and interest were not due until after graduation. New officers elected included: President, Mrs. N. B. Porter, Madison; Vice-President, Mrs. Lloyd Daniels, Aberdeen; and Secretary-Treasurer, Mrs. Bliss C. Wilson, Letcher. Afternoon events included playing golf at the Aberdeen Country Club. Thursday, the Auxiliary toured Siebrecht Greenhouse, where each guest was presented flowers.

SD Board of Pharmacy, 1930-1939

South Dakota pharmacy law stated it was "unlawful for any person other than a registered pharmacist to retail, compound, or dispense drugs, medicines or poisons." The law included patent medicines and poisons in the original packages. In 1924, however, the Legislature permitted lay persons to sell certain packaged poisons. Historically, the Board had difficulty enforcing the law, because they had no drug inspector. Persons violating the statute, however, were turned over to the states attorney for prosecution.

In 1927, P. E. Wood, Mitchell, was charged for selling some Watkins' Remedies without being a registered pharmacist. Municipal Judge Herbert ruled that the part of South Dakota pharmacy law, limiting the sale of packaged patent medicines and poisons to pharmacists, was unconstitutional. He explained his decision with this statement, "If a clerk in a drug store, without pharmacy instruction can sell patent medicines and other drugs already made up for sale, it seems only reasonable that grocery stores or any other parties who wish to enter the business of selling drugs in the original package, be permitted to do so."[9]

Pharmacists appealed the decision. Eventually, the case was carried to the South Dakota Supreme Court, who upheld the decision of the lower courts. The Association and the Board of Pharmacy, mindful of the Supreme Court's decision, decided to go to the 1931 State Legislature to change the pharmacy law.

Fortunately, there were four pharmacists serving in the 1931 Legislature. L. E. Highley, Hot Springs and L. G. France, Canistota both served in the Senate. Highley had also served in the 1929 Legislature. L. J. Laxson, Canton, and A. C. Thompson, Colton, both served in the House of Representatives. Thompson had also served in the 1929 Legislature. Highley was Chairperson of the Food and Drug Committee in the Senate, and Laxson was Chairperson of the same committee in the House.

Generally, there was a revamping of the South Dakota pharmacy law. The final bill that passed the Legislature contained these features:

- Limited future ownership of South Dakota pharmacies to registered pharmacists only. However, a grandfather clause permitted a corporation, whose owners were not registered pharmacists, to continue on as before. (At the time, all pharmacies were independently owned, except St. Luke's Hospital in Aberdeen, Walgreen Pharmacy in Sioux Falls, and two clinic pharmacies, one in Huron and one in Sioux Falls.) Non-pharmacist owners were permitted to sell their interests to registered pharmacists.
- New pharmacies could not be opened by non-registered pharmacists.
- For the first time, all pharmacies needed to be licensed, by paying a $10 fee to the Board of Pharmacy before July 1, 1931.
- All apprentice pharmacists must register their practical experience time with the Board of Pharmacy and pay a fee.
- Board of Pharmacy authorized to hire a full-time salaried pharmacist drug inspector.

A History of Pharmacy in South Dakota

- Illegal to use the words 'drug store' or 'pharmacy' in advertisements or signs, by any business unless it be by a licensed pharmacy.
- Four-year college of pharmacy degree and one year of practical experience required to take Board of Pharmacy examinations by July 1, 1933. (However, if a person was engaged in a pharmacy one year prior to this act, that person could register by examination under the old requirement of a high school diploma and three year's experience in a pharmacy under supervision of a registered pharmacist, but such registration must be before July 1, 1933).
- Lay persons could continue selling certain packaged poisons, with the skull and crossbones printed on the label, under a $1 license secured from the Board of Pharmacy. Each sale had to be recorded and signed for by the purchaser in a poison register. Registered pharmacists were required to follow the same procedures.

The matter of lay persons selling pre-packaged patent and proprietary medicines wasn't resolved until the 1933 Legislative Session. That year, the Legislature, to provide some state control, authorized persons, other than licensed pharmacists, to sell packaged Patent Medicines under a $1.00 license obtained from the Board of Pharmacy. Patent Medicine License holders were not authorized to sell any U.S.P. or N.F. items.

Administration of 1931 Pharmacy Law Amendments

All pharmacies in South Dakota needed to pay the $10 fee and be licensed by July 1, 1931. The location of the 331 pharmacies licensed by that date indicated: 203 were located in cities and towns that had more than one pharmacy, and 128 were in towns and cities with one pharmacy. Ownership of the 331 pharmacies was as follows: 327 independents; 1 in St. Luke's Hospital, Aberdeen; 1 in Walgreens, Sioux Falls; and 2 clinic pharmacies, 1 in Huron and 1 in Sioux Falls. Three hundred fifty-three $1 poison licenses were also issued by the Board.

On July 31, 1931, the Board of Pharmacy hired Pharmacist F.E. Briggs, Sioux Falls, as its first drug inspector at a salary of $1,500 per year. His 1932 report showed he had made 1,770 inspections since employed. He traveled 14,500 miles and was paid $.04 a mile, which was three cents less than the $.07 a mile allowed by the state. He said he had given out 100 poison registers and 60,000 poison labels to license holders. Briggs also noted there were 108 medicine peddlers operating in the state, however, only 60 had obtained a peddler's license issued by the State Sheriff. His inspection of the 331 pharmacies showed some minor infractions, which he ordered corrected. His total travel expense was $811. In 1933, Briggs inspected 340 drug stores, and 1,235 other license holders. His inspection included the holders of the new Patent Medicine License, of which 175 had been purchased before the July 1, 1933 deadline.

That same year, Secretary Rowland Jones, Jr., took two parties to court who had used in their advertisements, "Save on Drugs", a practice made illegal by the 1931 Legislature. Inspector Briggs' 1934 report showed he had made 1,979 inspections and had found 210 violations. A large percentage of the violations included the illegal sale of aspirin, asperline, and aspercin which could be sold by registered pharmacists only. By 1934, the Board of Pharmacy had issued 599 Patent Medicine Licenses and 527 Poison Licenses. Total Board of Pharmacy 1934 license fee revenue from drug stores, patent medicine dealers, poison dealers, examinations and other fees, plus a $750 grant from the South Dakota Pharmaceutical Association, totaled $6,589. The number of licenses issued for 1939-1940 included 338 pharmacies, 543 poison retailers, and 796 patent medicine retailers. Many hardware stores, grocery stores, etc., carried both the Patent Medicine License and Poison License.

On July 1, 1939 the Board of Pharmacy hired a new drug inspector, George W. Lloyd, Spencer.

SD College of Pharmacy, 1930-1939

Four-Year Pharmacy Course

Association President J. J. McKay, Pierre, had recommended to the 1930 convention that the pharmacy law be changed to require completion of a four-year pharmacy course to take the Board of Pharmacy examinations. This change would satisfy the requirements of the National Boards of Pharmacy. A resolution was adopted to support that concept before the 1931 Legislature. A law was passed requiring a four-year pharmacy course, plus one year of practical experience, effective July 1, 1933. The extra time permitted the Division of Pharmacy and its students to prepare for the new standard culminating in a B.S. degree. The three-year Ph.C. course, first offered in 1918, ended in 1930.

H. C. Christensen, president of APhA, told the pharmacists at the 1931 convention that thirty-eight states, including South Dakota, now require a four-year pharmacy course in order to take the Board examinations. He maintained:

"The four-year course is a real salvation of pharmacy. If we are to be classified as professionals, we must enforce professional standards. While the pharmacist may not be called on to compound drugs and medicines as frequently as a few years ago, he must know as much or more than ever if he is to remain a guardian of the public health and welfare.

"Remington gives the following definition for pharmacy: 'Pharmacy is the science which treats of medicinal substances. It embraces not only a knowledge of medicines and the art of preparing and dispensing them, but also of their identification, selection, preservation, combination, analysis, and standardization.' Pharmacy therefore is more than mixing a few ingredients and sticking a label on a bottle.

"We have lived through an era in which manufacturing and distribution have been taken away from small local units, and supplanted by mass production and mass distribution through large organizations. Machine-made products are taking the place of hand-made products. The retail pharmacist is dispensing the products of large pharmaceutical manufacturers instead of his own products, as he did some years ago. Modern medicine requires synthetic organic chemicals and biological products which no pharmacist can manufacture with his limited facilities, as these require specially equipped laboratories, research work, etc. But the fact that the retail pharmacist has survived in spite of all these changes proves that there is a field for him, although his service to the community may be along somewhat new lines. The problem is ours to work out."[10]

Dean Earl R. Serles, at the same 1931 convention, talked about the new era for pharmacy: "Shall we agree with the man who loudly proclaims that pharmacy is a lost art simply because physicians no longer prescribe tinctures, fluid extracts, ointments, powders, pills, and lotions but are using in their stead, tablet triturates, ampules, serums, vaccines, hypodermic solutions and are doing blood transfusions instead of blood letting, or shall we keep abreast of the times, modernize our prescription department, equipping it as a laboratory and continue to serve the physician in the new field which he has entered. The profession of pharmacy is today entering upon a new era. The practice of medicine has changed from the use of the old-time preparations, tinctures, and fluid extracts, to the administration of more scientifically prepared substances to give a definite result. I believe, positively, the future field of pharmacy will have an opportunity for the [pharmacist] to develop a service as laboratory assistant to that newer type of physician."[11]

Association President O. J. Tommeraason, Madison, talked about the old-fashioned drug store at the 1932 gathering in the Alonzo Ward Hotel, Aberdeen: "The old-fashioned drug store with the aroma of liquids, pills, and powders and the long rows of dusty bottles has been superseded by the modern department store which sells everything from sandwiches to radios. The modern pharmacist must...know the conditions that affect general merchandising as well as fulfill the duties of giving expert prescription service to the doctor and to the sick."[12]

Dean Earl R. Serles, in reference to the four-year course, said, "The prescription materials used today are changed very much from the simple inorganic chemicals, tinctures, and fluid extracts and in their places have come synthetic organic compounds, ampules, isotonic solutions, and intricate proprietaries. Serums and vaccines have been added to the list and a knowledge of their content is demanded, hence Bacteriology."[13] He also said that the new four-year college training requirement "has enabled the Division of Pharmacy to outline courses of training in three distinct fields: retail pharmacy, pharmaceutical research, and clinical and hospital pharmacy."[14]

The three fields of training at the Division of Pharmacy were activated in the fall of 1930. Bliss C. Wilson, Letcher, Chairperson of School of Pharmacy Association Committee, reported at the 1932 convention about the three fields of training. The curricula for the first two years were the same in all groups and provide training in Pharmacy, Pharmacognosy, Chemistry, Bacteriology, Physiology, and English. At the end of the sophomore year, the students elected their field of training. The remaining courses within the three fields were as follows:

Retail Pharmacy Field: Sign Writing, Window Display, Store Management, Business Law, Salesmanship, Business Mathematics, Economics, Sociology, and Entomology;

Pharmaceutical Research Field: Mathematics, Physics, Advanced Organic Chemistry, Toxicology, French or German, Drug Assay, and Pharmacology;

Clinical and Hospital Pharmacy Field: Bacteriology, Clinical Methods, Pharmacology, Pathology, and other research.[15]

C. A. Locke, Brookings, Chairperson, Association's Division of Pharmacy Committee in 1934, presented a summary of the Division of Pharmacy since 1888: 500 students had enrolled; 394 had received degrees; 148 are registered in South Dakota of which 74 operated their own drug store. Enrollment in the Division of Pharmacy was 86 in 1930-31; 62 in 1931-1932; and 100 in 1938-1939. Seventeen graduated with a B. S. degree in 1935, and 25 in 1939. Tuition and fees in 1931-1932 were $151 a student along with laboratory fees of $21 each.

Chairperson A. O. Bittner, Cresbard, Association's Division of Pharmacy Committee in 1936, explained why the enrollment had increased:

"The pharmacy course gives training to the student in clinical laboratory work including the use and operation of an X-ray. This enables the student to serve as a hospital pharmacist or be of service to physicians who use these practices in connection with the clinical studies; courses given in the Department of Entomology are so designed to acquaint the student with the use of insecticides and fumigants; courses taken in the Department of Veterinary Medicine offer an opportunity for information concerning contagious and non-contagious diseases of animals.

"These two latter department courses are of valuable aid to retail pharmacists located in agricultural areas. The drug garden...offers them opportunities for research work with various medicinal plants. The well-equipped laboratories offer unlimited opportunities to do research in such fields as Cosmetics, Drug Standardization, and Biological Assays. With the high enrollment of 100 students, additional laboratory space must be provided."[16]

In 1931, a bill was introduced by Senator J. S. Harkness, Mitchell, in the State Senate to establish a 'Greater University System'. One of the provisions of the bill would have moved the Division of Pharmacy to the Medical Department at the University of South Dakota. Both SDPhA and the Division of Pharmacy opposed the bill. It did not pass; however, the Legislature agreed to have the Board of Regents study the Montana system.

Student Loan Fund

This fund was established by Secretary E. C. Bent, after the Edison Company donated a phonograph which was raffled off for $450 at the 1921 convention. Secretary E. C. Bent donated another $50 to the fund. The Association gave $100 a year until the fund totaled $1,000. The Board of Pharmacy contributed another $200 bringing the total to $1,200. Between 1920 and 1934, 75 loans were made: 45 loans made and paid; 12 current; 9 past due; 4 paid on a past due basis; and nothing had been paid on 5 loans. Average loans amounted to $100 per year. After 1930, only seniors could borrow money from the fund. Between 1920 and 1939, 81 loans had been made.

Student Groups and Early Scholarships

In 1920, Secretary E. C. Bent, Dell Rapids, gave a $10 gold piece to the highest ranking pharmacy student, possibly the earliest pharmacy scholarship award. However, Chairperson C. A. Locke, Brookings, Association's Division of Pharmacy Committee reported at the 1935 convention, that the first pharmacy award established at the school was by Rowland Jones, Jr., Gettysburg, former secretary 1929-1935, who gave $50 for a Jones Scholarship Award. The award was granted to a junior pharmacy student who performed the best work in Practical Pharmacy.

Shortly after, Jewett Drug, Aberdeen, established the Jewett Drug Scholarship for $200. The award was given to a graduate who was best suited for graduate work.[17]

The Whitehead Chapter of SDPhA, established in 1923, was active throughout the year and had good programs at each of its bi-weekly meetings. Tau Chapter of Rho Chi Society, national honor society in pharmacy, was organized April 1931. Its objectives included the promotion of the profession of pharmacy and the pharmaceutical sciences by encouraging scholarship and good fellowship. Membership was open to students in the highest twenty percent of their class, who had a grade point average of 3.0, and had completed 100 hours of course work applicable to their degree. In 1934, the chapter had 52 alumni members and 11 active members.

Accreditation

A 1933 accreditation visit to the Division of Pharmacy by a representative of the American Association of Colleges of Pharmacy indicated: "The faculty was well trained and carried reasonable instructional loads. Buildings and laboratories adequate and well equipped. Drug Plant Garden a real adjunct to teaching and research."[18]

Representatives of the American Council on Pharmaceutical Education (ACPE), organized in 1932, visited the Division of Pharmacy, State College, Brookings on May 12-13, 1939. Their report indicated that Pharmacy was given 'full accreditment', but among the five recommendations for improvement of the College were suggestions for 'more adequate space' and for an 'additional instructor.' At the time, David F. Jones, Watertown, was one of the ten first members of the ACPE.[19]

Budgets

A.O. Bittner, Cresbard, chairperson, Association's Division of Pharmacy Committee presented twelve-year budget figures to the 1936 convention. Averages of his figures for State College's Division of Pharmacy are presented below:

- Enrollment: Between 1924-1929, the average enrollment per year was 72. Between 1930-1935, the average enrollment per year was 74. Low was 61 in 1930 and high 101 in 1935
- Total average salary money appropriated by state per year was $9,504. High in 1927 was $11,620 and low in 1933 was $7,401.
- Faculty: During the 12 year period, the average number of faculty on duty per year was 3.3, it was never below 3 and

never above 4. (Does not include 1 or 2 additional employees per year.)

- Salary: Average salary of faculty members was $2,880 per year
- College monies from tuition, fees, etc.: Average per year was $8,122
- Budget: from state appropriation for maintenance of laboratory, new equipment, care of drug garden etc. Average was $4085 per year. High in 1925 was $5,000, and low in 1934 was $3,725
- Supplies, Equipment and Breakage: Between 1924-1929 it averaged $3,948 per year. Between 1930-1935 it averaged $1,465 per year.[20]

Professor Clark Eidsmoe, commenting about the 1930s depression, said, "Legislative appropriations were kept at the barest minimum and salaries of personnel were drastically reduced. Under such conditions progress was difficult. Nevertheless, in the Division of Pharmacy, the faculty was kept intact and the quality of instruction was maintained at a high level. During this period...a Department of Pharmaceutical Chemistry, and one of Pharmacology and Pharmacognosy were created. These departments were headed by Professors Serles, LeBlanc, and Hiner respectively. In 1935, at the request of the State Nurses' Association, a Department of Nursing was established at South Dakota State College and for administrative purposes was attached to the Division of Pharmacy. This arrangement was continued until July 1, 1956."[21]

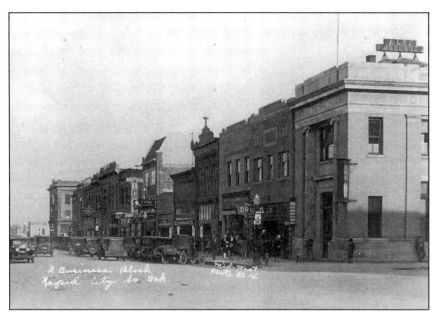

Three drug stores on one block in Rapid City, 1930:
C.M. Fallon Drug; Roy Doherty Drug; R.H. Ottmann Drugs
(Photo courtesy Robert Kolbe Collections, Sioux Falls, SD)

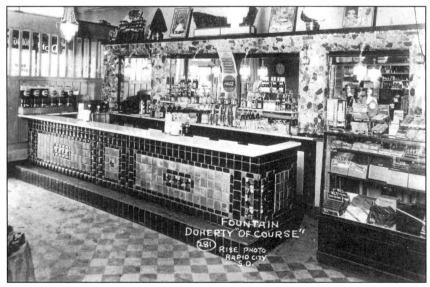

Roy Doherty Drug Fountain, Rapid City, circa 1935.

A History of Pharmacy in South Dakota

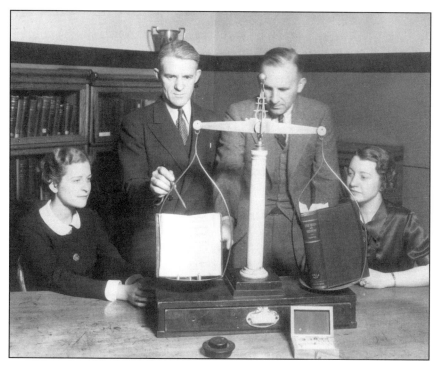

Official testing of the scale, left to right, student Dorothy Nelson, Prof. C.T. Eidsmoe, Dean Floyd LeBlanc, Secretary Helen Spomer, circa 1937.

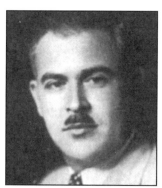
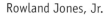
Rowland Jones, Jr.

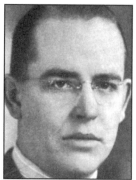
Kenneth Jones

Pharmacist Rowland Jones, Jr. Gettysburg, on the left, was secretary to the Association and Board 1929-1935, before leaving for Washinton, D.C. as NARD's Washinton Representative. His brother, Pharmacist Kenneth Jones, on the right, also from Gettysburg, was then named secretary to the Association and Board. He served until 1942, when he accepted a job with McKesson and Robbins in Sioux City. The Executive Committee then hired Pharmacist Bliss C. Wilson, Letcher, as secretary.

CHAPTER 7
1940-1949

SD Pharmaceutical Association (SDPhA), 1940-1949

Association Events

Pharmacists gathered at Deadwood Elks Lodge for the 1940 convention. At one of the business sessions, delegates learned the South Dakota Division of Taxation collected $10,000 a month from the three percent sales tax collected by pharmacies. The figures did not include taxes from the sales of liquor, cigarettes, and newspapers. Using their information, the gross pharmacy business in South Dakota totaled $4,000,000 a year. The average gross business for each of the 314 licensed drug stores was $12,738 per year.

Another speaker at the 1940 meeting, Dale Ruedig, Eli Lilly & Company, said that 60% of all sales came from three departments in a drug store, one of which is the prescription department. Overall, the prescription department produces twenty percent of the total business. The average prescription price was $.92 for the 165,000,000 prescriptions written annually. The average doctor wrote $1,000 of prescriptions per year; whereas the average family spent $40 in a drug store each year.[1]

President J. A. Clute, Murdo, expressed concern about competitors at the 1941 Madison meeting in the City Armory. He said, "There are ideas as to how to compete with chain stores, cut rate competition, and catalog houses. [He believed] we study their methods of merchandising and use a few of their ideas. We must merchandise now more than ever."[2] A speaker from the Store Equipment Company of Michigan said that in 1941, druggists spent $71,000,000 for remodeling and new equipment. Consequently, modernized pharmacies increased gross sales by an average of thirty-one percent. Following a banquet at the Madison City Armory, war correspondent Eric Sevareid spoke on "Europe's Last Front."

The 1942 Association convention met at Sioux Falls in the Cataract Hotel. George W. Lloyd, Spencer, a delegate to the August 1941 APhA convention in Detroit, reported that he was one of 1,225 delegates from forty-four states, and that membership had grown to 4,500.

A History of Pharmacy in South Dakota

World War II

Just before the war, Mills Drug Softball Team, Rapid City, was runner-up in the state tournament in Rapid City on September 1 and 2, 1940. Soon, World War II had a strong impact on pharmacies and pharmacists. Pharmacists had just begun to recover from the depression and hard times of the 1930s when the Japanese bombed Pearl Harbor on December 7, 1941. In a short time, America mobilized for war. An example of how the depression and war affected Harold W. Mills of Rapid City, is typical of others. In May 1929, Mills had opened a drug store in downtown Rapid City. After the 1929 stock market crash and the beginning of the depression, he began to sell malted milks for a dime each, to attract customers. His small store grew to an 11,900 square-foot store. Before World War II, thirty people worked in his soda fountain serving $.10 malted milks to 2,500 customers a day. After the War started, he had to close the fountain because of a shortage of materials. Mills continued with his pharmacy, and served on the Board of Pharmacy between 1951 and 1960.

Many pharmacists enlisted or were drafted for military duty. The Board of Pharmacy therefore, waived the $5.00 license renewal fee for them for the duration of the war. Federal officials asked that conventions be postponed, to save vital materials and ease the shortage of help. In March 1943, Association President Carl Anderson, Sioux Falls, and the Executive Committee voted to cancel that summer's Mitchell convention, as well as future conventions, for the duration of the war. To meet statutory requirements, however, the Association agreed to meet at least one afternoon each year, to handle business.

Because of shortages of gasoline and tires, it would have been difficult for pharmacists to attend a state convention. Gasoline was rationed by December 1942. A Class A ration book was good for three gallons of gas a week. Class B and C ration books were available for emergency needs. The statewide speed limit was thirty-five miles per hour. For a time in 1944, the Class A ration for gas was reduced from three gallons to two gallons a week. New tires, if available, were only provided for ambulances, fire trucks, fuel and food delivery trucks, farm tractors, and doctor's cars. For example, the state ration for February 1942 consisted of 352 new tires and 295 new tubes. The Office of Price Administration (OPA) was created in 1941 and was given authority to ration and set prices for food, fuel, tires, and other supplies.

Association officers, members of the Board of Pharmacy, and others met one afternoon in the spring of 1943 at Brookings. During this time, the Board of Pharmacy was giving Board examinations to eight candidates who had graduated March 15, 1943. NABP had approved an accelerated program whereby pharmacy students could take a four-year course in three years by attending summer school classes. At that short meeting, the Association approved a resolution supporting the creation of a Pharmacy Corps in the United States Army. Otho J. Jones, Redfield, was elected president.

The Association met in the Lutheran Church basement at Arlington on May 23, 1944. Thirty-six pharmacists and fifteen guests and speakers attended. They honored C. C. Maxwell of Arlington for sixty years of service to the pharmacy profession. Secretary Bliss Wilson reported the Board of Pharmacy had granted free license renewals to 101 South Dakota pharmacists who were serving in the Armed Forces. A. A. Jarratt, Colman was elected president. Despite the short meeting, the Constitution was amended creating a fourth vice-president, by a vote of 21 Yes and 5 No. The second, third, and fourth vice-presidents would form a permanent resolutions committee.

A short afternoon meeting was held by the Association in Mitchell, June 4, 1945. A roster of pharmacists who served in the Armed Forces during World War II up to that time was presented. One hundred and nineteen South Dakota pharmacists served in all branches of the service. Seven of the 119 pharmacists were killed in action: Lon Fischer Brown, Belle Fourche, Army; Ronald L. Helder, Palto Alto, CA., Army; Robert F. Holcomb, Aberdeen, Army; Harrison P. Klusmeier, Redfield, Marines; Robert E. Knorr, Marion, Army; Burton G. Tousley, Gettysburg, Army; and James H. Vogel, Pierre, Army. Free license renewals were given in 1945 to 112 pharmacists serving in the Armed Forces, two of whom were women: Crystal V. Rindahl, Watertown, WACS; and Annette C.L. Smith, Yankton, ANC.[3] The Association purchased a $2,000 War Bond.

President A. A. Jarratt, Colman, reminded the delegates at the 1945 meeting, that despite the war, "The practice of pharmacy has changed tremendously, and for the better, during the past twenty-five years. There was a time in years long past when the pharmacist made his fluid extracts, tinctures, elixirs, syrups, pills, and powders. Now most of these preparations are made by large and small pharmaceutical companies, where they are made in large quantities, by the latest and best scientific methods. The pharmacist of today uses standardized drugs made elsewhere, and combines or compounds them with skill into prescriptions, which enter the sick room or hospital, and at the same time, he is equally responsible with the physician for the safety of that prescription."[4]

SDPhA Presidents following the war were: Ted E. Hustead, Wall, 1946-1947; Richard W. Kendall, Brookings, 1947-1948; Roger F.

Eastman, Platte, 1948-1949; John H. Sidle, Alexandria, 1949-1950. In 1946, a full convention was held at Yankton in the Elks Club. The Association met in Rapid City in 1947 and Huron in 1948. At Huron, the Allied Drug Travelers hosted a buffet at the Elks in the Marvin Hughitt Hotel, and danced to Don Shaw's Band afterwards. Aberdeen hosted the convention in 1949.

Association membership was 701 in 1941, 660 in 1943, 724 in 1945, and 783 in 1949. A significant resolution approved in 1949 was opposition to a Compulsory National Health Insurance Program. Four points concerned the delegates: place medical care under political influence; lead to socialized medicine; hinder medical research; and be a burden on the taxpayer.

Veteran's Prescription Program

World War II veterans with a service connected disability were provided medical care and medicines at a veteran's hospital. The Veterans Administration (VA) and SDPhA worked out a program in 1946, whereby local pharmacists would provide prescriptions to eligible veterans. This would save the veteran a trip to a distant VA center. A local pharmacist, filling a prescription for an eligible veteran, sent the bill directly to the SDPhA office for payment. A ten percent service charge was added to the bill by the SDPhA office. Once a month, the office sent all bills to the VA.

Between November 11, 1946 and May 10, 1947, the SDPhA office received bills for 576 prescriptions which cost $945 for an average cost $1.64 each. This figure did not include the ten percent service charge added by the SDPhA office. In 1949, 1,891 prescriptions were filled for an average cost of $2.77 each. Secretary Bliss Wilson listed some of the problems with the service: carbon copy instead of original bill sent to office; no signature of veteran; and no date on prescription. However, no payment was denied. It simply took longer to correct the mistake before payment was made. In 1950, 1,372 prescriptions were filled costing $4,989 for an average cost of $3.64 each. The program was still operating in 1955, but by 1962, the VA began handling its prescription service for veterans from its VA offices.

New Board and Association Secretary

Kenneth Jones, Gettysburg, resigned the secretary's job August 8, 1942, and accepted a job with McKesson and Robbins in Sioux City. The Executive Committee employed Bliss C. Wilson, Letcher, as the new secretary the same date. Wilson, a graduate of SDSU College of Pharmacy, formerly of Frankfort, took the Board exams January 16, 1918 and became a registered pharmacist holding License 2011. At the time of his appointment, Secretary Wilson operated his drug store in Letcher. Secretary Wilson continued operating his pharmacy, the same as past secretaries. He continued both jobs in Letcher until July 1946, when the Executive Committee authorized him to move the office to Pierre. His salary would be $4200 a year, half paid by the Board and half by the Association.

In 1952, Secretary Wilson was paid $5,700 per year at $475 a month; $200 from the Board, $200 from the Association, and $75 from the Commercial and Legislative Section. Part-time secretarial help was also provided, however, in 1954 the Executive Committee authorized $2,000 a year for the employment of a full-time office assistant, $1,000 from the Board and $1,000 from the Association. Wilson's office was in a small Legislative office on the third floor of the capitol building. During the sixty-day Legislative Session, every two years, he moved his office to another location, usually a hallway, within the building.

Legislative Matters

President J. A. Clute appointed a three-member Legislative Committee for the 1941 Legislative Session: Chairperson Fred L. Vilas, Pierre; Floyd W. Brown, Lead; and R. L. Overholser, Selby. O. J. Tommeraason, Madison, served in the South Dakota Senate for both the 1941 and 1943 Legislative Sessions. Attorney Perry F. Loucks, Watertown, was the lobbyist for the pharmacists. The pharmacists rented space in the St. Charles Hotel for the session costing $300. Eleven bills were introduced affecting the pharmacy profession. A bill to increase the budget for the Division of Pharmacy at State College failed.

Two bills affecting the sale of liquor caused great concern for pharmacists who sold liquor as a part of their business. One bill required that an entire business be closed during hours that liquor could not be sold. Another stated that liquor could not be sold in conjunction with any other business except tobacco and its related products. Both liquor bills were defeated. H. B. 157 passed which raised the minimum wage for women from $12 to $15 a week in towns over 2,500 in population. But H. B. 161, which would have removed the maximum of 54 hours of work per week for women employees, was defeated. President Clute had appointed pharmacist captains in ten districts to provide local support for or against certain legislative bills.

Lobbyist Attorney Perry F. Loucks, Watertown, died during the summer of 1942, therefore the Executive Committee hired Attorney Karl Goldsmith, Pierre, to replace him. During the Legislative Session of 1945, the pharmacists shared a Saint Charles Hotel office with the South

A History of Pharmacy in South Dakota

Dakota Retail Merchants. In 1947, they shared space [usually a room or connecting rooms] in the hotel with the Hardware Dealers. One pharmacist bill that passed during the 1947 Legislative Session raised the appropriation for the Division of Pharmacy, SDSU, from $5,000 to $8,000 a year for a two-year period.

South Dakota Journal of Medicine and Pharmacy

Since 1901, Northwestern Druggist, Minneapolis, had been the official publication for SDPhA news. From time to time the Association Secretary, or someone appointed by the president, was the correspondent for the magazine. C. L. "Roy" Doherty, Rapid City, had been the correspondent to the magazine since 1945. In 1947, the Executive Committee voted to join with the *South Dakota Journal of Medicine* as the official publication of SDPhA. The name of the magazine was changed to *South Dakota Journal of Medicine and Pharmacy*, in 1948. All pharmacy news for the magazine was sent to Secretary Bliss Wilson for review before it was sent to the magazine. The Association requested that the printing type be of equal size for medicine and pharmacy.

The Association paid for 400 subscriptions in 1948, but only 266 pharmacists paid the $1.50 subscription cost. In 1949, the subscription was raised to $2.00 a year and collected on a voluntary basis. The following year, Charles F. Van De Walle, Sioux Falls, was named associate editor for the pharmacy part of the magazine. Collection for the subscription continued to be a problem. The Executive Committee recommended that $2.00 from each Commercial and Legislative member be applied to the subscription.

SD Board of Pharmacy, 1940-1949

Selling Packaged Drugs and Medicines

Pharmacies had been licensed since 1931. On July 1 of that year, 331 pharmacies were licensed in the state. All licenses were issued to independent pharmacies, except 1 to a hospital, 1 to a chain drug store, and 2 to clinics. In 1944, there were 290 licensed pharmacies in which 349 pharmacists practiced, a ratio of 1.2 pharmacists per pharmacy. Seventy-four of those pharmacies were in the ten larger South Dakota cities.

Of the 331 pharmacies that had been licensed in 1931 only 276 remained in 1949, 55 fewer pharmacies in eighteen years. Many changes were occurring in the retail drug business. H. L. Lewis, of Lewis Drug Co., Sioux Falls, was issued a license to operate a "Self-Service Drug Store" in Sioux Falls. SDPhA President H. L. Lewis, Sioux Falls, told the conventioneers meeting in the Cataract Hotel in 1942, "I applied for and received a legal license from the State Board of Pharmacy to operate a self-service drug store here in Sioux Falls. Self-service is not so radically different from the old, out-of-date method of conducting a drug store, except that the goods are all displayed and the customers allowed largely to make their own selections. Poisons are sold by registered pharmacists, prescriptions are filled by registered pharmacists. A registered pharmacist is on duty every hour of the day. All state and federal laws are complied with 100 percent."[5]

Also in 1931, the South Dakota Legislature had passed a law stating that only registered pharmacists could own pharmacies. In 1949, however, the United States Supreme Court ruled that a state law limiting ownership of fixtures and merchandise of a drug store to pharmacists only was unconstitutional. However, the Court also ruled that the "active management" of a drug store must be by a licensed pharmacist. As a result, the South Dakota Board of Pharmacy passed a regulation in 1950, requiring a non-pharmacist owner of a pharmacy to provide an affidavit delegating complete management authority of the pharmacy to a registered pharmacist.

Originally, South Dakota law limited all sales of drugs, medicines, patent medicines, and poisons to registered pharmacists. In 1924, the Legislature amended the law allowing lay persons to sell certain poisons in their original factory packages under a $1.00 Poison License. In 1927, the South Dakota Supreme Court ruled that the law limiting the sale of patent medicines in the original packages to registered pharmacists only was unconstitutional. The 1933 Legislature passed a law permitting lay persons to sell patent medicines in the original factory packages, under a $1.00 Patent Medicine License. Both the Poison License law and the Patent Medicine License law were administered by the Board of Pharmacy. In 1924, 340 Poison Licenses were issued, compared to 660 in 1949. In 1933, 175 Patent Medicine Licenses were issued, compared to 1,042 in 1949.

The United States Pharmacopoeia (U.S.P.) and the National Formulary (N.F.) were two books that contained the official list of drugs and medicines. They also contained the standard formulas and methods for the preparation of prescription medicines and drugs. The sale of any of these items, whether compounded into a prescription or in their original factory packages, was strictly limited to pharmacists. An example of a few of the original packaged U.S.P. and N.F. items that could only be sold by pharmacists were: aspirin, cod liver oil, glycerin, milk of magnesia, mineral oil, spirits of turpentine, tincture of iodine etc.

A bill was introduced in the 1945 Legislature, to permit lay persons to sell some of the U.S.P. and N.F. items in their original factory packages, under a $3.00 Household Remedy License. Supporters of the bill believed that making these items available for sale would be beneficial to people living in rural areas where there were no drug stores. Therefore, the Legislature wanted to expand the Patent Medicine License to include some of the U.S.P. and N.F. items. The bill introduced contained thirty-six U.S.P. and N.F. items that could be sold by a Household Remedy License holder. It passed the Senate with one dissenting vote, despite the protests from pharmacists. Pharmacists successfully amended the bill in the House with these changes: Board of Pharmacy would compile the list of U.S.P. and N.F. drugs which could be sold; a license holder had to be located eight miles from a licensed pharmacy; a seller had to pass an examination for each of the items sold; and items could only be sold in the original factory packages. The bill passed and became law July 1, 1945.

The Board of Pharmacy passed rules to administer the law, effective July 23, 1945. They approved twenty-one U.S.P. and N.F. items, which the license holder could sell in their original factory packages. The items included: alum, aspirin, camphorated oil, cod liver oil, cream of tartar, essence of peppermint, glauber salts, glycerin, hydrogen peroxide, milk of magnesia, milk sugar, mineral oil, olive oil, pine tar, raw linseed oil, saccharin, saltpeter, spirits of camphor, spirits of turpentine, sulfur flowers, tincture of iodine, and phenothiazine.

Between 1924 and 1945, the Legislature had greatly expanded the sale of factory packaged drugs and medicines by lay persons. In 1949, the following licenses were issued to lay persons by the Board of Pharmacy: 1,042 Patent Medicine; 660 Poison; and 62 Household Remedy. One pharmacist was concerned that a lay person with the Patent, Poison, and Household Remedy license could sell everything that a pharmacist sells in a pharmacy except prescriptions. Also in 1949, the Board of Pharmacy issued licenses to 276 pharmacies, that cost $10 each. Pharmacies could also sell patents, poisons, and household remedies under the regular pharmacy license.

Drug Inspectors
F. E. Briggs, Sioux Falls, was the first drug inspector, hired in 1931. By 1945, there were hundreds of license holders in hardware stores, grocery stores, variety stores, cafes, gas stations, and grain elevators. George W. Lloyd, Spencer, was hired to help Inspector Briggs during 1941 and part of 1942. After Lloyd's resignation, Harry L. Dow, Sioux Falls, worked for one year as a drug inspector for $1,800 per year. After Dow's resignation, John A. Clute, Rapid City, was hired and worked in 1943. Walter McMurdy, Mitchell, was hired in August 1945. F. E. Briggs, retired in December of 1945. Walter McMurdy continued until June 6,

1953 when the Board of Pharmacy hired Glenn Velau, Sioux Falls. Velau's salary was $3,300 per year plus traveling expenses.

Drug inspector's reports throughout the years show that they made many inspections. George W. Lloyd made 2,737 inspections in 1942 and found 42 violations, none of which needed court action. F. E. Briggs, in 1944, inspected all but two drug stores. He also found that some Patent Medicine License holders were selling U.S.P. and N. F. items. Walter McMurdy made 2,693 inspections in 1947 and found 218 violations. Some of the violations, which he corrected during the inspections were: some druggists were not keeping a proper poison register; fourteen cafes were selling aspirin with their Patent Medicine License, rather than with the Household Remedy License.

Not only was the Board of Pharmacy charged with enforcing various kinds of drug laws, they were also charged with interpreting existing laws and rules, as well as with the handling of new products. In 1940, a Circuit Court Judge ruled that only pharmacists could sell aspirin, which basically upheld the pharmacy law. However, in 1945, the Legislature allowed a lay person, holding a Household Remedy License, to sell aspirin along with twenty other U.S.P. and N.F. drugs.

Also in 1940, the Board of Pharmacy ruled that the sale of barbiturates and urea derivatives, sulfanilamide and its related products could only be sold with a prescription from a medical doctor. In June 1945, Attorney General George T. Mickelson gave an opinion to the Board of Pharmacy which stated, "serums, vaccines, and bacterins intended for the treatment of domestic animals, may not be sold at retail by merchants and that the retail of these animal biologicals is confined to duly licensed pharmacists and veterinarians."[6]

SD College of Pharmacy, 1940-1949

World War II and Enrollments

Dr. Earl R. Serles, Dean of the Division of Pharmacy, accepted a position as Dean of the College of Pharmacy, University of Illinois in 1940. Dr. Floyd J. LeBlanc was named Acting Dean by the Board of Regents. LeBlanc had joined the faculty in 1922 and earned his B.S. in pharmacy from State College in 1924 and a M. S. in pharmacy in 1927. He received his Ph.D. at Purdue in 1938. The Board of Regents on July 1, 1941, named LeBlanc Dean of the Division of Pharmacy, State College.

Except for military service, 1918-1919, Serles had served as Head of the Department of Pharmacy since the death of Professor Bower T. Whitehead in 1917. After a reorganization of the Department by the Board of Regents on January 24, 1924, Serles was named Dean of the newly formed Division of Pharmacy. Prior to his leaving State College, Serles served as president of the American Association of Colleges of Pharmacy in 1938-1939. In 1941, Serles said that graduates of the College of Pharmacy, University of Illinois, earned $22.50 a week. One of his achievements at the University of Illinois was serving as president of the American Pharmaceutical Association in 1946-1947.

Dean LeBlanc faced immediate challenges during the World War II years, 1941-1945, and the rapid expansion of the Division of Pharmacy which followed the war. Between 1941-1943, an average of nineteen graduated each year. In 1943, for example, the twelve men who graduated went to the Armed Forces, and the six women went to work in pharmacies. Those pharmacists going into the military were supposed to be commissioned as Second Lieutenants, however, some were assigned lower ranks. It was difficult for the United States Army to end the long standing practice of using enlisted men to dispense prescriptions. During the war, the Division of Pharmacy was on a four-quarter basis to speed up graduation. A student could finish a four-year pharmacy course in three years by attending summer school. Local draft boards had deferred some pharmacy seniors so they could graduate and take the Board examinations.

Only eleven graduated with their B. S. degree in 1944. Enrollment in the Division of Pharmacy that fall was only 28, the low point. State College President Lyman E. Jackson reported that State College enrollment in the fall of 1942 was 1,215 students. In January 1943 enrollment was down to 875, and by June 7, 1943 it was down to 150 students. The band, with 140 members in the fall of 1942, had only 18 members left a year later.

During World War II, some pharmacy students went into the service in the middle of their four-year pharmacy training. John Nelson, Arlington, for example, completed his sophomore year at the Division of Pharmacy, State College, Brookings, SD in 1942 before leaving for the U. S. Navy. He served as a Pharmacists Mate First Class in the Atlantic and the Pacific aboard a destroyer escort and a baby flattop carrier. He returned to classes for his junior year in the fall of 1945 and graduated from the Division of Pharmacy in the spring of 1947. John Nelson in a letter to the author, said that as a part of his pharmacy training he did learn to compound ointments, tinctures, suspensions, and emulsions. Nelson completed the following courses at the SD State College, Division of Pharmacy, for his B.S. degree:

Freshman 1940-1941, Military, Pharmacy Latin, English, Inorganic Chemistry, Business Math, Theoretical Pharmacy, and Practical Pharmacy

Sophomore 1941-1942, Theoretical Pharmacy, Practical Pharmacy, Organic Chemistry, Pharmacognosy, Physiology, Entomology, and Volumetric Analysis

Junior 1945-1946, Theoretical Pharmacy, Practical Pharmacy, Psychology, Toxicology, Contagious Diseases, Bacteriology, Drug Assay, Window Display, Economics, and Clinical Methods

Senior 1946-1947, Store Management, Pharmaceutical Research, Pharmacology, Genetics, and Jurisprudence.[7]

Nelson served as president of SDPhA in 1976-1977 and as a member of the South Dakota Board of Pharmacy 1981-1987.

The United States Army Air Force opened an Administration School on the campus during World War II. In January 1943, 800 enlisted men and fifty officers filled the empty dormitories and classrooms to attend a three-month course on Army Air Force Administration. (The author had the pleasure of attending that three-month Army Air Force Administration School during the summer of 1943. During basic training in Kearns, Utah, the commanding officer asked for volunteers who could operate a typewriter. I bravely raised my hand. A week later, I was on a train headed for Brookings, South Dakota to attend the Army Air Force Administration School. Some of the courses at the school included preparation of morning reports; compilation of requisitions for supplies; preparation of letters for different commands; maintaining stock control; completing payrolls; and handling enlisted men's records.

We attended classes in various campus buildings. I roomed in a former girls' dormitory on the west side of the campus. At retreat each evening before sundown, on a drill field in the northeast part of the campus, the whole command, with band playing, marched past the reviewing stand while the flag was being lowered. During the remainder of the war, stationed both in the United States and at Guam in the South Pacific with the 20th Army Air Force, I was always assigned to an Army Air Force Headquarters' Squadron, doing the things I had learned in Brookings.)

In the fall of 1946, the first year after the war, a record 124 pharmacy students enrolled in the Division of Pharmacy. Enrollment was limited to sixty-four freshmen. The 1946 record was broken in the fall of 1947 when 164 enrolled. That same year, the Legislature finally raised the appropriation from $5,000 to $8,000 a year. Also in 1947, the Board of Pharmacy approved six months of practical experience, for students who had served in an Armed Forces medical facility. Twenty-two pharmacy students graduated in June of 1948, however, enrollment that fall was still at 152. In 1949, thirty-four pharmacy seniors graduated, the largest class ever, up to that time. In 1948, nineteen candidates with B.S. degrees took the Board exams and all passed. In 1949, thirty took the Board exams and all passed.

Need for Pharmacy Building

In 1944, the SDPhA Executive Committee met with Governor M. Q. Sharpe in Huron, relative to a proposed new pharmacy building following the war. The Committee instructed the Association's lobbyist, Attorney Karl Goldsmith, Pierre, to meet with the Brookings County Legislators to introduce a separate bill in the 1945 Legislature authorizing the construction of a new pharmacy building at State College. Nothing happened in regard to these early proposals for a pharmacy building.

A space crisis developed following World War II, however, college officials promised the Division of Pharmacy more space in the Administration Building as soon as the new Agricultural Hall was completed. A. A. Jarratt, Colman, chairperson of the Association's Division of Pharmacy Committee, reported the Division of Pharmacy was in the north wing of the first floor of the Administration Building. If plans occur as agreed, the Division of Pharmacy would have the entire first floor when the Agricultural Hall was completed. It would provide needed space for laboratories and classrooms.

Pharmaceutical Institute

In 1938, the Division of Pharmacy conducted a pharmaceutical institute on the college campus. It consisted of three days of lectures and discussions. The institute was also described as a refresher course or as a short course for drug store owners. Institutes were held yearly, except during World War II. Attendance in 1949 was thirty. In 1950, thirty-seven attended the three-day April institute on the campus. Some of the courses included: Prescription Compounding Problems, Advances in Drug Therapy, Field of Insecticides, Animal Health Pharmacy, and National Laws Pertaining to Pharmacy. The banquet was held in the Union Ball Room, followed with entertainment including a film "As the Customers Like It." Twenty-eight attended the institute in 1956. SDPhA sponsored the institutes and usually a $5.00 attendance fee was charged. The institutes were discontinued in 1966 when faculty of the College of Pharmacy began a series of traveling circuit conferences.

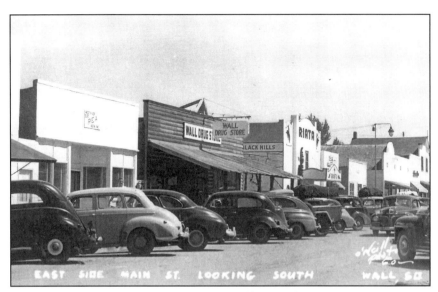
Ted and Dorothy Hustead's Wall Drug, circa 1940s.
(Photo courtesy of Robert Kolbe Collections, Sioux Falls, SD.)

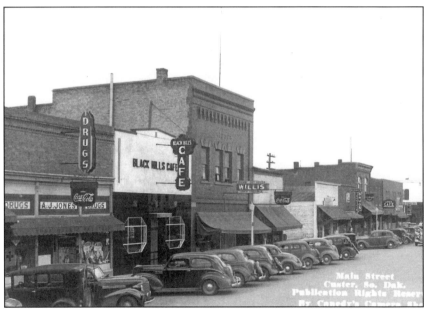
A.J. Jones Drug Store, left, and O.J. Sieler Drug Store, center, Custer, SD,
circa 1948. *(Photo courtesy of Robert Kolbe Collections, Sioux Falls, SD.)*

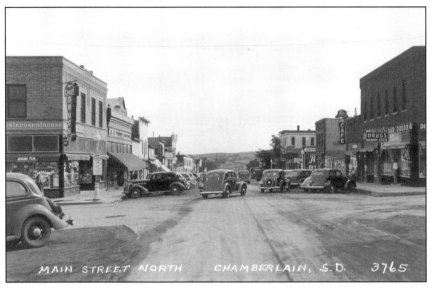

Joe Casey Drug Store, left, Neil Fuller Drug Store, right, Chamberlain, SD, circa 1940s. *(Photo courtesy of Terry Casey, Chamberlain, SD.)*

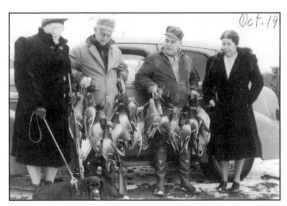

Earl and Daphne Serles, return to SD to hunt ducks with Herbert and Beth Crissman, Ipswich, SD. 1942.

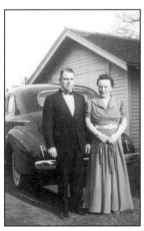

Mr. and Mrs. George Lloyd, Spencer, SD. Lloyd was SDPhA president, 1934-1935, and drug inspector 1941-1942, circa 1942.

CHAPTER 8
1950-1959

SD Pharmaceutical Association (SDPhA), 1950-1959

The Executive Committee in 1951 authorized the treasurer to destroy all Association records that had been audited and were more than six years old. This was a common practice for many groups. In the case of the Board and Association, the secretary's reports on the two groups were always read, discussed, and printed as a part of the annual proceedings of the convention. Many of the printed annual convention proceedings, between 1886 and 1972, have survived and are excellent resources for historical information. However, since 1973, all state departments and agencies were required to store annual records in their offices rather than printing them in expensive annual proceedings.

In 1954, the Executive Committee authorized Secretary Bliss Wilson to purchase a dictaphone, mimeograph, and adding machine for his office. The Board of Pharmacy paid half of the cost. Secretary Bliss Wilson's records show that pharmacist membership was 814 in 1950 which grew to 957 in 1961. In 1953, the pharmacist license renewal fee was raised from $5 to $10. Between 1950 and 1958, there were also two registered assistant pharmacists who paid their $1.00 annual renewal fee.

The delegates at the 1950 convention voted to create a Commercial and Legislative Section (C & L Section.) Its purpose was to help with legislative lobbying, and provide commercial services to the profession of pharmacy. Membership fees were $25 for wholesalers, $10 for pharmacies, and $5 for individual pharmacists. Other standing committees were: Finance, College of Pharmacy, Publicity, Prescription Pricing Schedule, and Legislative. LaVerne J. Mowell, Murdo, was president at the time. The Association participated in Muscular Dystrophy Week in June 1952. Pharmacists handed out envelopes to their customers who could send a contribution direct to MD national headquarters.

In 1951, Druggists Mutual Fire Insurance, which was organized by South Dakota Pharmacists in 1895, ceased doing business in South Dakota. Retail Druggists Mutual Insurance Association of Iowa began doing business in South Dakota in 1951. It was originally founded in

A History of Pharmacy in South Dakota

1909 by members of the Iowa Pharmaceutical Association. In 1992, the company name was changed to Pharmacists Mutual Insurance Company and continues to serve the South Dakota pharmacy industry. PMC Quality Commitment, Inc, a subsidiary of Pharmacists Mutual Insurance Company, located in Algona, Iowa, is an advertiser in *South Dakota Pharmacist*.

President J. C. Shirley, Brookings, in 1952, was concerned that only the Aberdeen and Rapid City districts had held meetings. At the time, there were fifteen districts within the Association, mostly inactive. A resolution passed at the 1953 Association convention added the immediate past president to the Executive Committee. J. C. Shirley, Brookings, was the past president. Newly elected president was Neil E. Fuller, Chamberlain, 1953-1954. Presidents elected after Fuller were: Charles F. Van De Walle, Sioux Falls, 1954-1955; Edward W. Peterson, Elk Point, 1955-1956; Alger D. Knutson, Clark, 1956-1957. President George A. Lehr, Rapid City, 1957-1958, and the Executive Committee supported a new Code of Ethics which was adopted at the 1957 convention. The first Code of Ethics was adopted at the 1886 convention.

The Interprofessional Committee consisting of Tom Haggar, Watertown; Tom Mills, Sioux Falls; and Welles C. Eernisse, Rapid City; met with the same committee from the South Dakota Medical Association. Their 1958 report to the Association convention indicated that the two committees agreed on the following:

- physicians discontinue giving free samples except for needy patients
- SDMA recommend discontinuance of physician dispensing and label it an unethical practice
- urge physicians to mark refill or no refill on prescriptions
- maintained that the AMA Code of Ethics prohibited doctor-owned clinic pharmacies [at the time there were three in SD]
- when clinic leases space to pharmacist, rent should not exceed by more than 25 percent that paid by doctors in area for like space.[1]

Convention Awards

President Vere Larsen, Alcester, and the Executive Committee in 1958, approved buying a past president pin and presenting it to retiring president George A. Lehr, Rapid City. It was agreed to make the presentation an annual event. The Committee also agreed to start a practice of presenting Fifty-Year Membership Certificates at the convention's Veteran's Breakfast. The Committee in 1958, asked for nominations for another new award called the Honorary President's Award. The award would be given to a pharmacist for outstanding contributions to the profession, but for one reason or another was never able to seek the office of president. The Executive Committee reviewed the nominations and selected R. E. Trumm, Hayti, as the first pharmacist to receive the award. It was presented at the 1958 convention held in Brookings.

In 1959, President Willis Hodson, Aberdeen, and the Executive Committee agreed to send a letter to all registered pharmacists asking for nominations for another new award called the Bowl of Hygeia. The award was given to a pharmacist for outstanding professional and community service, by A. H. Robbins Company. Floyd Cornwell, Webster, was selected by the Committee and was presented the first Bowl of Hygeia award at the 1959 convention held in Mitchell. In 1961, the Committee agreed to have special nominating forms for the Honorary President and the Bowl of Hygeia Awards, sent to all pharmacists four months before the convention. Nominations were reviewed by the Executive Committee who picked a person for each award.

Conventions

The official program of the June 1951 Association convention at Watertown has survived. LaVerne J. Mowell, Murdo, was president. The convention was co-sponsored by the Ladies' Auxiliary, President Mrs. Neil Fuller, Chamberlain; Vice-President Mrs. Roger Eastman, Tripp; and Secretary-Treasurer Mrs. Vere Larsen, Alcester. Allied Drug Travelers, President Ken Brolyer, was also a sponsor. General Convention Chairperson was Loran F. Thomes, Watertown. Convention committees included: Program, Registration, Reception, Housing, Banquet and Dance, Veteran's Luncheon, Sports, Prizes, and Women's Activities. The program contained a list of eighty-six donors of merchandise for prize drawings and nine who made cash contributions. The Tuesday smorgasbord was hosted by Brown Drug Company, Sioux Falls. Allied Drug Travelers hosted a mixer and buffet at the Flamingo Club that evening. On Wednesday, Jewett Drug Company, Aberdeen, hosted the ladies' breakfast at the Grand Hotel. A Ladies' Auxiliary luncheon and bridge party was hosted by McKesson Robbins Company, Minneapolis, on Thursday.

Convention events on Tuesday included an address by Dr. E. J. Pankow, President of South Dakota Medical Association. Wednesday's program included "Modern Merchandising" by W. L. Mickelson, Walgreen Agency; "Antibiotics Today and Tomorrow," Dr. John Erlich, Parke, Davis & Company; "Limitations of the Experimental Method," Dr. H. C. Batson, University of Illinois, College of Medicine. At the third general session on Wednesday, talks were presented by J. C. Sheve, Lederle Labs, "Veterinary Sales Through the Drug Store"; Roy L. Sanford, APhA, "Pharmacy and the APhA"; and Benjamin A. Smith, Eli Lilly, "Professional Pharmacy." At the Thursday morning session, Malcom Solberg, talked about the "Office of Price Stabilization."

President A. O. Bittner, Aberdeen, attended the NARD convention at Minneapolis in October 1952. Over 6,500 attended and heard United States Senator Karl E. Mundt, Madison, speak for an hour on "What Price Freedom." At the first Executive Committee meeting following the 1958 convention in Brookings, George A. Lehr, Rapid City, made a motion that hereafter the entire Executive Committee be introduced at the convention. The motion was seconded by L. B. Urton, Sturgis, and carried.

Journal of Medicine and Pharmacy

The magazine, which had been designated the official publication of SDPhA in 1948, was not receiving good support by South Dakota pharmacists. The Executive Committee decided in 1950 that the Association would no longer subsidize it. Each pharmacist must be a separate subscriber. President J. C. Shirley, Brookings, in 1952, recommended that each pharmacy pay the $2.00 subscription. Hopefully, if there were enough subscribers, the Association could dispense with sending a monthly bulletin to pharmacists. Some of the speeches presented at the annual convention were printed in the Journal, to save some of the cost of printing the annual convention proceedings.

In June 1953, Charles F. Van De Walle, Sioux Falls, resigned the position of associate editor for the pharmacy section carried in the magazine. Van De Walle was elected Association president in 1954. Dr. Harold S. Bailey, Brookings, was appointed associate editor, and by agreement of the Executive Committee, he was paid a salary of $50 per month. In 1961, Dr. Bailey resigned and Dr. Guilford C. Gross, Brookings, was named associate editor at the same salary.

Legislative Matters

The newly formed Commercial and Legislative Section became an active force in spearheading legislative matters before the Legislature. In 1950, President LaVerne J. Mowell, Murdo, appointed the following members to the Section: Royce L. Overholser, Selby; Neil E. Fuller, Chamberlain; and Fred L. Vilas, Pierre. In 1951, pharmacies and pharmacists paid in a total of $2,235. C & L Funds were used to pay $75 a month to Secretary Bliss Wilson, as part of his salary. The 151 pharmacies who had paid the $10 membership received a free subscription of the *Journal of Medicine and Pharmacy*. The Association had recommended the fee be raised for both the Patent and Poison Licenses. However, after testing the Legislative climate at the 1951 session, it was agreed not to pursue the matter.

President John H. Sidle, Alexandria, was a South Dakota delegate to the 1949 NARD convention. He had attended a Fair Trade panel-discussion where he was given a Fair Trade Kit to promote Fair Trade at home. Vice-President Albin Barkley spoke strongly for the Fair Trade Act. Nationwide delegates told Sidle that food stores are strong competitors to pharmacies in their states. One of the Association's goals in 1951, was to continue support for the Fair Trade Act. The Act had existed for fifteen years in the state. Fair Trade Act helped preserve small businesses, and pharmacists resolved not to let it die without a fight. Under the Act, a retailer would not sell a product below the minimum price printed on the package. A bill to repeal the South Dakota Fair Trade Act was killed in a Legislative Committee in 1957, due to strong lobbying by members of the C & L Section. Association President Vere A. Larsen, Alcester, and the members of C & L Section took a very active role in 1959, favoring national legislation to continue the Fair Trade Act. Bills which passed in 1953 raised the pharmacist license renewal fee from $5 to $10, and the pharmacy license from $10 to $25. A bill to license drug clerks in the 1957 Legislature was put on hold until a later Legislature.

Pharmacy Statistics and Trends

A representative of E. R. Squibb Company reported to the 1952 convention at Aberdeen that the average sales per pharmacy in 1939, was $37,028 compared to $78,859 in 1951. I. D. Harvey, Abbot Labs, spoke at the 1953 convention at Brookings saying the average prescription price was $.94 in 1939 compared to $2.10 in 1952. In 1954, convention delegates learned that the average sales per square foot in United States pharmacies was $70, however, the Walgreen chain averaged from $100 to $125 per square foot. A 1954 Eli Lilly study showed that 24.9% of sales came from the prescription department, and that the average prescription price was $2.27.

A 1956 South Dakota prescription survey completed by the Division of Pharmacy, State College showed that in 1956, 5.9% of the prescriptions were compounded and that 94.1% were dispensed. The average prescription price was $2.68. Total prescription income per pharmacy per year was $29,145; $15,195 from new prescriptions and $13,950 from refilled prescriptions. Total prescriptions per pharmacy per year were 10,875, about 50% new and about 50% refills.

SD Board of Pharmacy, 1950-1959

Administration and Licensing

In 1950, there were 269 licensed pharmacies in the state, compared to 239 in 1961. The number of Poison License holders during the period averaged 617. Household Remedy License holders, under which persons could sell twenty-one U.S.P. and N. F. items in original factory packages, grew from 80 in 1950 to 129 in 1961. Those selling patent medicines in the original factory packages, grew from 1,101 in 1950 to 2,306 in 1961. Comparatively, in 1942, there were only 177 people with a Patent Medicine License. A 1951 Board of Pharmacy regulation required wholesalers selling patent medicines and poisons to determine if the purchaser had a license before making the sale.

During the Korean War, the Board of Pharmacy waived the pharmacist license renewal fee for those in the Armed Forces. The Legislature raised licensing fees as follows: poison from $1 to $3 in 1951; pharmacist from $5 to $10 and pharmacy from $10 to $25 in 1953. The license fee for selling Household Remedies and Patent Medicines remained at $3.00 each. Drug Inspector Glenn Velau was kept busy inspecting hundreds of license holders and non-license holders. In 1953, he made 1,860 inspections of all types of business such as grocery stores, cafes, hatcheries, pool halls, etc., including 265 pharmacies. Velau said, "When I go into a town, I go to all stores likely to handle patent medicines and drugs."[2]

The Board of Pharmacy in 1954 hired Inspector N. F. Jones, Canton, on a part-time basis, to help Inspector Velau complete a backlog of inspections. In 1956, Glenn Velau reported that he had traveled 28,304 miles and had made 2,888 inspections. His salary was $4,000 a year plus travel expenses. That same year, N. F. Jones traveled 9,719 miles and made 1,063 inspections. His salary for five months was $1375. N. F. Jones resigned that year. Velau's salary increased to $4,800 a year in 1959. Comparatively, Secretary Bliss Wilson was paid $3,250 from the Board and $2,400 from the Association for a total of $5,650.

Apprentices, Graduates, and Examinations

After January 1, 1948, pharmacy students needed to register their earned apprentice time with the Board of Pharmacy. In 1954, there were 145 registered apprentices. They needed to work fifty-two average work weeks under the supervision of a registered pharmacist and not concurrent with time spent attending college classes. Although there was no fee, a candidate had to register each period of time worked as well as for each location. Beginning March 1, 1956, candidates registering their apprentice time, needed to pay a $1.00 fee. That year, eighty-six were registered, which grew to 132 in 1957.

Examinations in 1954, were conducted by Board members Harold L. Tisher, Yankton; Milford L. Schwartz, Huron; and Harold W. Mills, Rapid City. Written examination subjects included Materia Medica, Pharmacology, Chemistry, Pharmacy, Pharmaceutical Mathematics, Toxicology, and Jurisprudence. A Practical exam was also given to the candidates. At the time, the Board permitted candidates with their four-year B.S. degrees, to take the written part of the exam before going into the field and finishing their one year of practical experience. Fifty-seven candidates, of which thirty-six were recent graduates, appeared at Brookings for the Board exams in May 1954. A number of candidates only took the written part of the examination because they had not yet completed their one year of practical experience.

A 1955 South Dakota Law created a position called Pharmacy Intern. The Board could issue an intern certificate to a person who had completed a B.S. degree, and obtained an average grade of 75% or more in the written Board examinations, but who had not completed the one year of practical experience. While working for practical experience, that Pharmacy Intern, working under the supervision of a registered pharmacist, was permitted to take charge of the pharmacy for two days, in the absence of the registered pharmacist. Other students earning practical experience before obtaining a B.S. degree were called apprentices.

In 1957, forty-seven took the examinations, and thirty-one were licensed. Seventy with B.S. degrees appeared for the examinations in 1959. At the 1959 meeting, the Board passed a regulation ending the so-called 'split exams.' Consequently, that ended the title Pharmacy Intern, because a candidate needed to have completed the practical experience before the examinations. In 1960, for the first time in many years, candidates wanting to take the Board exams, had to have completed their one year of practical experience as well as their B.S. degree. Terry Casey, Chamberlain, was one of the candidates for the 1960 examinations which took three days: one for written exams, one for compounding, and most of the third day for interviews by the Board. In 1961, twenty-seven took the exams and all passed.

Non-pharmacist Owners and Pharmacies Within a Department Store

In 1949, the United States Supreme Court ruled that a state law limiting ownership of a pharmacy to a registered pharmacist, was unconstitutional. South Dakota's 1931 law did limit ownership of a pharmacy to a registered pharmacist. The United States Supreme Court, however, also ruled that a pharmacist must be in active management of the pharmacy.

Therefore, the Board of Pharmacy in 1950, passed a regulation that stated that if the merchandise and fixtures of a pharmacy were owned by a non-pharmacist owner, that owner must delegate full and complete authority to a registered pharmacist to be in active management of the pharmacy. Following implementation of the new regulation, ownership of the 269 South Dakota pharmacies in 1950 was as follows: independent 247, hospital 6, clinic 4, college 1, Walgreen 3, and Rexall 8.

On January 31, 1954, the Board of Pharmacy issued a pharmacy license to pharmacist James A. Cameron, 'Pharmacy Department-Chaffin Self Service.' The new pharmacy department was located within the Chaffin Self-Service Variety Store in Aberdeen. The Board directed that Cameron keep a registered pharmacist on duty in the pharmacy department at all times the store was open to the public. This was the first time the Board of Pharmacy approved a pharmacy license to operate within another established business.

The concept was a problem for many pharmacists who were concerned with corporate ownership of large chain stores. A number of pharmacists met with the Board of Pharmacy at a special meeting in Huron on February 7, 1954. After much discussion the Board reminded the group that they had issued the license upon the advice of the Board Attorney Karl Goldsmith.

The Board of Pharmacy, however, was also concerned about placing a pharmacy within a department store or clinic, even if the non-pharmacist owner had delegated complete authority and active management to a registered pharmacist. To regulate how a corporation, partnership, or non-pharmacist owner could locate a pharmacy within a large store or clinic, the Board passed a new rule on November 7, 1954. The regulation, effective January 1, 1955, stated that space for a pharmacy within another established business, must follow these guidelines:

(1) the space must have an entrance which affords the public direct access from the street

(2) the space must be separated from the remainder of the building in which it is located, by walls extended from the floor to the ceiling. The walls must contain doors to the interior of the building which shall be closed and locked when the pharmacist is not on duty

(3) the space must contain not less than 400 square feet.

The regulation did not apply to any pharmacy which had been registered prior to the effective date of the new rule.[3]

In general, non-pharmacist owners needed to delegate complete authority to a registered pharmacist to operate a pharmacy. If such pharmacy was within a building of another existing business, the Board further defined the size and shape of that pharmacy. [Those regulations are still in force.]

Secretary Bliss Wilson in 1954 listed the ownership status of South Dakota's 266 pharmacies:

Individual or partnership and pharmacist controlled 212
Individual or partnership and non-pharmacist controlled ..11
Corporations and SD pharmacist controlled 25
Corporations and out-of-state pharmacist controlled............2
Corporations and Hospital Association controlled 7
Corporations and non-pharmacist controlled......................5
Corporations and physician controlled 3
State of SD 1

Restricted Drug Area in a Pharmacy

Pharmacists were generally concerned about the unregulated and unrestricted self-service sales by the holders of Patent Medicine and Poison Licenses. Secretary Bliss Wilson told the delegates to the 1952 convention in Aberdeen, "The pharmacist must assume responsibility in making the sale and warn the public against any danger and refuse to sell whenever it is in the interest of the public health. Unregulated and unrestricted self-service sales in a drug store may be just as harmful as unregulated sales by other retail outlets."[4]

In 1954, the Association members passed a resolution asking the Board of Pharmacy to pass a regulation governing the retailing of factory packaged drugs, medicines, and poisons within a registered pharmacy, for the protection of public health. Members favored a regulation strict enough to protect the user "by an oral warning and refusal to sell where health might be endangered."[5]

The concept was to eliminate the self-service sale of factory packaged drugs, medicines, and poisons in a drug store. It wasn't until 1958, however, that the Board of Pharmacy passed Section H-Anti-Self-Service Regulations. The regulation required that each pharmacy segregate the sales display of factory packaged drugs, medicines, and poisons from any sales display of general merchandise. The regulation pertained to non-prescription drugs and medicines.

The regulation required that no factory packaged drug, medicine, or poison could be so displayed that a customer could pick up and examine the package. Those articles could only be displayed in a Restricted Drug Area adjoining the prescription department. All sales from a Restricted Drug Area could only be made by a pharmacist or by trained personnel over sixteen years of age, who were acting under the immediate supervision of the pharmacist. The pharmacist and the trained personnel were required to follow strict selling guidelines to warn the public against any danger, so as not to endanger the public health. The drug inspector was required to inspect the Restricted Drug Area as part of the pharmacy inspection. Owners were required to state on the pharmacy license renewal form that the pharmacy had a Restricted Drug Area.

Substitution of Drugs Prohibited

In 1952, the United States Congress passed the Durham-Humphrey law. The law stated that any drug product bearing the prescription legend, could only be dispensed by a registered pharmacist and not be sold over-the-counter. A pharmacist could not refill any legend drug prescription unless specifically authorized by the doctor, either on the face of the prescription or by later phone or written instructions. The federal government had the right to audit pharmacy records.

The Board of Pharmacy on April 24, 1955 passed a strict regulation prohibiting the substitution of drugs by a pharmacist. In general, the regulation stated that dispensing a different drug than the one prescribed, without permission of the prescriber or the purchaser, "shall be evidence [that the pharmacist] is incompetent...and shall constitute grounds for revocation of a certificate of registration."

However, the Association expressed a different position in respect to generic drugs in a 1955 convention resolution: "The use of generic names is approved by pharmacy colleges, public health service, hospitals, clinics, and it is agreed by all...that the generic names mean the common, chemical name of drugs or the names recognized in the U.S.P. and N.F....the use of generic names is in keeping with the highest ethical standard of the medical and pharmaceutical professions. Therefore, it is resolved that SDPhA go on record as favoring use of generic names in writing prescriptions by physicians."[6]

SD College of Pharmacy, 1950-1959

Dean Floyd J. Le Blanc reported that 57 students graduated with their B. S. degrees in 1950, 49 men and 8 women. Up to that time, it was the largest graduating class in the history of the College of Pharmacy. Of the 57, 42 accepted jobs in South Dakota pharmacies and 15 accepted jobs in other states. Total enrollment in the College of Pharmacy in 1949-1950 was 142.

Forty graduated in 1951, 36 men and 4 women. Some entered the Armed Forces to serve during the Korean War. The College of Pharmacy staff in 1954 consisted of four with a Ph.D. degree and two with a M.S. degree, all registered pharmacists. The faculty changed to six with a Ph.D.

degree and one with a M.S. degree in 1956. In 1957, 250 were enrolled in the College of Pharmacy, and fifty-one earned their B.S. degrees. There were 240 enrolled in 1959 and seventy earned their B.S. degrees.

Dr. Guilford C. Gross in a speech on the 'Trend of Pharmaceutical Education' informed those at the 1954 convention that the American Association of Colleges of Pharmacy (AACP) would act whether to approve a five-year pharmacy program in August. The concept had been rejected in 1951 by the colleges. Thirteen schools already had more than a four-year program. If approved, the five-year program would be mandatory on and after April 1, 1965. The College of Pharmacy with the present four-year program required, exclusive of electives, 206 quarter hours. If the program would be extended to a five-year program, the plan called for two years pre-professional and three years of professional training. Some however, favored one year pre-professional and four years professional.[7] The five-year program was approved by the AACP. Those who enrolled in the fall of 1960 enrolled for the five-year course. The purpose of the additional year would allow students to enlarge their scope of professional training and broaden their cultural background.[8]

Compounding

Wiley Vogt, Mitchell, graduated from the College of Pharmacy, University of Nebraska, in 1951. He recalled that he had one year in compounding. "We compounded nearly everything: fluid extracts, solutions, tinctures, lotions, assorted mixtures, syrups, ointments/creams, suppositories, pills, sterile and non-sterile ophthalmic medications, and capsules. [When] I became a registered pharmacist in 1951, about 40% of prescriptions had a statement that stated 'mix and make according to the art.'"[9]

Terry Casey, Chamberlain, graduated from the SDSU College of Pharmacy in the spring of 1960 and remembered a part of his training under Professor Clark Eidsmoe. It included "compounding suppositories, pills, powders, capsules, liquids of all types, and external creams and ointments."[10]

Space, Faculty, and Accreditation

In 1919, the College of Pharmacy moved from the old Chemistry Building to the first floor of the Administration Building. With bulging enrollments during the 1950s, more space was needed for classrooms and laboratories. After an accreditation visit by American Council of Pharmaceutical Education (ACPE) officials in 1950, the College of Pharmacy was given a B rating, because the staff and curriculum were in need of critical attention. State College officials had promised Dean

LeBlanc more space in the Administration Building upon completion of Agricultural Hall.

Finally, in 1952 Dean LeBlanc reported that all of the first floor of the Administration Building, except room 116, had been allocated to the College of Pharmacy. It doubled the floor space and permitted establishing three laboratories: dispensing, pharmacology, bionucleonics and manufacturing. The Legislature had provided $70,000 to remodel and equip the Administration Building. Following a 1952 College of Pharmacy accreditation inspection by ACPE, the report stated, "with the addition of Dr. Kenneth Redman and Dr. Harold S. Bailey to the staff in 1951...and the space to be made available and the revision of the curriculum resulted in a restored Class A rating."[11] In 1953, the College of Pharmacy took over the space in the Administration Building which had been vacated by units of the Division of Agriculture.

A report by the ACPE committee in 1953 stated, "The staff appears to be well-balanced, to have a good morale and genuine interest in the progress of the Division." The report also took into account that Dr. Guilford Gross, who had returned with a Ph.D. degree, rejoined the staff. Dr. Norval E. Webb joined the same year. Other members joining the staff during the period were: Dr. Conald Abler, 1950; Dr. Winthrop Lange, 1955; Dr. Gary Omodt, 1958; and Dr. Stanley Shaw, 1960.

Student Societies, Tuition, and Scholarships

In 1956, Chi Chapter of Kappa Epsilon Pharmaceutical Society was formed on the campus. Its purpose was to unite women students of pharmacy, to stimulate a desire for high scholarship, to foster a professional consciousness, and to provide a bond of lasting friendship. Kappa Epsilon was open to sophomore women students in pharmacy who had a grade point average of 2.0. The Ladies' Auxiliary to SDPhA contributed $150 to the new society.

Gamma Kappa Chapter of Kappa Psi Pharmaceutical Fraternity was organized in 1958. Its purpose was to advance the profession of pharmacy, educationally and socially; to instill fellowship and high ideals in its members; and to foster scholarship and research. Membership in Kappa Psi was open to sophomore men students with a grade point average of 2.2.

The Whitehead Chapter SDPhA, established in 1923, became the South Dakota Chapter of Student APhA in 1954.

The Student Loan Fund, formed in 1921, had made 89 loans up to 1949. Only two loans were still outstanding, one of which was a $175 loan, granted in 1925, that still had $53 unpaid. In 1950, the fund had $1,581 in its treasury. In 1957, the Student Loan Fund was transferred to the Earl R. Serles Memorial, Scholarship and Loan Fund. The assets of the new fund in 1959 totaled $3,722. That year, $986 was contributed from memorials.

Between 1951 and 1956, the Board and the Association each contributed a $75 scholarship to eligible students at the College of Pharmacy. Dean LeBlanc said they needed more scholarships. In 1957, tuition for the College of Pharmacy was raised from $84 a year to $108. The next year it grew to $150. Throughout the years, both the Board and the Association provided one scholarship each. In 1959, tuition was raised again to $198, so the Board and the Association again provided one scholarship each for $198.

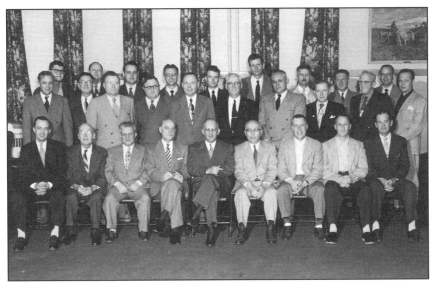

1954 Institute at College of Pharmacy, Brookings, SD.

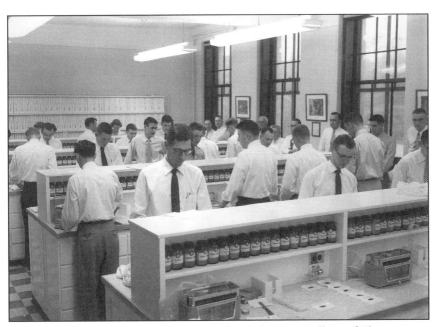

Candidates performing practical part of Board Exams, College of Pharmacy, Brookings, SD 1954

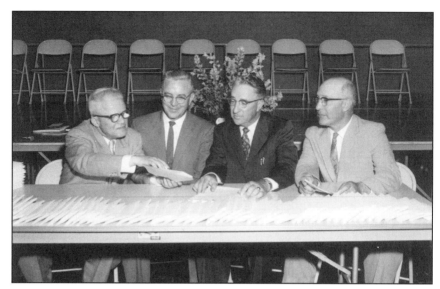

Secretary Bliss Wilson, Board members Roger Eastman, Harold Mills, and Tom Haggar, directing 1959 Board of Pharmacy examinations in Brookings.

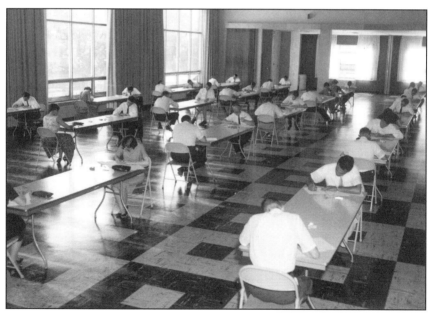

Candidates taking Board of Pharmacy examinations in Brookings, SD. 1959

A History of Pharmacy in South Dakota

CHAPTER 9
1960-1969

SD Pharmaceutical Association (SDPhA), 1960-1969

New Secretary Harold H. Schuler

At a meeting of the Executive Committee February 10, 1963, held in Pierre when the Legislature was meeting, President L.B. Urton, Sturgis, and other officers talked about pharmacy public relations. The Committee wanted an individual to handle publicity for pharmacy, "perhaps one who is not a pharmacist. It was thought for the good of pharmacy that a competent public relations person would help us through the legislative years, as well as to keep us informed with monthly reports, etc."[1]

President Urton asked Roger Eastman, Platte, to contact Harold H. Schuler of Pierre. Schuler had just spent eight years as an assistant to United States Senator Francis Case both in his Washington and Pierre offices. Senator Case died in June of 1962. Schuler had entered business in Pierre, SD by purchasing the Hughes County Abstract Company. After a discussion with Eastman, Schuler agreed to the proposal. On March 24, 1963 the Executive Committee met again and hired Harold H. Schuler as director of public relations at $125 a month. He would work part-time with Secretary Bliss Wilson.

In June of 1963, Schuler's job was expanded to include director of the Commercial and Legislative Section at a salary of $200 a month. In August, the funds of the Commercial and Legislative Section were transferred to Schuler's office. At a November 1963 meeting of the Executive Committee, Earle Crissman, Ipswich, made a motion to hire Schuler as Association lobbyist for the 1964 Legislature. It was seconded by Carv Thompson, Faith, and passed. The Committee directed that bills be introduced to raise the Patent Medicine and Poison Licenses from $3 to $6. President Wayne Shanholtz, Mitchell, appointed Roger Eastman, Platte; Tom Haggar, Watertown; and Melvin Holm, Redfield, to work with Schuler. The bills to raise the license fees passed the Legislature.

Secretary Bliss Wilson, who had ably served the Association and Board since 1942, resigned effective December 31, 1963. Wilson, had received his certificate of pharmacy registration No. 2011 in 1918. He had owned a pharmacy in Letcher, when he became secretary to the Association and Board of Pharmacy in 1942. After disposing of his pharmacy in 1946, Wilson moved the office to Pierre. He was elected President of the National Association of Boards of Pharmacy in 1963. Wilson was presented with a special plaque honoring his twenty-two years of service as secretary to the Association and the Board of Pharmacy at the 1965 convention.

The Executive Committee met January 5, 1964 and hired Harold H. Schuler as secretary to the Board of Pharmacy and Association at a salary of $7,500 per year. Schuler moved the pharmacy office from a basement hallway of the capitol to an office next to his Hughes County Abstract Company. He continued his business in Pierre as well as serving as Association and Board Secretary. Schuler, originally from Tripp, served in the United States Army Air Force in the South Pacific in World War II. He graduated from the University of South Dakota with a B.A. degree in government in 1950 and an M.Ed. in 1951.

Association Business

The numbers of in-state and out-state registered pharmacists were similar throughout the period with 956 in 1962 and 912 in 1969. A breakdown of the 1966 list showed 499 in-state pharmacists and 489 out-state pharmacists. The license renewal fee which had been $10 per year was raised to $20 in 1968.

Attendance at conventions between 1964 and 1972 averaged 170 people. The high year was 200 in 1969. Convention profits varied from $300 in 1969 to $1,100 in 1971. A breakdown of attendance at the 1969 convention events in Rapid City, where 200 had registered and paid the $20 fee, was as follows: Saturday night banquet 171, Sunday luncheon 131, wholesaler luncheon 146, and veteran's breakfast 29.

Albert H. Zarecky, Pierre, served as president 1960-1961. Conventions usually opened with a prayer by a local minister, followed by a talk from the mayor, welcome from the local pharmacists, summary of convention activities by the local chairperson, followed with a speech by the Association president. The 1961 convention in the Sheraton-Johnson Hotel at Rapid City, was opened by Father Kelley whose prayer had particular significance for pharmacists: "Oh God, who in thy Fatherly love, has granted that plants and herbs should be useful, not only as food, but as medicine and as a safeguard against sickness and suffering, guide these pharmacists in their task and help them to be exact and conscientious and efficient in their work."[2]

At the same convention, George Smith, Regional Sales Manager with Parke Davis presented a statistical summary on Medicine Development up to that time. His list of new drugs included: penicillin in 1940; strepto-mycin in 1946; antihistamines in 1947; antibiotics and corticosteroids in 1940-1950; polio vaccine in 1955; and 63 new drugs in 1959. In 1960, seven-hundred million prescriptions were filled: half of the drugs used were not available in 1955, and 75% were unknown in 1950. He told the group that the average prescription price in 1961 was $3.00 and that only 1.5% of the prescriptions cost over $10 each. Smith reported that only nineteen million people were covered by health insurance in 1951 com-pared to one-hundred and twenty-seven million (72% of the population) in 1959.[3]

President Phil Case, Parker, was concerned about the decline in phar-macies from 269 in 1950 to 239 in 1961. He believed that pharmacies must modernize to keep current with business trends. "In 1950, I felt our drug stores were behind other retail outlets in regard to modern equip-ment and merchandising methods; today that situation has changed. Remodeling is the rule rather than the exception. Merchandise lines have been expanded and new merchandising methods have been adopted. We have definitely moved forward. Prescription departments are now fea-tured with pride, rather than being hidden in the back room. Prescription filling has become our most important function."[4]

M. F. McCameron, Manager Omaha District, Eli Lilly Company expressed his views pertaining to Prescription Trends at the 1964 gather-ing in Mitchell. He maintained that "prescription trends are undergoing dramatic changes and that forces presently at work will eventually require different planning." Trends he presented are summarized as follows:

- growing number of one-stop shopping stores, selling front-end merchandise of drug stores
- hospital pharmacies seeking outpatients
- growing nursing home pharmacy service
- growing government welfare programs
- changing trends of medical practice and clinic pharmacies.

McCameron stated, "The future belongs to those who are aware of these trends."[5]

A South Dakota study in 1964, listed the average prescription cost at $3.21 and the average total gross sales per pharmacy at $102,600. The prescription business was 31% of gross sales.

One highlight of the 1962 convention at the Sioux Falls Sheraton-Cataract was a speech by United States Senator Hubert H. Humphrey Jr., who was introduced by Al Bittner, Aberdeen. Humphrey was born at Wallace, SD in 1911 where his father ran a drug store. In 1913, the family moved to Doland and then to Huron. Humphrey graduated from the

Denver College of Pharmacy in March 1933, and returned to Huron to work at his father's drug store. He became a South Dakota registered pharmacist in May 1933, holding License No. 2652. Later he returned to college and graduated from the University of Minnesota in 1939. He taught at Macalester College in St. Paul before being elected mayor of Minneapolis in 1945. He was elected to the United States Senate in 1948 and reelected in 1954 and 1960. In 1964, he was elected Vice-President along with Lyndon B. Johnson as President. In 1968, Humphrey ran for President on the Democratic ticket but lost to Richard Nixon.

In the summer of 1965, Vice-President Humphrey contacted Secretary Harold H. Schuler, Board of Pharmacy, and asked for a new registration certificate because his original had been damaged beyond repair. Schuler, who was acquainted with the United States Senate, discussed this with both Board and Association officers and it was decided to present Humphrey the new certificate in person at the October NARD convention to be held in the nation's capital. The following Association officers: President Nina Lund, Rapid City; Earle Crissman, Ipswich; Lloyd Wagner, Marion; and Board of Pharmacy member, Carveth Thompson, Faith, and Secretary Harold H. Schuler made the presentation of the new certificate to Humphrey in his Ceremonial Vice-President's Office in the United States Capitol in mid-October 1965. Joining the presentation were Senators Karl E. Mundt and George McGovern.

Federal Trade Commissioner and former Governor, Sigurd Anderson spoke at the 1963 convention in Pierre. Also at the Pierre gathering, the Ladies' Auxiliary attended a tea at the Governor's mansion, hosted by Mrs. Archie Gubbrud. At the 1964 Mitchell convention, when Melvin C. Holm, Redfield, was the president, Governor Archie Gubbrud was the speaker. Governor Nils Boe addressed the delegates at the 1960 Aberdeen convention, and Governor Frank Farrar spoke at the 1969 gathering in Rapid City.

Earle T. Crissman, Ipswich, was elected Association president in 1966. His father, Herbert S. Crissman, Ipswich, served as president in 1939-1940. In 1952, Earle purchased his father's drug store. In 1996, Earle sold the pharmacy to his daughter Judy, who is working on her pharmacy degree. His daughter, Jody, who with her husband Brian Volinske, both pharmacists, own a pharmacy in Williston, ND. Earle has attended every SDPhA convention for the past fifty-two years.

Lloyd Wagner, Marion was elected Association president in 1967. His father, Joe F. Wagner, Garden City and Conde, had served as president 1911-1912. Robert W. Ehrke, Rapid City; Clayton Scott, Sioux Falls; and Lloyd Wagner, Marion; attended the NARD convention at Boston in

A History of Pharmacy in South Dakota

October 1968. Association President Robert W. Ehrke reported at the 1969 SDPhA convention at the Alex-Johnson Hotel and said, "Among the problems repeatedly discussed at the NARD convention were prepaid prescription plans, pharmacy technicians, government intervention in pharmacy, welfare programs, discriminatory pricing by drug companies, and physician dispensing."[6] In his president's address, Ehrke reiterated "our goal: wherever drugs are dispensed, they will be dispensed by a pharmacist."[7] Board of Pharmacy member Carveth Thompson, Faith, expressed similar views: "Our Board adopted a goal that 'whenever drugs are stored, dispensed, or used, a licensed South Dakota pharmacist would be in charge and responsible."[8]

Legislative Matters

A Veterinary Committee was added to the various committees of SDPhA at the 1961 convention. That same year, a mail ballot was sent to all pharmacists asking if they favored expanding the Restricted Drug Area of a pharmacy to include certain pre-packaged veterinary medicines. It was supported by a vote of 127 Yes and 21 No. The matter was discussed again at the 1962 convention in Sioux Falls.

The idea was further discussed and consequently the Board of Pharmacy passed a new Section K, Regulation No. 8, Patent Medicines. The Board of Pharmacy would issue a special license to lay persons, to sell packaged animal medicines of the non-prescription type. However, that person had to pass an examination on animal medicines, conducted by the Board. Attorney Karl Goldsmith, Pierre, represented the Association at the time, for an annual retainer of $150.

The Association had been working with livestock groups on the matter, however, the above regulation was strongly opposed by those groups. Consequently, Senate Bill 26 was introduced in the 1963 Legislative Session. The bill would have required the Secretary of Agriculture to license all persons who wanted to sell packaged drugs and medicines for the care of animal health, and repeal all laws which heretofore restricted such sales. The bill would have repealed much of South Dakota Pharmacy Law as it pertained to Patent Medicines, Poisons, and Household Remedies. After negotiations between the Board of Pharmacy and the supporters of S.B. 26, the parties agreed to compromise. The Board of Pharmacy met during the Legislative Session and repealed that part of Section K, Regulation No. 8, pertaining to animal medicines. S.B. 26 then died in committee.

During the period a number of pharmacists served in the South Dakota Legislature. Bill Hustead, Vice-president of Wall Drug, Wall, served in the House of Representatives 1963-1966, and two years in the

Senate 1967-1968. Tom Mills, Mills Drug, Sioux Falls, served in the House of Representatives 1967-1970, and in the Senate 1971-1974.

Lobbyists for the Legislature included Pierre Attorney Karl Goldsmith. Pierre Attorney Tom Adam followed Goldsmith, however Adam resigned in 1966. The Association then hired Pierre Attorney Donald A. Haggar, a former member of the 1959 House of Representatives, representing Minnehaha County, to be a lobbyist for the Association. He was paid $600 plus travel and expenses, half by the Board of Pharmacy and half by the Association. However, a 1961 Attorney General's opinion stated that no state funds could be used to hire an attorney or lobbyist. So one-half of Haggar's salary was paid by the Commercial and Legislative Section and the other half by the Association. Harold H. Schuler also served as a lobbyist during the 1964 Legislative Session. Considering that he was paid half his salary by the State Board of Pharmacy, the Executive Committee felt that they should continue the practice of hiring an attorney to be their lobbyist and not the Board secretary. Secretary Schuler worked with Attorney Haggar and could also testify in Legislative Committees on either Board or Association matters.

It was apparent that the voice of pharmacy must be heard in the Legislature. The Executive Committee therefore, at a November 1967 meeting, approved a buffet-social for the entire Legislature at the Pierre Elks Lodge on January 2, 1968. Each of the districts selected three pharmacists to attend the affair. District members and Association officers made up a group of 35 to 40 pharmacists who attended the first buffet-social to mingle with the Legislators. The buffet-social, funded by the C & L Section, was so successful that President Clayton Scott and the Executive Committee voted to have the function again at the 1969 meeting of the Legislature.

Legislative Accomplishments, 1964-1969

Association Presidents Wayne C. Shanholtz, Mitchell; Melvin C. Holm, Redfield; Mrs. Nina D. Lund, Rapid City; Earle T. Crissman, Ipswich; Lloyd E. Wagner, Marion; Robert W. Ehrke, Rapid City; Clayton Scott, Sioux Falls; other Association officers, members, lobbyists, and Secretary Harold H. Schuler worked for the passage of the following laws:

- Raised license fees: Patent and Poison License from $3.00 to $6.00; Pharmacy License from $25 to $50; and Pharmacist License from $10 to $20; all of which helped Board and Association finances

- Unlawful to purchase or have in possession more than six grains of codeine except pursuant to lawful prescription
- Placing pharmacist on State Board of Health. Vere Larsen, Alcester, was appointed to the post
- SD Narcotic Law and Drug Abuse Act in 1968, both patterned after federal laws
- Placed a pharmacist on the State Public Health Advisory Committee. Bill Hoch, Tyndall, was appointed to the post
- Placing pharmacist on Medicaid Advisory Committee of SD State Welfare Department. Earle Crissman, Ipswich, was appointed to the post
- Placing pharmacist on State Comprehensive Health Planning Agency. Roger Eastman, Platte, was appointed to the post
- A new recodified pharmacy law in 1967. Prior to the Legislative Session, a draft of the proposed law was reviewed in each of the twelve district meetings in October and November. Suggested changes, after passage by a majority vote, were sent to Secretary Harold H. Schuler and to Attorney Donald A. Haggar for consideration by the Executive Committee.

Association Changes

Publicity

In 1962, President Phil Case, Parker, said, "we need a newsletter on a monthly basis to keep our members informed."[9] At the time, Dr. Guilford C. Gross was associate editor of the pharmacy section of the *South Dakota Journal of Medicine and Pharmacy*. He had replaced Dr. Harold S. Bailey in 1961. In 1964, Dr. Gary Omodt replaced Dr. Gross as associate editor. That same year, new Secretary Harold H. Schuler prepared a bi-monthly four-page newsletter that was mailed to all pharmacists. In 1965, only fifty-five pharmacies subscribed to the journal. The 12-page section on pharmacy cost the Association $2,600 a year. The Executive Committee ended the connection with the *Journal of Medicine and Pharmacy* on March 1, 1965.

Creation of District Organizations

From time to time, throughout the years, Association presidents appointed captains in areas or districts around the state to help during Legislative Sessions. Secretary Schuler believed that a permanent district organization would be of help to promote the profession of pharmacy. The Executive Committee in early 1964 agreed and approved a district set-up which divided the state into twelve districts. Each district was so arranged to include from eighteen to twenty-five pharmacies. However, there was some disparity, for example, the Sioux Falls District had thirty-eight pharmacies compared to ten in the Rosebud District. Each district was required to meet twice a year, sometime in April and sometime in October.

Over 500 pharmacists, spouses, and friends, attended the twelve district organizational meetings in October and November 1964. Seventy percent of the pharmacies were represented at the meetings. Each district elected a president, vice-president, and secretary-treasurer and adopted $5.00 district dues. A minuteman phone system for any legislative emergency was also created. Speaking at the meetings according to their proximity were: Secretary Harold H. Schuler; Drug Inspector Harry Lee; Board members Tom Haggar, Roger Eastman, and Carveth Thompson; Association officers Mel Holm, Nina Lund, Lloyd Wagner, Earle Crissman, Robert Ehrke, J. C. Shirley; and College of Pharmacy faculty Dean Guilford Gross, Dr. Gary Omodt, and Dr. Kenneth Redman.

Newly elected district presidents were as follows: Pierre District, Franklin Underhill, Pierre; Brookings District, Gerrit Heida, Brookings; Mitchell District, Harold Bittner, Tripp; Northern Hills District, Red Urton, Sturgis; Mobridge District, Jack Dady, Mobridge; Huron District, J. C. Jones, Miller; Watertown District, Dean Gackstetter, Watertown; Southern Hills District, Bernard Tennyson, Custer; Aberdeen District, Dick Angerhofer, Aberdeen; Winner District, Maurice E. Hiatt, White River; Sioux Falls District, Phil Von Fischer, Sioux Falls; and Yankton District, Russ Ahern, Yankton.

The district agenda for the 1968 October meetings indicated the various types of business to be performed by the districts:

1. Association officer report
2. Election of district officers
3. Select three delegates to send to the Legislative social-buffet in Pierre
4. Make plans for National Pharmacy Week
5. Review Allied Drug Travelers relationship with SDPhA
6. Nominate a person for Bowl of Hygeia
7. Nominate a person for Honorary President
8. Adopt resolutions to present to convention
9. Recommend names for the election of Association officers
10. Recommend names to the Governor for the Board of Pharmacy

A History of Pharmacy in South Dakota

In 1969 each district was also asked to nominate the best salesperson of the year from their district. That person was presented the award at the annual state convention.

Association Accomplishments, 1964-1969

Lobbyist attorneys Karl Goldsmith, Tom Adam, and Donald Haggar; Association officers; pharmacist members, and staff all worked to accomplish the following:

- Provided two scholarships of $198 each, for students at College of Pharmacy
- Established twelve district organizations
- Issued thirty-six newsletters in five years, about seven a year. Released news stories from time to time, for example, forty news stories were released in 1964
- Survey showed average prescription price in SD was $3.21
- Subscribed to SDSU newspaper clipping service to keep posted on all pharmacy activities
- Expended $1,500 in 1968 to promote National Pharmacy Week and National Poison Week. One paid Poison Week ad on KELO-TV, resulted in over 200 letters asking for Poison Counterdose Charts
- Conducted high school poster and essay contest on combating drug abuse. A $100 cash prize was awarded to a winner of each category
- Expended $1,000 on radio time to promote the profession
- Districts nominated candidates for Bowl of Hygeia and Honorary President Awards. Executive Committee made final selection
- Endorsed $2.00 professional fee in regard to any proposed state funded drug program
- Hired full-time administrative assistant in pharmacy office in 1967, to help Secretary Schuler. The salary was $390 per month, half paid by the Association and half by the Board. For example, the workload between December 18, 1968 and April 18, 1969, included the mailing of 5,034 pieces of mail including licenses, newsletters, notices to pharmacies and pharmacists, legislative bulletins, and preparing replies to 370 letters
- Reinstated fifty-year certificates honoring fifty year registrants

- Supported and promoted College of Pharmacy's program conducting institutes, seminars, and traveling circuit conferences for pharmacists
- Expended $500 to sponsor educational TV programs on pharmacy as produced by the Philadelphia College of Pharmacy and the SDSU College of Pharmacy
- Complete recodification of South Dakota Pharmacy Law in 1967.

SD Board of Pharmacy, 1960-1969

In the Interest of Public Health

The South Dakota Board of Pharmacy was guided by the principle that they worked in the 'interest of public health.' Board member Roger Eastman, Platte, told the pharmacists at the 1961 Rapid City convention, "It has been the policy of the Board to enforce the laws pertaining to pharmacy in the *interest of public health* and to the best of our ability."[10]

Board member Carveth Thompson, Faith, expressed the same sentiment at the 1965 Huron convention, "I don't think we have to be afraid of competition. It comes and goes, but most of all I feel the pharmacist has the professional responsibility of protecting the public health and I think we all feel this way whether it is in the field of human or animal medicines."[11]

The Board in October 1965 passed a new regulation on *Free Choice of Pharmacy*. The regulation required that each pharmacy erect a sign stating that principle. The Board believed that any person has the right to have their prescription filled in the pharmacy of their choice. The Board sent out reminders for the protection of public health, from time to time, reminding pharmacists of things they can and cannot do:

- cannot accept the return of unused portions of prescriptions
- cannot refill a prescription without authority of the prescriber
- fee-splitting and paying a percentage of rent in any form is illegal
- only a pharmacist can fill a prescription
- a restricted drug area must be properly set up and managed at all times
- every sale of exempt narcotics and poisons must be registered.

Accomplishments of the Board of Pharmacy, 1964-1969

Board of Pharmacy members Carveth Thompson, Faith; Tom Haggar, Watertown; Melvin Holm, Redfield; Roger Eastman, Platte; Robert

A History of Pharmacy in South Dakota

Ehrke, Rapid City; and Allen Pfeifle, Sioux Falls, lobbyists and staff all worked to accomplish the following:

- Employed two full-time drug inspectors
- Legislature raised Patent and Poison Licenses from $3 to $6
- Regulation prohibiting any advertising on prescription blanks
- Compiled jurisprudence exam which was given to all candidates taking board examinations and to those registering by reciprocity
- Helped Health Department develop regulations for use of drugs in Nursing Homes and Homes for the Aged.

Accomplishments also included the recodification of the South Dakota Pharmacy Law in 1967. Some of the main provisions of Senate Bill No. 121 passed by the Legislature were:

- Pharmacy declared professional practice (Not in old law)
- Defined dispensing
- Listed who can prescribe drugs
- Changed physician exemption in pharmacy law, "nothing shall...prevent him from supplying, *under his supervision*, to his patients such drugs as may seem to him proper" (Italics new)
- Binding Code of Ethics
- Unlawful to solicit drugs through the mail
- Non-pharmacist owners of pharmacy must delegate active management to a pharmacist
- Authority to raise pharmacist and pharmacy license fees by rule
- Board can grant intern credit for time served in military
- Association can recommend any pharmacist to Governor for appointment to Board of Pharmacy, rather than just those doing retail drug business
- Authorized part-time limited pharmacies in hospitals and nursing homes
- Board can pass regulation on animal medicines which are patent medicines, provided such regulation is subject to approval of the Livestock Sanitary Board
- Board can issue regulations to conform with new law

Board of Pharmacy Activities

In 1962, the Board of Pharmacy lost $761. With increased license fees the Board had a surplus of $24,347 in 1969. The Board issued 3,326 licenses in 1961 compared to 3,407 in 1968. This does not include about

900 pharmacists, who were licensed by the Board, however, the income from the pharmacist license fees went to the Association.

In 1965, District 5, NABP, consisting of Boards of Pharmacy members and Colleges of Pharmacy faculty within the district, met in Watertown. It was the twenty-eighth meeting of the group which was formed in 1937. Dr. Kenneth Redman, College of Pharmacy, Brookings, was elected secretary in 1964. Hand-written exams were given by the Board in January and early June. Those dates were tied in with graduation at the College of Pharmacy, SDSU. In June 1966, exams were given to sixteen pharmacy graduates, all of whom passed. In January 1968, seven took the exams and all passed. In June, eight took the exams and two failed.

In 1968, NABP members began preparing a National Board Examination for use in all states. A Blue-Ribbon Committee was formed to study the matter. Board of Pharmacy member Allen Pfeifle, Sioux Falls was appointed to the Committee. He attended his first meeting at Chicago in December 1968. The purpose of the meeting was to establish criteria for a National Board Examination, and compose test questions. Four subjects would be covered by the examination: Pharmacy, Mathematics, Chemistry, and Pharmacology. It was hoped the examination would be available for optional use by June 1969.

In January 1970, Pfeifle went to Chicago again. At this meeting the theoretical examinations that had been given were corrected and improved for the coming year. Study for a national practical examination was also started. The National Board Examination called NABPLEX was given for the first time by the South Dakota Board of Pharmacy in June 1976.

Drug Inspector Glenn Velau, Sioux Falls, resigned his job in 1960. That same year, Harry Lee, Alcester, was hired as drug inspector. He was paid $400 a month plus state travel expenses. At the next year's convention Lee reported that he had inspected elevators, feed stores, produce stations, hardware stores, grocery stores, cafes, bars, truck stops, and drug stores. Lee said, "in hardware stores I have taken off sale any mouse seed containing strychnine, informing them it's strictly a drug store item and a Class A Poison."[12] In his 1962 report he said, "I caught up with a salesman on Highway 18. He had been selling for five years without a license. If you have a medicine peddler in your area, notify the secretary."[13] In 1965, the board hired Larry J. Wieland to cover the western part of the state, who served one year. In 1966, Glenn E. Velau, Rapid City, was rehired at $550 a month. Harry Lee, Alcester, continued in his position.

The state was divided into two territories, one for Glenn E. Velau and one for Harry Lee.

Part-Time Pharmacies in Hospitals and Nursing Homes

In 1964, the Board of Pharmacy worked with the Department of Health to establish regulations for nursing homes and homes for the aged. New Department of Health regulations required: drugs must be stored in locked storage; all drugs must be kept in the original prescription containers; any discontinued prescription must be destroyed, unless the doctor authorized that it can be taken with the discharged patient; homes wishing to stock bulk prescription drugs, must employ a pharmacist either on a full or part-time basis. The federal government was soon expected to require that all nursing homes and hospitals contain either a full-time or part-time pharmacy.

To meet the need of placing pharmaceutical service in nursing homes and hospitals, the Association and Board of Pharmacy supported that concept in the new 1967 Pharmacy Law. It contained provisions for hospitals and nursing homes to obtain a part-time limited pharmacy license. The new part-time license would be limited to in-patients, and the pharmacy would need to be placed in a separate room. If bulk drugs were stored at nursing stations in hospitals or intensive care nursing homes, the facility needed an organized medical staff. A pharmacist could own drugs and fixtures in a nursing home but must be designated as the permittee on the part-time license.

The first part-time pharmacy license was issued to Memorial Hospital in Sturgis. Merle Walker of Walker Pharmacy was contracted to manage the hospital's part-time pharmacy for in-patients only. Pharmacist Walker said, "This will give much better control of medications and relieve the nursing staff of trips to a pharmacy for medications. In addition, it will relieve the administrative staff of ordering drugs and seeing drug company representatives, and place the responsibility of dispensing in the hands of a qualified pharmacist."[14]

St. Joseph's Hospital, Mitchell, was the next to receive a part-time pharmacy license. In 1967, there were sixty-one hospitals in South Dakota: eleven with regular pharmacies, and two with part-time pharmacies. The remaining forty-eight hospitals had no pharmacy. The Winner Nursing Home installed a Brewer Medication Cart that had fifty-six drawers for storage of patient prescription containers. The portable cart could be moved from room to room. In 1969, the Board of Pharmacy issued regulations pertaining to an automated mechanical device for use in hospitals. The hospital pharmacist was responsible for the inventory and stocking of drugs in the device.

In 1968, the Board of Pharmacy issued twenty-one part-time pharmacy licenses that grew to forty-three in 1969. The fee for the license was $25.

SD College of Pharmacy, 1960-1969

New Name, New Deans

The South Dakota Legislature passed a law effective July 1, 1964, that the name South Dakota State College be changed to South Dakota State University. At the same time, the Division of Pharmacy was changed to College of Pharmacy. Dean Floyd Le Blanc retired at the end of the 1963-1964 school year. Clark T. Eidsmoe said, "of Dean LeBlanc, it must be said he has been a diligent worker for, and has shown an unremitting interest in the development of pharmacy at SDSU. His connection with the College of Pharmacy has been longer than that of any other individual in its history, and his influence is reflected in the large number of graduates who have taken their places as useful and productive citizens of the communities in which they live. His tenure was marked by steady progress and expansion. An enrollment of more than three times that of the year in which he assumed the deanship made it necessary to enlarge faculty and physical plant."[15]

The Board of Regents named Dr. Guilford C. Gross as Dean of the College of Pharmacy July 1, 1964. Dr. Gross became the first dean for the new College of Pharmacy. He had earned his B.S. and M.S. from SDSU and his Ph.D. from University of Florida. Dr.Gross had been on the faculty since 1940, except for service in the Navy during World War II.

Because of health reasons, Dean Gross resigned August 31, 1965. The Board of Regents appointed former Dean LeBlanc as acting dean while a search was made for a new dean. Dr. Raymond E. Hopponen was named Dean of the College of Pharmacy February 1, 1966. Hopponen had received his B.S. (1943) and his Ph.D. (1950) from the University of Minnesota. Since 1950, he had served as assistant dean and professor of pharmacy at the College of Pharmacy, University of Kansas. Dr. Gross returned to the faculty in 1967 as professor of pharmacy.

Off Campus Seminars and Television Programs

In 1938, Dean Earl Serles started conducting a pharmaceutical institute on the campus. The annual three-day program of lectures and discussions continued until 1966. That year, Dean Ray Hopponen instituted traveling circuit conferences for extra educational opportunities for practicing pharmacists. Three meetings were held around the state on Sunday afternoons. Generally, two meetings were in the eastern part of the state and one in the western part. One circuit was held in the spring and one in the fall with an average attendance of 45-50 pharmacists at each meeting. College of Pharmacy faculty presented three one-hour programs followed by dinner.

The conferences in October 1967 were held in Aberdeen, Rapid City, and Sioux Falls. Speakers for each of the programs and their topics were: Dr. Gary Omodt, "Atherosclerosis", Dr. B. K. Rao, "Drugs for Peptic Ulcer", and Dr. Raymond Hopponen, "Coughs, Causes, and Correctives."

Clark T. Eidsmoe described another outreach program on educational television. "In the spring of 1969, an experimental television series produced by the Philadelphia College of Pharmacy and Science was used. This series, which consisted of five one-half hour programs, was telecast on Monday evenings at 7:30 over Channel 2, Vermillion and Channel 8, Brookings, and was re-broadcast at 7:30 on Wednesday evening over Channel 9 in Rapid City. The success of this venture led to discussions with the Director of Extension Services at the University of Minnesota College of Pharmacy who was preparing closed circuit television programs for use by Minnesota pharmacists. As a result a cooperative effort including a number of groups was established. Minnesota produced the program, and South Dakota and Nebraska broadcast them jointly and simultaneously."[16] The South Dakota Pharmaceutical Association contributed $500 to help with the sponsorship of the programs.

Enrollment, Graduates, and Space

The five-year pharmacy program began in the fall of 1960. That class would graduate in June 1965. The last of the four-year students graduated in the spring of 1963, consequently, there was no graduation class in 1964. In 1962, forty-three pharmacy students received their four-year B.S. degrees. In 1967, thirty-nine received their five-year B.S. degrees.

In 1953, the College of Pharmacy had received all of the space of the first floor of the Administration Building, except room 116. In 1959, enrollment in the College of Pharmacy was 240. Enrollment in the College of Pharmacy 1967-1968 was 333, and in 1968-1969 it was 312. Space was needed again. The new Science Building (Shepard Hall) was ready for occupancy in September 1964. The College of Pharmacy was allocated the third floor and a suite of rooms on the lower floor for work on bionucleonics, in the new Science Building. It also retained most of its space in the Administration Building.

Following the visit of the American Council on Pharmaceutical Education in 1968, the College of Pharmacy was placed on the list of accredited colleges of pharmacy. At the time, there were eight on the staff. The report about their 1970 visit, revealed eight full-time and eight part-time faculty. This report also stated, "unaccreditable status was threatened if a new building was neglected."[17] Dean Hopponen told pharmacists at the 1969 convention in Rapid City, that a new pharmacy building ranked second on the priority list of the Board of Regents. In October 1968, an architect had been appointed to draft preliminary plans. Money for a new building was requested at the 1969 Legislature, but the bill died in committee.

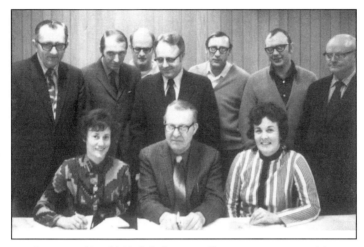

Secretary Harold H. Schuler, standing center, meets with
Mitchell committee in preparation for 1964 convention.
Wayne Shanholtz, far right, was SDPhA president.

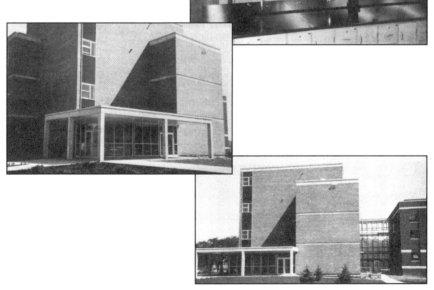

Views of new Shepard Hall opened in 1965. The entire third floor and some
other rooms were occupied by the College of Pharmacy. Top right photo shows
third floor chemistry laboratory.

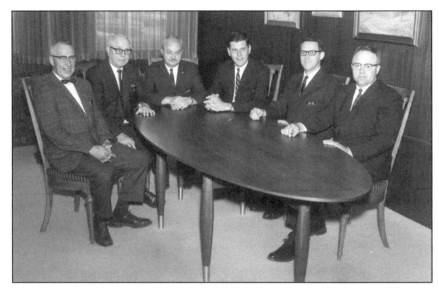

Board of Pharmacy meeting at College of Pharmacy before 1968 Board examinations. From left to right, Glenn Velau and Harry Lee, inspectors; Melvin Holm, Carveth Thompson, and Al Pfeifle, Board members; and Secretary Harold H. Schuler.

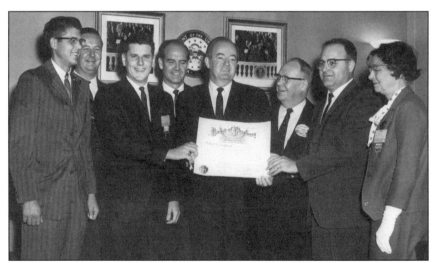

Presenting Vice-President Hubert Humphrey a new S. D. registration certificate to replace his damaged old one, in his U.S. Capitol office. Appearing at this 1968 event were, left to right, Earle Crissman, Lloyd Wagner, Carveth Thompson, Senator George McGovern, Vice-President Hubert Humphrey, Senator Karl Mundt, Harold H. Schuler, and Nina Lund.

A History of Pharmacy in South Dakota

CHAPTER 10
1970-1979

SD Pharmaceutical Association (SDPhA), 1970-1979

The Ladies' Auxiliary elected the following officers at the June 1970 Sioux Falls convention: President, Mrs. James Rogers, Watertown; Vice-President, Mrs. Patrick Lynn, Huron; Secretary, Mrs. George Tibbs, Rapid City; and Treasurer, Mrs. Lloyd Jones, Aberdeen. The treasurer reported that the balance on hand was $608. Ione Larsen, Alcester, was named historian for the Auxiliary.

At the 1970 meeting, the matter of pharmacy assistants was discussed. President Clayton Scott, Sioux Falls, reported that in 1926, thirty-eight states recognized the right of assistant pharmacists. In 1969, there was still one registered assistant pharmacist in South Dakota. That person by law, was permitted to relicense since 1926, when the state stopped licensing assistant pharmacists. Scott said, "I believe it unwise to bring back a practice that was discontinued years ago."[1] In 1971, during the term of President James Rogers, Watertown, a convention resolution was approved as follows: "In the interest of public health and welfare, we continue opposition to use of technicians in the practice of pharmacy."

President George Tibbs, Rapid City, and Vice-President Lloyd Jones, Aberdeen, attended the NARD Legislative Conference in the nation's capital. They brought news to the 1972 convention in Mitchell, about a new system of health care in the country, called Health Maintenance Organization (HMO). John T. Fay, McKesson and Robbins, one of the speakers at the NARD conference, talked about HMO's-The Phantom Army. Tibbs told the South Dakota pharmacists that Fay warned, "The greatest danger to pharmacy in this program is exclusion. Nowhere, so far, within the framework of HMO's is there any place for pharmacy."[2] The South Dakota Legislature passed House Bill 732 in 1974, which created authority to set up a HMO in the state. SDPhA took no position on the bill, which was signed into law by Governor Richard F. Kneip. Lloyd Jones also reported that NARD was fighting against Senator Ted Kennedy's bill for national health insurance.

President Wiley Vogt, Mitchell, at the 1973 Watertown convention, said, "This past year I visited approximately 50% of the pharmacies in the state, and conversed with another 15% of pharmacy owners, traveled over 9,500 miles and spent all or part of forty-one days on behalf of the Association."[3] Treasurer Jack Dady, Mobridge, reported that the books of the Board and Association are audited each year by a CPA firm, Wohlenberg and Gage, of Pierre. April 30 balances for the three groups were: Board of Pharmacy cash on hand $4,201 plus $3,500 in savings; Association cash on hand $11,219 plus $5,000 in savings; and C and L Section cash on hand $1,584 plus $2,000 in savings.

The Public Relations Committee consisting of Wiley Vogt, Mitchell, John Radeke, Milbank, and Robert L. Gregg, Chamberlain, reported in 1973 that $1,000 was expended to print and distribute two pamphlets to all pharmacies: "What You Always Wanted To Know About Prescriptions And Were Afraid To Ask" and "Pharmacy Facts." Copies were sent to each of the pharmacies for distribution to their customers. "Pharmacy Facts" was prefaced with this statement, It's not only the cost of that little pill, it is also the cost of [thirty-five other items]. Some of the cost items were: license, labor, delivery, advertising, telephone, freight, bad debts, utilities, insurance, interest, theft, inventory spoilage, income tax, depreciation, bad checks, and many more. The committee also had created a speaker's bureau. That same year, President M. Lloyd Jones, Aberdeen, and Vice-President Cliff Thomas, Belle Fourche, attended the NARD convention in the nation's capital. Their duties included a visit to the offices of Congressmen James Abdnor and Frank Denholm, and Senators George McGovern and James Abourezk.

In 1974, President Phil Von Fischer, Sioux Falls, and the Executive Committee voted to discontinue printing the annual proceedings, usually about 150 pages long. Their decision was based upon the fact that the Governor Kneip Administration no longer required it be printed. Therefore, the 1973 issue was the last printed annual proceedings of both the Board and Association. A yearly summary of financial activities, convention resolutions, Executive Committee minutes etc., were to be kept on file in the office. That same year, an Aberdeen convention resolution removed Board of Pharmacy members from the Association's Executive Committee.

One of the resolutions which failed, at the 1975 convention in Sioux Falls, was to elect officers by a mail ballot rather than by convention vote. A resolution which passed was "The Association commends Secretary Harold H. Schuler for the fine job he is doing as Secretary." Awards presented at the banquet included Milton Swenson, Lake Preston, Bowl of

Hygeia, and Shirley Vail, Gettysburg, Honorary President. Congressman Larry Pressler spoke at the wholesalers' luncheon at the Airport Holiday Inn. Robert Ehrke, Class of 1954, was named SDSU Distinguished Alumnus for 1975.

The 1976 convention at the Northern Black Hills Holiday Inn, Spearfish, was chaired by President Cliff Thomas, Belle Fourche. Cliff Thomas, a NDSU pharmacy graduate in 1949, served three years in the Eighth Air Force in England as a radio operator and waist gunner on a B-24 bomber crew during World War II. Thomas purchased a pharmacy at Belle Fourche in 1964 and sold it in 1985 to pharmacists Ron and Marilyn Schwans. Ron served as SDPhA president in 1979-1980. Marilyn served in that same capacity in 1989-1990. Cliff then joined the South Dakota Board of Pharmacy as a drug inspector. He also became "The Philosophical Pharmacist", and served as an after-dinner speaker at over 600 pharmacy gatherings around the state and nation. His book, *Humor in Pharmacy*, Nemo Publishing Company, Belle Fourche, SD was released for sale in 1998.

Full and partial registration for the Spearfish convention totaled 272. Attendance figures at various events included: opening ceremonies, 160; first open session, 120; first business session, 96; continuing education, 87; smorgasbord, 229; veterans' breakfast, 124; memorial hour, 110; second open session, 105; wholesalers' luncheon, 226; second business session, 92; final business session, 96; and president's banquet, 241. Brown Drug Co., Jewett Drug Co., Davis Bros. Inc., and Northwestern Drug hosted the hospitality hour and the luncheon. An Institutional Pharmacy Committee was created at the 1976 convention. At the time, there were thirty-five full-time pharmacists and fifty-five part-time pharmacists working in hospitals. There were also many pharmacists serving as consultant pharmacists in nursing homes. The committee reviewed problems of pharmacy practice in institutions and reported them to the Association.

Following a recommendation by President John Nelson, Arlington, and the Executive Committee, the 1976 convention approved a resolution to select a person for Lay Person of the Year Award, for outstanding contribution to pharmacy. It would be given annually when warranted. Nominations would be made at the districts with the final selection by the Executive Committee. Dick Brown, Brown Drug, Sioux Falls, and Harvey Jewett III, Jewett Drug, Aberdeen, were the first two winners and their awards were presented to them at the 1977 convention in Brookings.

There were some changes in the makeup of the Association districts which had been reduced from twelve to nine. The procedure for district resolutions was changed in 1977, during the term of President Jack Dady, Mobridge. District resolutions needed to be approved by a majority vote of those attending the meeting. The approved resolutions were placed on a prescribed form and signed by the district president, who sent them to the Association office. The Association secretary mailed the district resolutions to all pharmacists in advance of the convention. At the time of the convention, the district resolutions, as written, were placed on the floor by the resolutions chairperson for discussion and vote.

The district meeting agenda for 1978 included a report by an Association officer, and nominations for the following: Bowl of Hygeia, Honorary President, Salesperson of the Year, and Outstanding Lay Person. Nominations were also made for Association officers and a member of the Board of Pharmacy. Approving or rejecting resolutions, electing officers, and discussing district business matters, were also on the agenda. They selected three pharmacists to attend the buffet-social at the 1979 Legislature.

Congressman James Abdnor was the main speaker at the President's Banquet at the 1978 Pierre convention. Professor Gary Omodt, SDSU College of Pharmacy, was the Master of Ceremonies. Officers attending national conventions that year included: President Ed Swanson, Madison, Ron Schwans, Hoven, and Harold H. Schuler, Pierre, to the NARD Legislative Conference in Washington, D.C.; Ron Huether to APhA convention in Anaheim, California; and President Ron Schwans, Hoven, and Ron Huether, Sioux Falls, to NARD convention in Las Vegas, Nevada. SDPhA Association Committees included: College of Pharmacy, Finance, Peer Review, Inter-professional, Publicity, Serles Memorial, Veterinary, and Institutional Pharmacy.

Ed Swanson, Madison, said, "the most important problem during my term as SDPhA president, 1978-1979, was the differential prices that manufacturers were charging hospitals, independent pharmacies, and discount (mass merchandiser pharmacies). Former SDPhA President Phil Von Fischer, Sioux Falls, and I went to Washington, D.C. and discussed these problems with our Congressmen."[4]

Legislation

Pharmacist Legislators

During the period a number of pharmacists served in the South Dakota Legislature. Tom Mills, Sioux Falls, who had served in the House 1967-1970 was elected to the State Senate in the fall of 1970, where he served until 1974. His Senate assignments included serving as

Chairperson of the Transportation Committee and Vice-Chairperson of the Senate Health and Welfare Committee.

Carveth Thompson, Faith, a member of the South Dakota Board of Pharmacy, 1963-1969, was appointed by Governor Frank Farrar in 1969 to the House of Representatives. He ran for election in 1970, and served in the House 1971-1972. Thompson ran for Governor and won the Republican Party primary election in June 1972. In the fall general election for Governor he lost to incumbent Governor Richard F. Kneip. Governor William Janklow appointed Thompson to the State Fair Commission where he served thirteen years. In 1958, pharmacist Carveth Thompson had purchased Thompson Drug in Faith from his father, pharmacist Odin Thompson. Odin had been connected with the pharmacy since 1916. Carv and two other Faith businessmen in 1976, opened the Prairie Oasis Mall, a block-long nine-store shopping center on Faith's Main Street. It may be the smallest town in America with a shopping mall. One of the stores in the mall was Thompson Drug. Throughout the years, Carv and his wife, Margaret, expanded their business. At one time they owned drug stores, all Walgreen franchises, in Faith and six other towns in western South Dakota. In 2001, after selling his businesses, Carv Thompson retired, selling Thompson Drug in Faith to Jim Stephens, of Pierre.

James Hersrud, Keystone, served in the House of Representatives, representing Pennington County, 1973-1974. Governor Kneip appointed Hersrud to the Board of Pharmacy in 1978 where he served until 1981. Kenneth B. Jones, Yankton, resigned his position as vice-president of SDPhA when he was elected to the South Dakota Senate in 1974. He served in the Senate 1975-1978. In 1979, Governor William Janklow appointed Ken Jones to the board of directors of the Milwaukee Railroad. Ken Jones, a member of the Board of Pharmacy 1981-1985, was named Distinguished Alumnus by SDSU College of Pharmacy in 2002. O. J. Tommeraason, Madison, who had served in the South Dakota Senate 1941-1944 and 1957-1958, died in 1977. Mrs. Ione E. Larsen, Alcester, spouse of Vere Larsen, ran for the United States Congress in the 1974 Republican primary election. She lost to Larry Pressler. Ione Larsen served as historian for the Ladies' Auxiliary for many years.

Other pharmacists connected with state government, at the time, included Marlyn Christensen, Mitchell, who was appointed by Governor Kneip, as the pharmacist member of the newly created Drugs and Controlled Substances Advisory Board. Charles Reinders, Sioux Falls, was appointed to the South Dakota Foundation of Medical Care. Robert

Ehrke, Rapid City, was president of the Health Systems Agency of South Dakota.

Legislative Buffet-Social Continues

The Legislative buffet-social in Pierre, which had started in January 1968, continued throughout the entire period. Each of the nine districts elected three pharmacist representatives and paid their expenses to the event. The buffet-social was held at the Elks Lodge between 1968 and 1974, when it was moved to the Kings Inn in downtown Pierre. Attorney Keith Tidball, Pierre, was hired as the Association attorney and lobbyist in 1970. Attendance at the Elks for the 1973 buffet-social totaled thirty-five pharmacists and spouses and ninety-five Legislators out of a total of 110. The record attendance for the Legislative buffet-social was in 1977 at the Kings Inn, where thirty-nine pharmacists and spouses and ninety-seven Legislators out of 105 attended.

The usual format for the day of the buffet-social in Pierre, included a noon luncheon for pharmacists and spouses. At the luncheon, lobbyist Donald Haggar, Keith Tidball beginning in 1970, and Secretary Harold Schuler reviewed all the legislation affecting the pharmacy profession. The Association, districts, and the Executive Committee had made prior decisions on various bills, and the pharmacists were asked to support the decisions and lobby the Legislators. If a pharmacist representative had a strong disagreement with the Association position, it was certainly discussed at the luncheon. With the Executive Committee present, the matter could have been changed, if necessary. Legislation, at times, was a fast moving thing, and a bill detrimental to the profession could have been introduced the day of the buffet-social. In the afternoon, the pharmacists visited the Legislative halls to talk with their Legislators. About 6:00 p.m. they all returned for the buffet-social at the Pierre Elks Lodge, at the King's Inn after 1973, and further socialized with the Legislators. There were no head tables, no speeches, just good food and good sociability.

Why All The Legislation?

The pharmacy profession is regulated by law. South Dakota law 36-11-1 states, "The practice of pharmacy in South Dakota is hereby declared to be a professional practice affecting the public health, safety, and welfare and is subject to regulation in the public interest. The practice of pharmacy means the interpretation and evaluation of prescription drug orders and dispensing in the patient's best interest." Because the pharmacy profession is regulated, many things in the health care field can affect the profession. The health care field involves doctors, dentists, pharmacists, nurses, and other specialists. The entire health care field was changing from day to day, consequently much of the change is accomplished by legislation. Some of the changes are as follows:

- pharmacy retail practice
- government programs involving drugs and medicines
- new drug treatment methods
- prepaid prescription drug programs
- drug programs funded by insurance companies
- overlapping health care with other professions
- new laws such as part-time pharmacies in hospitals and nursing homes
- Health Maintenance Organizations
- medicaid program providing drugs to indigent
- paying professional fee rather than the customary price markup.

To establish any of the above programs requires change and it was the Association's belief that pharmacists should be involved in the change for the protection of the profession and public health. For example, when the Legislature created a State Board of Health, it was the Association's position that a pharmacist should be a member of that board and they supported legislation calling for the inclusion of a pharmacist. The pharmacists approach to legislation was best summarized by Association President Robert Ehrke in his speech to the convention at Rapid City in 1969: "wherever drugs are dispensed, they will be dispensed by a pharmacist."[5]

Legislation Affecting the Profession in the 1970s

- Supported law permitting counties to match federal funds to be used to pay drug costs of persons on welfare (A forerunner to Title 19 Drug Program).
- Supported law permitting Board of Pharmacy to determine an intern training program by regulation.
- Defeated a bill which required the illness be typed on the prescription container.
- Favored law calling for a four-year medical school.
- Adds pharmacist to Advisory Board of Office of Controlled Drugs and Substances.
- Supported law permitting pharmacists to fill prescriptions from out-of-state doctors.
- Killed bill permitting unlimited advertising of drugs and their prices.
- Defeated a bill making it mandatory that aspirin could be sold under the Household Remedy Law. Sponsor of bill was

informed that aspirin could already be sold under the Household Remedy Law, so the Legislator asked that the bill be tabled.

- Repealed sales tax on prescription drugs.
- Supported a bill authorizing money for a pharmacy addition to Shepard Hall at SDSU, and for five extra pharmacy faculty.
- Favored amendment to Certified Nurse Practitioner law, that nothing in the law authorizes them to practice pharmacy.

1970s Legislation Attempting Separation of Association and Board

Background

The Legislature in 1890 created the South Dakota Pharmaceutical Association and the South Dakota Board of Pharmacy. Although two separate entities, the secretary of the Association was also the secretary of the Board of Pharmacy and maintained one office. A pharmacist paid the license renewal fee to the secretary of the Board of Pharmacy, who in turn issued the license to the pharmacist and deposited the money to the Board of Pharmacy account. The pharmacist was automatically a member of the Association.

The law was changed in 1893. A pharmacist paid a $2.00 renewal fee to the secretary of the Board of Pharmacy, who in turn issued the license to the pharmacist; however, the renewal fee was deposited to the account of the South Dakota Pharmaceutical Association. The Board of Pharmacy survived financially with other license fees, whereas the Association depended on the renewal fees for its survival. This concept was completely reinstated in the 1967 recodification of the South Dakota Pharmacy Law. The concept continued until the 1970s when there was a determined effort to separate the two groups.

In 1972, South Dakota voters supported a change in the State's Constitution. One change created twenty-five departments in the executive branch of government. Shortly after the 1972 election, a Citizens Commission on Executive Reorganization met in Pierre. Representatives of the Board and the Association testified before the group as to duties of the Board of Pharmacy. In January 1973, Governor Richard Kneip submitted his plan to reorganize the government pursuant to the Constitutional Amendment. Under his plan the Board of Pharmacy was transferred to the new Department of Commerce and Consumer Affairs, and under the Division of Professional and Occupational Licensing. Nineteen other examining boards were also transferred to Commerce and Consumer Affairs. Those boards would report to the new department on

A History of Pharmacy in South Dakota

July 1, 1973 but would continue the same as before. However, the department secretary had to submit a plan by January 1, 1974, to centralize all twenty examining boards into one centralized board.

In December 1974, the department secretary conducted a hearing on his plan to consolidate the examining boards. President Lloyd Jones, Attorney Keith Tidball, and Secretary Harold H. Schuler appeared at the hearing and strongly opposed the plan. All examining boards opposed the plan. The plan failed.

During the next five years different Legislators attempted to pick apart the relationship of the Association and the Board by introducing separate bills. All the bills were opposed either by convention resolution or action of the Executive Committee, and all were defeated in the Legislature, either in Committee or on the Legislative floor. Here is a summary of the various bills which in effect, would have separated the Board from the Association:

- 1975 • H. B. 775. Give the $25 Association renewal fee to the Board of Pharmacy. Defeated.
- 1978 • H. B. 1131. All state Boards deposit license and fee money with the State Treasurer. Defeated.
  - S.B. 281. Required all Boards and Associations to have separate offices with no sharing of employees. It did pass in the House but it was defeated in the Senate.
  - S.B. 227. Repeal part of law where Secretary of an Association is also Secretary to a State Board. Defeated.
  - H. B. 1282. Increase Board of Pharmacy to five members: three pharmacists; one lay person; and one employee of State Health Department. Defeated in House 39 to 28.
- 1979 • H.B. 1312. Required Boards to place money in State Treasurer account and not in private banks. Defeated.
- 1980 • H. B. 1093. Sunset [terminate] State Board of Pharmacy and four other state Boards. Defeated.

Title 19 Drug Program

Historically South Dakota counties paid for prescription drugs for persons on county welfare. In 1961, the Legislature appropriated money for medical care for Old Age Assistance. An Advisory Committee of health care professionals plus three lay persons was created to help with the program. Governor Richard Kneip appointed Joe Cholik, Pierre, as the pharmacist representative. Pharmacists argued successfully that any reimbursement for prescriptions be based upon a 1958 price schedule, less a 10% discount. But little money was provided for the program, so it was delayed and the counties continued paying for prescriptions for welfare patients.

In anticipation of more government programs to pay for drug costs of those on public welfare, the pharmacists in 1965 passed a resolution, that when state institutions provide free drugs to their patients, staffs must be excluded from such free services. At the 1968 SDPhA convention, a resolution was passed that pharmacists be paid a $2.00 professional fee when filling a prescription for a government agency. In 1970, State Representative Ellen Bliss, Sioux Falls, introduced a bill that would have permitted Boards of County Commissioners to match federal funds to pay for drugs for persons on state public assistance. But again little money was provided, so the counties continued paying drug bills.

The State Welfare Department agreed to start a Title 19 Drug Program January 1, 1971, however, the Legislature had to fund the program. It wasn't until 1974 that the Legislature approved a Title 19 Drug Program, with the following provisions:

- State will match $800,000 federal money with $400,000 state money
- An I.D. card will be provided to 39,000 eligible recipients, who can present it and the prescription at a pharmacy of their choice
- A full-time consultant pharmacist and seven employees will manage the program
- Pharmacies will submit monthly claims to the State Department of Social Services, which will be placed on a computer. After computation, checks will be prepared by the computer
- A $2.00 professional fee will be paid the pharmacists for each prescription.

Willis Hodson, Aberdeen, was hired as the consultant pharmacist at a salary of $14,120 a year. Hodson, a 1942 graduate of SD State College of Pharmacy, began his career in a Spearfish pharmacy earning $25 a week. In 1943, he started working at Walgreen Drug, 202 South Main, Aberdeen, at a salary of $37.50 a week. Later, he went to Minneapolis for the company, but returned to Aberdeen in 1947 as a store manager at Walgreen Drug. Hodson also recalled that he had earned some apprentice time in 1941, at Crissman Drug, Ipswich, earning $2.00 a day. But it was much better than the $1.00 a day he had earned doing other odd jobs during the summer.[6]

Over 4,500 claims were filed by July 31, 1974. All claims were processed by computer and were paid by September 20, 1974. The August 31 claims were paid by October 4, 1974, a thirty-four day turn around. After a study, the fee was raised to $2.25. By 1981, Governor Kneip's budget called for a professional fee of $3.00. Willis Hodson retired in 1981 and he and his wife moved to their cabin in the Black Hills. Don Mahannah, Chamberlain was hired as the consultant pharmacist. In 1991, Consultant Pharmacist Don Mahannah reminded pharmacists to submit medicaid claims electronically to the Department of Social Services, because they are processed in one week, compared to three weeks for paper claims. Mahannah retired in 1994.

Drug Product Selection

Pharmacists were prohibited by law and regulation to dispense a different drug than the one prescribed, without permission of the prescriber and the purchaser. For example, a 1958 Board of Pharmacy regulation stated that anyone violating the law or regulations, "shall be evidence [that the pharmacist] is incompetent...and shall constitute grounds for revocation of a certificate of registration."

However, it was believed that the pharmacist should have more to say about the matter, considering the availability of more approved generic drugs, more years of College of Pharmacy training, and different practices within the pharmaceutical industry. A 1976 convention resolution urged the passage of a drug product selection law by the Legislature. The SDPhA Executive Committee at an October 10, 1976 meeting agreed to support a bill at the 1977 Legislature which called for Drug Product Selection provided, however:

"that a pharmacist filling a prescription order for a drug product prescribed by its trade or brand name may select another drug product with the same active chemical ingredients of the same strength, quantity, dosage, and of the same generic drug type as defined in Par.1, unless the physician has expressly forbidden such selection on the prescription form. Par. 1 'Generic Drug Type' means the chemical or generic name, as determined by the United States Adopted Names (USAN) and accepted by FDA, of those drug products having the same active ingredients."[7]

After meeting with representatives of the South Dakota Medical Association, the doctors preferred some language relieving them of all liability when the pharmacists used Drug Product Selection. However, no action was taken by the 1977 Legislature. Later that year, the doctors and the pharmacists agreed to a dual line signature prescription form. There was considerable discussion whether 'Dispense as Written' should be on the left side or on the right side of the bottom of the prescription form. At a later meeting, the Executive Committee agreed with Legislation that placed at the bottom of the prescription form the language: 'Dispense as Written' on the right side, and 'Substitution Permitted' on the left side.

The 1978 Legislature approved a Drug Product Selection law, the procedure as follows:

- Generic drug type means the chemical name, generic name as determined by the USAN, published for the year 1976, for those drug products having the same active chemical ingredients
- The physician communicates instructions to the pharmacist by signing either the left side or the right side of the prescription form. No prescription is valid without the signature of the physician
- If authorization for substitution is given, the pharmacist may select another drug product with the same active chemical ingredients of the same strength, quantity and dosage, and of the same generic drug type
- A pharmacist may not substitute a drug product unless it has been manufactured with the following minimum manufacturing standards: marked tablets with identification code or monogram; expiration date shown on the label; policy to accept return goods that have passed their expiration date; records maintained for product information; and recall capabilities as available for unsafe or defective drugs.

Continuing Education (CE)

The College of Pharmacy had conducted pharmaceutical institutes on the campus between 1938 and 1966. Dean Ray Hopponen changed the format in 1966 and instituted traveling circuit conferences. A few television series were also conducted. There were also good educational programs presented at conventions. The programs were all on a voluntary basis.

Pharmacists at the 1975 convention, by a vote of 63 Yes and 15 No, favored the passage of a law calling for mandatory continuing education. The matter was favorably reaffirmed at the 1976 convention. Senator Kenneth Jones, pharmacist from Yankton, introduced a bill in the 1977 Legislature calling for mandatory continuing education for pharmacists. The law would be effective October 1, 1980 and the program would be determined by regulation of the Board of Pharmacy. Approved programs of continuing education hours could be obtained at conventions, lectures, TV programs, pharmaceutical journals, etc.

Not all pharmacists were in favor of the proposed law, in fact, many contacted their Legislators to oppose the bill. The Legislative history shows that the bill had many supporters as well as opponents as it worked its way through the Legislature. The floor action is reviewed below to show how difficult it can be, at times, to obtain passage of a bill in the Legislature.

House Commerce Committee—at a hearing, there was some opposition to the bill because it might be difficult for retired pharmacists to obtain the CE hours. The Committee, by a vote of 7 Yes and 5 No, sent the bill to the House floor.

Floor of the House of Representatives—The bill was amended to apply only to active pharmacists. It passed the House by a vote of 58 Yes and 3 No, and was sent to the Senate.

Senate Commerce Committee—The bill met heavy resistance in the Committee. Some Legislators were concerned that the Board of Pharmacy would make standards so high that it would drive some pharmacists from the profession. After several Committee votes, Senator Jones was able to have the bill sent to the Senate floor without recommendation.

Floor of the Senate—Many pharmacists called their Legislators to support the bill and many called to oppose the bill. After much debate the bill passed in the Senate with a vote of 22 Yes and 12 No and 1 absent. It was signed into law by Governor Richard Kneip. Senator Kenneth Jones of Yankton, was given much credit for securing passage of the bill. Lobbyist Keith Tidball and Executive Secretary Harold H. Schuler also worked with Jones on the matter.

The main provisions of the law, requiring mandatory continuing education for pharmacists to renew their license, were as follows:

- Effective October 1, 1980
- Board of Pharmacy authorized to approve regulations for CE programs, not to exceed twelve hours in length in any one year
- Establishment of an Advisory Council to the Board, consisting of two pharmacists appointed by the Board; two pharmacists appointed by the College of Pharmacy; and four pharmacists appointed by SDPhA.

The Board of Pharmacy held a hearing on proposed rules in January 1978. Some of the regulations were: twelve hours of CE needed to renew the pharmacist's license by October 1, 1980; pharmacists keep their own records; CE time transferable from other states; all CE programs must be approved in advance by the Board; types of programs could be cassettes, seminars, College of Pharmacy courses; TV series; professional society programs, etc.

Pharmacy Facts 1973-1979

Board of Pharmacy Survey 1973 and 1978

Total in-state pharmacists in 1973 were 455, of which 380 were men and 73 were women. Median age for men was 42 and 34 for women. Pharmacy education with less than four years 53; four years 233; five years 139; six years 1; no degree 21; and not reported 8. Pharmacy degree from SDSU 322; NDSU 22; Creighton 21; U of Minn. 14; others 48; and not reported 28. Principal place of pharmacy practice: independent community, men 206, women 32; chain community, men 59, women 8; hospitals and nursing homes, men 19, women 14; manufacturing, men 7, women none; government, teaching, men 20, women none, and not reported 69 men and 19 women.[8]

A Board of Pharmacy census of pharmacy in 1978 showed there were 596 in-state pharmacists and 513 out-state pharmacists. Of the 596 in-state pharmacists: 361 practiced in retail; 78 in hospitals; other 51; retired or otherwise engaged 106. Of the in-state pharmacists 163 were under 30 years of age; 135 between 30 and 39; 112 between 40 and 49; 69 between 50 and 59; 29 between 60 and 64; over 65 years 66; and not reporting 31. There were 446 men and 150 women pharmacists.

1979 Lilly Digest Community Pharmacy Survey

Using their national survey of 851 community pharmacies in 1978, *Lilly Digest* listed the average sales per pharmacy at $355,000; prescription sales amounted to $181,000 or 51% and other sales $174,000 or 49%. The cost of goods sold totaled $232,000 or 65%, leaving a gross margin of $123,000 or 35%.

Expenses totaled $111,784 or 31%, leaving a net profit before taxes of $11,399 or 3.2%. Total income, including the manager's salary of $23,900, was $35,329 or 9.9%. Annual rate of turnover of inventory was four times. New prescriptions dispensed totaled 13,558 or 48.5%, renewed totaled 14,394 or 51.5%. Average prescription charge in 1978 was $6.50.[9] Comparatively, in-state and out-state surveys showed that the average prescription charge was $.94 in 1939; $1.30 in 1946; $2.10 in 1952; and $3.00 in 1961.

SD Board of Pharmacy, 1970-1979

Board Business

In 1968, Board member Al Pfeifle, Sioux Falls, was appointed to a Blue Ribbon Committee of the National Association of Boards of

Pharmacy, to develop a national examination for use by the Boards. He made a number of trips to NABP headquarters in Chicago to edit, refine, and compose new questions for the national standardized examination. The nationally prepared test would be a great improvement over the old method where Board members in each state prepared their own tests. It would also provide a national measurement for reciprocating grades between the states for registration by reciprocity.

Board Chairman Robert Ehrke, Rapid City, and members T.C. Rutherford, Winner, and Allen Pfeifle, Sioux Falls, met ten times in 1971. They approved the registration of thirteen reciprocity candidates and gave the Board exams to sixteen candidates, two of whom failed. Licenses issued by the Board in 1971 included: 215 pharmacies, 55 part-time pharmacies in hospitals, 717 poison, 1,860 patents, 212 household remedy, and 891 registered pharmacists of which 440 were in-state. The Board of Pharmacy hosted the District V, NABP and AACP meeting in Rapid City in 1972. Board members and College of Pharmacy professors from Iowa, Manitoba, Minnesota, Nebraska, North Dakota, and South Dakota participated in the event.

Al Pfeifle, Chairman of the Board of Pharmacy outlined the work and responsibilities of the Board in his 1973 report. He said, "throughout the year the Board has acted on the usual [matters] which must be taken at any given time in the fields of licensure, disciplinary action, public relations, education, governmental, legislative, and personal assistance to pharmacists. [The Board] accomplished its assigned task of protecting the public health of the people of South Dakota."[10]

The Board approved new practical experience regulations, effective January 1, 1973, which conformed with NABP standards. A new title of intern replaced the old title of apprentice. A student needed to have completed two years of college work towards a pharmacy degree before registering for intern time. Each student had to complete 1,500 hours of intern time, 400 hours of which could be earned concurrent with college work. The 400 hours of externship and clinical training would be handled by the SDSU College of Pharmacy.

The Board met in Brookings and gave the exams in June and October of 1972 and in May 1973. Forty-six new pharmacists were registered by examination, and ten by reciprocity. The Board began using the NABP national paper examinations called, NABPLEX, in the spring of 1976.

A part of Governor Richard Kneip's government reorganization program included naming a lay person to serve on each of the state's twenty examining boards. In July 1973, he appointed Donna Burns, Brookings, to a three-year term as the lay person on the Board of Pharmacy. The

Board was composed of three pharmacists and one lay person. Terry Casey, Casey Drug, Chamberlain, was also appointed by Governor Kneip. Casey said "I went on the board the same time as the first lay member, Donna Burns. Lay membership gave us a wonderful insight into our profession."[11] Shirley Heitland, Brookings, was appointed by Governor Kneip as the lay person succeeding Donna Burns. Shirley Heitland served between 1976 and 1988.

In 1973, Harry Lee, Alcester, retired as drug inspector for the Board. He had served since 1960. Lee worked the eastern part of the state and Glenn Velau worked the western part. At the 1973 SDPhA convention, a resolution was approved extending to Lee "our sincere appreciation...for untiring efforts to further the profession." Al Pfeifle, Sioux Falls, in his Board report said, "The Board wishes to take this official report to note and publicly commend Harry Lee for his many years of dedicated service."[12] He was presented a watch for his outstanding service to the profession of pharmacy. Executive Secretary Harold H. Schuler also praised Harry Lee's fine work as a drug inspector and said, "We will greatly miss him."

Advertising of Drug Prices

In 1957, the Board of Pharmacy passed Regulation E-13, prohibiting pharmacies from advertising prices or discounts for prescriptions. This same prohibition was reinstated in the 1967 new pharmacy law approved by the South Dakota Legislature. Following the 1967 Legislature, the Board passed Regulation E-13 again. Carveth Thompson, Faith, a member of the Board 1963-1969, said "One of the biggest issues the Board of Pharmacy faced those years was the matter of 'advertising prescription prices.' Board of Pharmacy rules at that time, prohibited advertising using the words 'discount', 'sale', 'cut-rate', etc. Anything that advertised that any prices were lower than other pharmacies was prohibited by Board of Pharmacy rules [and law]."[13] That prohibition against advertising prices or discounts for prescriptions had a rocky road for the next ten years. The following is presented as another example of the legislative process and why it is important to have a lobbyist representing the Association at the South Dakota Legislature. It also shows the history of advertising and non-advertising of drug prices in the state.

Following a federal program to control prices during an inflationary period, the Federal Trade Commission in 1971, issued regulations requiring all pharmacies to post prices for the forty prescription drugs which had the highest sales volume. Posting was permitted in the pharmacy department only and could be done by sign, typewritten sheet, or notebook. However, South Dakota's regulation and law prohibiting advertising of drug prices was still in effect.

In 1972, a bill was introduced which would have repealed Regulation E-13, but it was tabled in Committee. Legislators in 1973, passed Senate Bill 72, which permitted pharmacists to voluntarily post prescription prices in the pharmacy department. It was still illegal to advertise drug prices. A bill in the 1974 Legislature would have barred the Board of Pharmacy from passing any regulation which would stop a pharmacy from advertising of drug prices. It was tabled in Committee.

Bills were introduced in the House and Senate, in 1975, to repeal Board of Pharmacy regulations which prohibited advertising of drug prices. They were all defeated. At the end of the 1975 Legislative Session, the law stated that pharmacists could voluntarily post prescription prices in the pharmacy, however a pharmacist could not refuse to quote the price of a prescription drug when asked. It was still illegal to advertise prices or discounts of prescription drugs.

When the U. S. Supreme Court ruled that a state could not bar the advertising of prescription prices, the South Dakota Legislature in 1977 repealed 36-11-47, the law which prohibited discount sales and advertising of drug prices. The Board of Pharmacy also repealed the regulation pertaining to posting of drug prices in the pharmacy. A pharmacist, however, according to South Dakota law, cannot refuse to quote the price of a prescription drug when asked.

SD College of Pharmacy, 1970-1979

Accreditation and a New Pharmacy Building

Although the College of Pharmacy had been a member of the American Association of Colleges of Pharmacy since 1908, the first inspection for accreditation was made in 1928. The College of Pharmacy was given an affirmative report. At the time, the pharmacy staff consisted of Dean Earl R. Serles, Karl H. Rang, Floyd J. LeBlanc, and Clark T. Eidsmoe. Finn Bernhart was a half-time member of the staff.

Between 1928 and 1977, the College was inspected ten times. Since 1939, representatives of the American Council on Pharmaceutical Education (ACPE) had conducted the inspections. Dr. Kenneth Redman said that space "was considered adequate only three times, 1928, 1933, and 1953." He also said that in printed reports of the accreditation visits between 1956-1977, "the suggestions that pharmacy needed a new building became increasingly stronger."[14] "Finally, the ACPE report for January 23, 1978 stated '...it was determined that the deficiencies of the program were of such a serious character that the baccalaureate program in pharmacy be placed on probation.' Faculty and staff, finances, and physical facilities were also the basis for the action."[15] More faculty and more space were needed to meet the ACPE standards. For example, between 1888 and 1974, the College of Pharmacy had been housed in five different buildings on the campus.

Members of the College of Pharmacy, South Dakota Pharmaceutical Association, and Board of Regents pitched in to help restore the accreditation status of the College of Pharmacy. The 1979 Legislature, with the urging of various supporters, approved an additional $119,700 to hire five new full-time faculty members. They also approved House Bill 1074 authorizing the South Dakota Building Authority to sell $500,000 in bonds to build a College of Pharmacy addition to Shepard Hall. The building would actually cost $636,927, however, to obtain Legislative approval, supporters agreed to raise $136,927 privately. JoAnn Long, Huron, chaired a sixteen-member Pharmacy Building Steering Committee, which raised the extra money through donations. Six plaques, located on the wall opposite the Dean's office within the new building, contain the names of 328 contributors, which includes pharmacists, pharmacies, pharmaceutical companies, organizations, and individuals.

Dean Ray Hopponen reported that ACPE lifted probationary status and restored the College of Pharmacy's accredited program July 1, 1979. Money for additional faculty, as well as the approved addition to Shepard Hall, met ACPE's accreditation requirements. At long last, pharmacy facilities and faculty would be located in one building.

Pharmacists at the June 1980 convention passed a resolution to name the new building, Guilford C. Gross Pharmacy Building. The SDSU pharmacy faculty, at an August 20, 1980 meeting, endorsed the SDPhA resolution. Dr. Gross had served the College of Pharmacy thirty-four years, both as professor and as dean. Construction of the pharmacy addition to Shepard Hall at SDSU began in the spring of 1980, with completion expected in the spring of 1981. An ACPE October 1981 report stated, "Between Shepard Hall (the entire third floor) and the new addition (approximately 7,800 square feet) a total of 13,000 net square feet of contiguous space is available to the College of Pharmacy. The new wing includes administrative and faculty offices, teaching laboratories, a classroom, a student study area, animal holding area, and other service and storage areas."[16] An open house for SDSU faculty and staff was held January 23, 1981. The new building was dedicated September 19,1981.

Students, Awards, and Scholarships

The E.R. Serles Memorial Fund was changed to Earl R. and Daphne C. Serles Memorial Fund in 1970, by SDPhA convention resolution. The fund grew to $11,115 by 1973. Scholarships were granted to pharmacy students selected by a Scholarship Committee of the College of Pharmacy. Three scholarships were awarded in amounts of $250 each for the year 1973-1974: Dale Gullickson, 5th year student from Roslyn; Shelia Knapp, 3rd year student from Eureka; and Ann Foley, 1st year student from Rapid City. SDPhA delegates at the 1978 convention voted to have the SDSU Alumni Association continue to manage the $15,000 fund.

In February 1973, pharmacy students conducted a successful Sunday Heart Fund Drive, in Brookings. Students from the Student American Pharmaceutical Association, Kappa Psi Pharmaceutical Fraternity, Rho Chi Pharmaceutical Honor Society, and Kappa Epsilon Pharmaceutical Fraternity participated in the drive. The Pharmacy Dinner Dance was held at the Staurolite Inn March 25, 1977. Two hundred and forty people were served at the event. Many awards and scholarships were given to the students.

The 1976 pharmacy float, 'Peace-Everyone's Dream' won first place at SDSU's Hobo Day homecoming parade. 'Rambling Rose' won first place in 1978. SDPhA had contributed $50 to the float fund in 1979. SAPhA-APhA chapter published the first edition of *Pharmic Focus* in January 1976 and an *All Pharmacy Directory* in 1982. The Lilly Senior trip to Indianapolis to tour Eli Lilly's research and manufacturing facilities was held in March 1978. Professors Gary W. Omodt and Joye A. Billow made the arrangements for the trip.

Faculty, Enrollments, Graduations

Budgets for the College of Pharmacy were as follows: 1975-1976, $162,000; 1977-1978, $264, 757 with a total of ten faculty; 1981-1982, $424,123 with a total of thirteen faculty—8 with a Ph.D., 3 with a Pharm.D., 1 with a M.S., and 1 with a B.S.

Dr. Kenneth Redman, who joined the faculty in 1951, retired in 1973. Delegates to the 1973 SDPhA convention passed a resolution praising him for "his untiring efforts for pharmacy." One of his contributions to the profession of pharmacy was authoring the book, *History of the South Dakota State University College of Pharmacy, 1975-1982.*

Enrollments in the College of Pharmacy were 277 in 1964 and 312 in 1970. Dean Raymond Hopponen told pharmacists at the 1971 SDPhA convention that 74% of the practicing pharmacists in South Dakota have graduated from the College of Pharmacy, SDSU. Between 1965 and 1971, for example, 75 out of 210 graduating pharmacists from SDSU remained in South Dakota to practice.

There were 361 undergraduates during the 1975-1976 school year. Board of Pharmacy member Terry Casey, Chamberlain, administered the Pharmacist's Oath to sixty-six pharmacy graduates in the spring of 1976. Dean Ray Hopponen reported that pharmacy graduates from SDSU scored in the 91st percentile out of 74 schools in the 1977 NABPLEX Chemistry exams. Of the 9,500 who took the national exams, SDSU pharmacy students scored as follows: 82nd percentile in both Pharmacy and Mathematics; 70th percentile in Pharmacology; and 69th percentile in the Practice of Pharmacy. The enrollment for the 1976-1977 year was 344, with nine on the faculty. The faculty was next to the smallest of the colleges of pharmacy in the nation.

When the College of Pharmacy was placed on probation in January 1978, there were 362 enrolled. Despite the fact that accreditation was restored in July 1, 1979, enrollment was down to 236. In 1980-1981 enrollment was 214 with a faculty of thirteen. The new Guilford C. Gross Building was opened in January 1981. At the 1981 graduation, Board of Pharmacy member Shirley Heitland, Brookings, gave the Pharmacist's Oath to twenty-six men and seventeen women graduates. Enrollment in 1981-1982 was 193. In the spring of 1982, thirteen men and thirteen women graduated. Dr. Kenneth Redman administered the Pharmacist's Oath to the graduates in the Christy ballroom.

The College Dispensary was moved from the Administration Building to the former Brookings Hospital in 1976. Jean Bibby, Brookings, was the pharmacist at the dispensary. School opened in the fall of 1978 with 293 pharmacy students, with a limit of fifty each for the second and the third-year class. The second-year class of forty, was the first class to start the 1-4 program [one-year prepatory, four-year professional], a change from the old 2-3 program. A grade point average (GPA) of 2.5 minimum was required to enter the third-year class. Sixty-seven students were selected for the third-year class for the fall of 1978. There were nine full-time faculty members during the school year of 1978-1979. That same year, Peter J. Cascella was named teacher of the year for pharmacy, and Gary C. Van Riper was appointed assistant to the Dean of Pharmacy.

Clark T. Eidsmoe presented a summary of the students who graduated from the SDSU College of Pharmacy between 1895, the first year a Ph.G. was given, through the year 1974. Of the total 1,862 who graduated, 1,583 were men and 279 women. The degrees granted were as follows; 290 Ph.G.; 118 Ph.C.; and 1,442 B.S. Those with the B.S. degree included 483 with the five-year program. The class of 1965 was the first class graduating with the five-year program.[17]

Practical Experience Needed to Pass Board Examinations

<u>*Background, 1890-1972*</u>

Practical experience in a licensed pharmacy had been one of the needed requirements to take the Board of Pharmacy examinations since the first South Dakota Pharmacy Law in 1890. Candidates without a college degree could take the Board examinations if they had completed three years of practical experience in a pharmacy. However, those with a College of Pharmacy degree were also eligible to take the exams.

State College began graduating pharmacy students with a Ph.G. degree in 1895. The Legislature in 1903, specifically listed how much practical experience those students needed to take the Board exams. Those who held a Ph.G. needed one year of practical experience in a drug store, before or after graduation. Those who had only completed one year of pharmacy courses at State College, along with two years of practical experience in a drug store, could also take the Board examinations.

The Board of Pharmacy in 1909, also required a high school diploma as part of the requirements to take the Board examinations. About that same time, the Department of Pharmacy, State College required a high school diploma to enroll in the pharmacy course.

Throughout the years, the requirements to take the Board examinations included two groups: those who held a College of Pharmacy degree with some practical experience, as well as those without a degree but who had completed three years of practical experience in a drug store.

Those two groups were evident in a review of the Board examinations given in October 1930 and May 1931 at the College of Pharmacy, Brookings. Fifty-four candidates qualified to take the Board examinations. Thirty candidates qualified to register as pharmacists by examination. Of the thirty who passed the examinations: 17 had a Ph. C. degree; 1 had a B.S. degree; and 12 had no degree but had completed three years of practical experience in a pharmacy.

Board of Pharmacy Chairperson, George Sherman, Huron, commenting on the 1930 and 1931 examinations said, "after correcting Board exams for the last three years of those graduates of schools of pharmacy, and [those who were] not college men, we certainly noticed the difference. The college graduates give intelligent answers to every one of the questions, but that was not the case with many others."[18]

The 1931 Legislature passed a new law, effective July 1, 1933, requiring pharmacy students to have a four-year B.S. degree from a College of Pharmacy, plus one year of practical experience in a pharmacy, to be eligible to take the Board examinations. The practice of taking the

Board exams with three years of practical experience, without any college training, was eliminated with the passage of the new law.

The one year of practical experience could be earned before or after graduation but not concurrent with attending classes in the College of Pharmacy. The Board of Pharmacy in their 1948 regulations stated that an apprentice in pharmacy needed to have completed fifty-two average work weeks of practical experience under the supervision of a registered pharmacist, which could not be concurrent with time spent in college. Such apprentice time had to be registered with the Board of Pharmacy.

Practical Experience at the College of Pharmacy

A clinical pharmacy program was established at the College of Pharmacy in 1968. A pharmacy student could learn practical experience at retail and hospital pharmacies. Clark T. Eidsmoe wrote that the program "consists of two phases, with retail pharmacists and hospital pharmacists acting as clinical instructors."[19] The program consisted of Clinical Pharmacy I and Clinical Pharmacy II.

Clinical Pharmacy I

Clinical Pharmacy I was required for all fifth-year pharmacy students. Pharmacy students working in the following settings gained practical experience: two students per day at Student Health Service Dispensary; two students per day at the Brookings Municipal Hospital Pharmacy; and two students worked one-half day per week at each of the four Brookings pharmacies. Students were directed by clinical instructors at each location.

Clinical Pharmacy II

Clinical Pharmacy II, an elective course, was performed in large hospitals. Students worked five days studying patient drug response. "Clinical instructors, all on courtesy appointments or non-college funds as of March 1974, were: Jean F. Bibby, Donald A. Strahl, Lester W. Hetager, Linus C. Werner, Ronald Huether, Betty Lindsay, Ronald Nelson, John Moriarty, Gary Ploeger, and Jay Drury."[20]

Clinical Pharmacy I and II were so-called "in-house courses" and did not qualify for the required fifty-two weeks of apprentice time by the Board of Pharmacy, thirteen weeks of which must follow graduation from a College of Pharmacy. In other words, up to 1972, all apprentice time needed to meet the requirements for the Board exams, had to be earned away from the College of Pharmacy and not concurrent while attending classes.

A History of Pharmacy in South Dakota

Extern and Clinical Pharmacy Programs

Practical Experience Concurrent with Attendance at the College of Pharmacy

Originally, pharmacy educators believed that apprenticeship should be earned after graduation. Dr. Kenneth Redman said that after 1945 AACP and ACPE both, "reversed themselves...insisting on students applying their classroom learning with the practice of pharmacy in a contemporary setting in the externship and clinical clerkship programs."[21] Dr. Kenneth Redman further states that the results of two national studies in the mid-1970s, "concluded that the pharmacist should be patient oriented in addition to being product oriented."[22] To meet that new concept, ACPE, NABP, and others recommended that at least 400 hours of intern time be gained in an externship and clinical pharmacy program under the direction of the Colleges of Pharmacy.

Up until 1972, the fifty-two weeks of apprentice time had to be earned in a registered pharmacy, not concurrent with time spent in college. However, the Board of Pharmacy, consisting of Al Pfeifle, Sioux Falls, Robert Ehrke, Rapid City, and Joe Cholik, Pierre, were formulating new rules which permitted pharmacy students to earn intern time concurrent with attendance in a College of Pharmacy. To comply with NABP standards, in order to facilitate reciprocity of South Dakota pharmacists, the Board of Pharmacy passed new intern regulations effective January 1, 1973.

New regulations required 1,500 hours of practical experience time, of which 400 hours could be acquired concurrent with attendance at a College of Pharmacy. The 400 hours consisted of an extern program and a clinical pharmacy program. Students in the program, classed as interns instead of apprentices, had to complete two years of College of Pharmacy courses before becoming eligible for the extern and clinical pharmacy programs. A 1981 curriculum in pharmacy listed six hours of Externship, PHA 515, and six hours of Clinical Pharmacy, PHA 513. A Tri-Partite Committee, one from the College of Pharmacy, one from the Board of Pharmacy, and one from the South Dakota Pharmaceutical Association, helped shape the programs.

Generally, the students in the extern program gained practical experience in registered retail pharmacies. Those students in the clinical program gained their time in clinical settings with registered pharmacies in hospitals. However, only 400 hours could be earned in those programs. A student still needed to earn 1,100 hours time in licensed pharmacies not concurrent with attendance in the College of Pharmacy.

In 1976, the extern program had seventy-two preceptors in licensed pharmacies for seventy interns, licensed by the Board of Pharmacy. The extern program in 1979 included thirty-six senior pharmacy students learning the practical side of pharmacy in fourteen hospitals and twenty community pharmacies, during the second half of the 1979 spring semester. The extern program was designed for any eight-week period with a minimum of forty hours per week.

Clinical pharmacy instructors from the College of Pharmacy staffed positions at Sioux Valley Hospital, Sioux Falls; McKennan Hospital, Sioux Falls; Sacred Heart Hospital, Yankton; and the VA Hospital in Sioux Falls.

In 1981, the Board expanded the regulations permitting students in the College of Pharmacy Extern Program to earn up to 640 hours under the College of Pharmacy rather than 400 hours. The other 860 hours had to be earned not concurrent with enrollment in the College of Pharmacy. Bernard D. Hendricks, SDSU College of Pharmacy graduate in 1977 with a B. S. degree, was appointed externship coordinator at the main campus in 1982.

By 1983 students could select a training period at ninety approved community and hospital pharmacies. Students were required to have five weeks each in a hospital and community pharmacy. They also needed four weeks clinical clerkship in one of three South Dakota hospitals supervised by College of Pharmacy staff with Pharm.D. degrees. Students also needed to complete one week in a Poison Control Center; one day in Public Health Nursing Center; two days of consultant pharmacist training in a nursing home. The total was 640 hours of training. In 1983, the College of Pharmacy awarded its first "Preceptor of the Year Award." Ron Nelson, Director of Pharmacy, St. Joseph's Hospital in Mitchell was the winner.

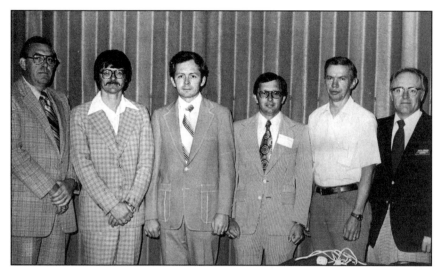

Newly elected 1977-1978 SDPhA officers at the Brookings convention, left to right, President Jack Dady, Ed Swanson, Ron Schwans, Ron Huether, Gerrit Heida, and Secretary Harold H. Schuler.

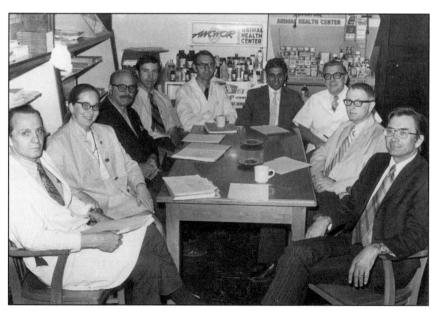

The College of Pharmacy faculty in 1972 included, from left to right, Bernard Hietbrink, Joye Billow, Kenneth Redman, George Brenner, Gary Omodt, Vispi Bhavnagri, Guilford Gross, Gary Van Riper, and Dean Ray Hopponen.

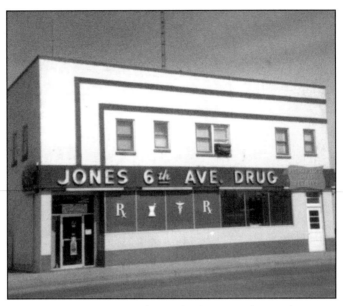

Jones 6th Ave. Drug, Aberdeen, Lloyd Jones, pharmacist, 1973.

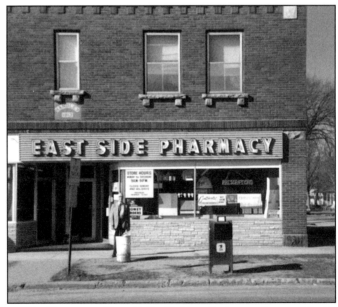

East Side Pharmacy, Sioux Falls, Weldon Norberg, pharmacist, 1973

A History of Pharmacy in South Dakota

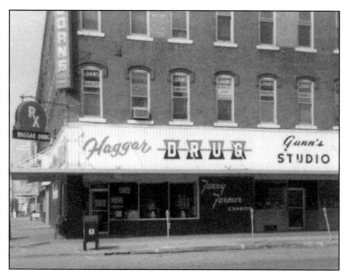

Haggar Drug, Watertown, Dean Gackstetter, pharmacist, 1973.

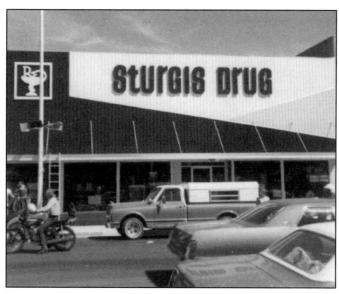

Sturgis Drug, Sturgis, Dale Stroschein and Terry Setera, pharmacists, 1972.

CHAPTER 11
1980-1989

SD Pharmaceutical Association (SDPhA), 1980-1989

New Secretary for SDPhA

In July 1985, Executive Secretary Harold H. Schuler, Pierre, gave notice that he would like to retire, but would serve until a new executive secretary was hired. In August, Administrative Assistant Gladys Pugh, Pierre, who had ably served in that capacity thirteen years, announced her resignation because she and her husband Merlyn, were moving to Sioux Falls. The Executive Committee, meeting in late August, agreed to hire a new administrative assistant by October 15, 1985 and a new executive secretary by December 1, 1985. Pam Stotz was hired as administrative assistant.

The Executive Committee made a public announcement seeking an executive secretary for the Association and the Board. After interviewing candidates in November 1985 and January 1986, they agreed to hire Galen Jordre of Gettysburg. Galen and his wife Ann, also a pharmacist, owned Jordre Community Drug in Gettysburg. Galen, from Veblen, graduated from SDSU College of Pharmacy in 1968. He served in the U. S. Army as a pharmacy officer from 1969 to 1974. After serving as head pharmacist at the Redfield State Hospital from 1974-1977, he and Ann purchased the drug store in Gettysburg. Secretary Schuler worked with Jordre until February 28, 1986. As one of his last functions, Schuler attended pharmacist George Tibbs' retirement dinner in Rapid City, February 27, 1986. The next day, February 28, on his return to Pierre, he stopped at Wall Drug and had a good visit with his old friend Ted Hustead. It was Schuler's last official act.

Schuler was employed as a public relations person for the Commercial and Legislative Section during the 1963 Legislative Session, and continued with that section the remainder of the year. Later, Executive Secretary Bliss Wilson, after twenty-two years of service, retired, and Schuler was named SDPhA executive secretary January 1, 1964. Including his service with the C and L Section, Schuler served twenty-three years with the Association and the Board of Pharmacy. Only Secretary E. C. Bent, Dell Rapids, served longer at twenty-six years.

Schuler in his last newsletter, recalled that when he came to the Association and Board of Pharmacy, "there was no newsletter, no district organization, no office secretary, and both the Board and Association were poorly funded. We all pitched in and throughout the years made progress. A few of those accomplishments included: recodified the SD Pharmacy Law in 1967; secured a favorable result 100 times and only lost once in opposing or supporting bills in the Legislature; passed law requiring hospitals to have a pharmacy license (In 1967, only 10 of 67 hospitals had a pharmacy license); passed the first drug substitution law [Drug Product Selection Law]; passed a continuing education law for pharmacists; secured an appropriation for a pharmacy building at SDSU; and raised dues and licenses to properly fund the Board and Association.

"One of the items transferred to new Executive Secretary Jordre was custody of $40,000 surplus Association certificates of deposits. What a thrill to work for such a fine profession for all those years. I worked with 23 Association presidents and 18 Board of Pharmacy members, and three deans of the College of Pharmacy. In 1985 I wrote a book, *The S.D. Capitol in Pierre* and will continue writing."[1] Between that time and 2002, Schuler had authored nine published books on South Dakota history.

Association Business

The president, two vice-presidents, secretary, treasurer, and immediate past president form the SDPhA Executive Committee. That Committee was authorized by the Constitution to conduct official business between conventions. The job of being an officer is a demanding responsibility. In the late 1970s, the committee began meeting at a two-day retreat for the officers. Among the many items on the agenda, the officers reviewed the nominations from the nine districts and made the final selection for the Bowl of Hygeia and Honorary President awards. One and sometimes two of the officers attended yearly national meetings of APhA and NARD.

The Auxiliary of the South Dakota Pharmaceutical Association was formed at the 1980 convention in Aberdeen. It replaced the Ladies' Auxiliary which had been created in 1902 at Flandreau. The purpose of the new Auxiliary was to unite socially and professionally the families of those interested in the practice of pharmacy. Membership, for a $2.00 fee, was open to any person who was a member or directly related to members of SDPhA or Allied Drug Travelers. Officers consisted of a president, vice-president, secretary, and treasurer. The new group would continue a student loan fund for women in the SDSU College of Pharmacy. Mrs.

Mary Ann Stroschein, Sturgis, was elected as president of the new Auxiliary.

The 1981 convention at the Mitchell Holiday Inn included eleven hours of continuing education. Registration for the complete convention for one person was $37 or $70 for a couple. Fifty year certificates, salespersons of the year, and district president's appreciation certificates were presented at the Sunday, June 14th Wholesaler's Luncheon, courtesy of Jewett Drug, Northwestern Drug, McKesson & Robbins, and Brown Drug. The Bowl of Hygeia, Honorary President, and other awards were presented at the Sunday president's banquet. Ron Huether, Sioux Falls, was president. Dale Stroschein, Sturgis, was elected president for the year 1981-1982. A constitutional amendment was approved allowing those pharmacists, who no longer wish to practice, to be associate members and be called pharmacist emeritus.

Over 150 pharmacists attended the nine district meetings held in October 1982. Jack Halbkat Jr., Webster, was elected president for the year 1982-1983 at the Rapid City convention. James Stephens, Pierre was elected president at the 1983-1984 convention at Watertown. A new set of district by-laws was adopted at the 1985 convention, chaired by President Allen Pfeifle, Sioux Falls. At that convention, held in the Ramada Inn, Sioux Falls, United States Senator James Abdnor spoke and was presented a special recognition plaque for outstanding service to the profession of pharmacy. Special awards were also presented to retiring drug inspectors, Glenn Velau, Rapid City, and Les Hetager, Sioux Falls. SDPhA President Allen Pfeifle, Sioux Falls, presented the Lay Person of the Year Award to retiring Secretary Harold H. Schuler. The Executive Committee, chaired by President Robert Gregg, Chamberlain, at an April 1986 meeting, recommended a constitutional change calling for two vice-presidents instead of three, which was approved at the June 1986 convention.

A new Pharm-Assist Program was also approved at the 1986 convention. Its objective was to render aid to and help the chemically impaired pharmacist/pharmacy student in the event of drug/alcohol misuse. David Kuper, Sioux Falls, was named chairperson of the Pharm-Assist Committee. The Auxiliary asked pharmacists to bring craft or related items to the next convention for a silent auction, the proceeds of which would be given to the committee. A new award, Distinguished Young Pharmacist Award, sponsored by Marion, was approved by the Executive Committee in 1987, for a pharmacist, who received a degree less than ten years ago and was active in the profession. The first winner was Mark A. Zwaska, Brookings, who was presented the award at the 1987 convention in Yankton.

A History of Pharmacy in South Dakota

A Ted and Dorothy Hustead Pharmacist of the Year Award was approved by the Executive Committee in April 1988. The award was given to a person who had made a significant contribution to pharmacy, not solely based upon community service. It was agreed that Ted Hustead, Wall, be named as the first recipient. President Mary Kuper, Sioux Falls, arranged for its presentation at the 1988 convention held in Sioux Falls.

Ad Hoc Historical Committee

In 1988, the convention approved a new Ad Hoc Historical Preservation Committee. Later, President Arvid Liebe, Milbank, appointed the following pharmacists to the Historical Committee: Roger Eastman, Platte; Pat Lynn, Sioux Falls; Harold Tisher, Yankton; Cliff Thomas, Belle Fourche; and Shirley Vail, Gettysburg. President Liebe said, "The committee wants information on several categories dealing with the history of pharmacy in South Dakota. Let's all get involved and re-live a little of our special heritage."[2] The new committee met at Pierre in March 1989 and decided to promote a pharmacy display somewhere in South Dakota, something like the late Joe Cholik's collection of pharmacy items, now permanently displayed in Louie Van Roekel's The Medicine Shoppe at Pierre.

One of the goals of the original committee, was to obtain a written history of the Association while records were still available. In 2002, Cliff Thomas and other members of the committee, supported such a compilation by Harold H. Schuler, former executive secretary.

Computers in Pharmacy

Pharmacists became more interested in computers, shortly after IBM introduced its personal computer in 1981. The Association scheduled two continuing education programs on computers at the 1982 convention in Rapid City: Computer Costs in a Pharmacy; and Computer and Pharmacy Law. The Executive Committee asked Secretary Harold H. Schuler to explore if a computer could be used in the pharmacy office. However, it wasn't until September 1986 that the Executive Committee authorized Secretary Galen Jordre to buy a computer, the cost to be shared by the Association and the Board of Pharmacy.

Ed Swanson, Swanson Drug, Madison, said, "our first and current computer system is NDC, [obtained in June 1986]. It took weeks to get the bugs out of the system. There is absolutely no comparison to pharmacy today as it was before the computer. I can remember figuring the prices with a pencil, writing down the patient information in a ledger. Pharmacy would be impossible today without the computer."[3]

Terry Casey, Casey Drug, Chamberlain, said, "we computerized in the spring of 1988. We had an IBM/PC with software through National Data Corporation (NDC). Doing the end of the year tax print outs for patients was then done so easily, it was wonderful."[4]

1994-1995 SDPhA President Margaret Zard, Mitchell, said, "I was dragged kicking and screaming into the computer age—gone was my familiar typewriter and my continuous roll of press-apply labels. In its place was a key board with too many keys, and a bright green screen with a cursor that wouldn't stop flashing. But I was made of stern stuff, and I moved forward valiantly—one hand on the keyboard, the other grasping my user's manual. Then I found myself speaking a new language—software, download, pixel, downtime, co-ax, dot matrix. But this, too, became familiar to me, and I gradually made a realization-at some point...I changed. I liked this system. I could access profiles at the stroke of a key—I could compare medical histories on dual screens—E-mail was a stroke away. I was traveling the information superhighway with my fingertips. Take my computer away, go back to a manual system? Never."[5]

Public Relations

Secretary Harold H. Schuler started an Association newsletter, *South Dakota Pharmacy Newsletter* in 1964. New Secretary Galen Jordre continued sending a publication to pharmacists, but in a different form. He published the first issue of *South Dakota Pharmacist* in November 1986. The magazine was printed every two months and mailed to pharmacists, pharmacist emeritus, student members, and advertisers. The magazine was taken to the printer in a camera ready form. The issue contained pharmacy news, advertisements, and a buy, sell, and jobs wanted page. It also contained two pages paid by the Society of Hospital Pharmacists, to provide information to their members. Ad rates in 1989 were $300 a page, $285 a page if an annual contract.

SDPhA President Dave Helgeland, Brookings, reported in the November 1986 *South Dakota Pharmacist*, that the new journal would carry continuing education programs throughout the year. Originally, Merrell Dow provided an educational grant to the *South Dakota Pharmacist* and sponsored a five-page CE program along with a quiz page. They continued sponsoring the CE program until January 1, 1991 when Searle Drug Co. provided the CE program. One hour and a half CE credit, managed by the College of Pharmacy, could be obtained at a cost of $3.50 for each program. In recent years, Pharmacia has provided the educational grant and sponsored a CE program. The Third and Fourth Quarter 2002 issue of *South Dakota Pharmacist*, for example, contains a program on Patient Counseling: Management of Sore Throat, conducted by Thomas A. Gossel, Professor of Pharmacology and Toxicology, Ohio Northern University, and Professor J. Richard Wuest, University of Cincinnati.

In 1989, there was no longer a charge for the hospital pharmacists for their two pages. Also in that year, the Association purchased desktop publishing software for its computer, as well as a laser printer.

To help pharmacists with their understanding of the laws and regulations affecting the profession, the Association in 1987, published a looseleaf notebook containing such information as South Dakota Laws, Regulations of the Board of Pharmacy, DEA information, Medicaid Rules, etc. The price for the notebook was $25 and $10 for the annual supplement.

In 1988, the Association participated in a national publicity program,Talk about Prescriptions and Communicate Before You Medicate, was the theme. The program stressed the important role communication plays between the pharmacist and the patients. An 8 x 11 poster was available which stated that whenever medicine is prescribed, tell your pharmacist the names of the other medicines you are taking as well as any problems you are having with your medicine. Another helpful program for pharmacists in 1989, was three videotapes which could be purchased from APhA. The twenty-five minute tapes permitted the viewer to participate in self-testing questions on: national medication awareness; self medication awareness; and managing needs of older people.

A resolution was passed at the 1982 convention for pharmacists to support a statewide charity day. Each pharmacist would contribute $1.00 for each prescription filled that day. The Executive Committee set April 6, 1983 as Pharmacists for Charity Day in South Dakota. They also designated the South Dakota Cancer Society as the recipient of all proceeds collected that day. Eighty-six pharmacies joined in the first charity day. After that day, one lump sum was sent to the Cancer Society.

By 1986, $3,750 was raised on Pharmacists Charity Day. The proceeds, after minor expenses, were distributed as follows: $1,415 to River Park in Pierre and $1,625 to SDPhA to use by its Impaired Pharmacist's Committee. Association President Mary Kuper, Sioux Falls, reported in November 1987 that one-half of the money was contributed to the Pharmacist-Assist for impaired pharmacists and one-half to Association Districts for substance abuse programs within their area. In 1988, members of the SDPhA convention voted to discontinue annual Pharmacists Charity Day and let each pharmacy determine the charity of their choice.

Pharmacists on the Move

In 1980, Joseph F. Statz, Parkston, started Tele-RX, the first mail order pharmacy in South Dakota. Later he changed the name to Tel-Drug. Joseph F. had purchased Statz Drug in 1960. His father, Joseph H. Statz had purchased the store in 1915. After Joseph F. died in 1988, his wife Anne and two pharmacist sons, Joseph M. Statz and Stephen R. Statz continued the businesses. Tel-Drug business was moved to Sioux Falls in 1989 and sold to Cigna Insurance Companies of Hartford, CT in 1993. The drug stores at Parkston, Mitchell, and Huron were sold in 1999. Stephen is a pharmacist at McKennan Hospital in Sioux Falls and a member of the South Dakota Board of Pharmacy. Joseph M. is a pharmacist with Tel-Drug, and his spouse Linda is a pharmacist at Sioux Valley Drug, both in Sioux Falls.

Ted and Bill Hustead, Wall Drug, were featured on the NBC Today Show in the fall of 1981. It was referred to as one of the largest drug stores in the country with 200 employees. Bill Hustead, who had been appointed to the South Dakota Transportation Board, was reappointed by Governor William Janklow in 1983. Bill was elected chairperson of the Transportation Board that year. Vice President Al Pfeifle, Sioux Falls, and Secretary Harold H. Schuler, Pierre, attended the 1983 NARD Legislative Conference in Washington, D.C. They had lunch with Senator James Abdnor in the United States Capitol dining room.

Carveth Thompson, who had been appointed to the State Fair Board by Governor William Janklow, was named chairperson of the Board in 1984. SDPhA officer Terry Casey, Chamberlain, and Secretary Galen Jordre, attended the 1987 Quad-State Meeting in Bismarck, North Dakota. In 1988, South Dakota hosted the group which consisted of Association officers from Montana, Wyoming, North Dakota, and South Dakota. (The Quad-State meeting was disbanded in 1994.) Stan Petrik, Rapid City, a member of the 147th Field Artillery, South Dakota National Guard since 1960, was named Assistant Adjutant General, and promoted to brigadier general.

Professional Concerns

In 1980, SDPhA President Ron Schwans, Hoven, expressed concern about FDA's proposed regulations pertaining to mandatory patient package inserts (PPI). Schwans said, "the talk of PPI has caused panic in every health profession. At the recent 1980 NARD Legislative Conference, Dr. Goyan, Commissioner of FDA, said that FDA did not have a single complaint from a consumer. NARD's position is...favoring patient drug information, but feels that PPI is not the way to inform the patient. The pharmacist is in the best position...to provide patient drug information. FDA is ready to mandate PPI's by legislation or regulation. Will the pharmacist act now or react later?"[6]

Another significant change for the profession was on January 1, 1982, when South Dakota's new law requiring a code imprint on all solid dosage drugs became effective. The law simply stated that manufacturers can't sell; wholesalers can't distribute; and pharmacists can't dispense any legend drug in solid dosage form without the code imprint identifying the drug and the manufacturer. The Board of Pharmacy cleared up some labeling questions in 1985 about substitution when it notified all pharmacists, that the general rule about labeling is that the name of the drug in the container should be the name that is placed on the label. If the prescribing doctor authorizes substitution, the name of the drug that the pharmacist selects, is the name of the drug which is placed on the label.

So many changes were happening that President David Helgeland reminded pharmacists in 1986 that "SDPhA must act as a watchdog over legislative, bureaucratic, and third parties affecting our profession."[7] Meanwhile, in 1987, the Board of Pharmacy took the first steps in the rule making process requiring pharmacists to keep a patient profile and to counsel the patient about a prescription. However, it wasn't until 1992 that these concepts became regulations.

The problem of multi-tiered pricing [discriminatory pricing] surfaced again at the 1988 SDPhA convention in Sioux Falls. A resolution was passed asking new President Arvid Liebe, Milbank to appoint a committee to study multi-tiered pricing of pharmaceuticals as well as acting to stop multi-tiered pricing favoring institutions. If the practice can't be stopped, the resolution favored a law limiting institutions to only selling drugs to their patients. Gerrit Heida, Aberdeen, was appointed chairperson of the committee. Later, the committee reported that they favored support of NARD's Pharmacy Freedom Fund.

In 1989, both APhA and NARD supported the Pharmacy Freedom Fund and led a drive to raise $240,000 to eliminate discriminatory pricing by federal legislation. "The discriminatory prices, once limited to nonprofit hospitals, are now common for mail-order pharmacies, managed health care pharmacies, and dispensing physicians. In the opinion of the courts, [they are legal], thus congressional action to amend the Robinson-Patman Act is the only way to stop them. The SDPhA C & L Section, has become a member of the Freedom Fund to support the national cause."[8]

Secretary Galen Jordre, explained the Prescription Drug Marketing Act, pertaining to drug samples. Some of the provisions of the new Act were: selling or trading of drug samples is prohibited; pharmacists and physicians may obtain samples only by a written request; manufacturers must store samples under conditions that will maintain their potency; audits will be made to assure that samples were actually delivered; and violators will be punished.[9]

Legislation

The Executive Committee, because of limited funds, voted not to hold the Legislative Social-Buffet during the 1981 Legislative Session. They did agree, however, to rehire Attorney Keith Tidball as the lobbyist to represent the profession before the Legislature. They also agreed to a format to contact Legislators at the State Capitol, called Pharmacist's Legislative Days. Three or four pharmacists from each district, were asked to meet in Pierre for a noon luncheon in the capitol. Some Legislators and governmental people would be invited as speakers. After the lunch, pharmacists would walk the Legislative halls and contact Legislators about bills affecting the profession. Thirty pharmacists did attend the January 19, 1982 noon luncheon in the capitol to hear Senator Homer Harding, Pierre, and Secretary Jim Ellenbecker, Department of Social Services. Thirty-three pharmacists, representing nine districts, attended the February 1, 1983 noon luncheon to hear Attorney General Mark Meierhenry.

Some pharmacists believed that the old method of having a social-buffet for all the Legislators should be reinstated. Ted Hustead, Wall, made a motion at the 1983 convention to reinstate a buffet-social for Legislators. It was defeated. The new format continued successfully, with Attorney Keith Tidball as lobbyist, until 1989, when pharmacists changed the format again, and hosted an Old Fashioned Ice Cream Social in the Capitol Rotunda. A soda fountain was set up in the rotunda where pharmacists served ice cream and sundaes. Attorney Robert Riter,Jr., was hired as the lobbyist for the 1990 Legislative Session. The format was changed again by serving a continental breakfast to the Legislators at the 1990 Legislative Day. Three or four pharmacists from each of the districts attended Legislative Day. The new format was well received by Legislators.

The matter of separating the Association from the Board of Pharmacy continued to be of concern to some of the Legislators. House Bill 1093 was introduced in the 1980 Session to sunset [discontinue] the Board of Pharmacy. It was defeated. Later that year, Attorney General Mark Meierhenry issued an Attorney General's Opinion about the close-connectedness of the South Dakota Pharmaceutical Association and the Board of Pharmacy. In summary, he said if the Legislature wants to set out a bifurcated [two separate units] mechanism to regulate the profession of pharmacy in the interest of public health, safety, and welfare of its citizens, they may do so. He added, "I find none of the authorized functions to be contrary to any state or federal policy or law. The Board and Association should be cognizant, however, that their functions are restricted to those statutorily authorized."[10]

In 1981, the Attorney General ruled that the Association was a state agency. Consequently, Association Attorney Keith Tidball, advised the Executive Committee that there must be a complete separation of Commercial and Legislative Section funds from Association funds. C & L Section expenses could only be used for lobbying, travel expense to NARD, Pharmacist's Legislative Day, etc. Fortunately, the C & L Section was strongly supported by pharmacists. Receipts for the 1987-1988 year were $8,850 from pharmacies; $3,550 from individuals; plus sums from other sources totaled $14,658. Expenses included lobbying $1,452, Legislative Day $905, per diem $3,515, plus other expenses for a total of $10,287. There was also $17,063 in savings.

In the 1984 Legislature, a bill to separate the Board from the Association failed on the House floor. In the 1989 Legislature, House Bill 1242 would have separated the Board and the Association, but it failed in committee. Some pharmacists believed that the time had come to split the two entities. A resolution at the 1989 convention in Watertown called for President Marilyn Schwans, Belle Fourche, to appoint a task force to investigate splitting the two groups and develop a plan for the Association to continue as a voluntary professional organization. It died because there was no second. However, a resolution to study the matter passed. A straw poll, at the 1989 convention of the South Dakota Society of Hospital Pharmacists showed the following vote: 11 to separate; 7 to keep status quo; and 4 were neutral. SDSHP President Thomas Wolff, Sioux Falls recommended the group study the manner and explore possible alternatives.

The Title 19 professional fee was raised by the Legislature as follows: to $3.00 in 1982; to $3.25 in 1984; and to $4.25 in 1987. Lloyd Jones, Aberdeen, represented the pharmacists on the Medicaid Advisory Committee of the Department of Social Services.

Doctor of Pharmacy (P.D.)

Graduates from the five-year program of SDSU College of Pharmacy were awarded a B.S. degree. But many pharmacists in 1982 believed that the title Doctor of Pharmacy, P.D. "more correctly identified the level of expertise associated with the education and experience required of a South Dakota licensed pharmacist." A resolution was presented at the

1982 convention to amend the Constitution authorizing the change and also asking the Board of Pharmacy to adopt the P.D. designation. If necessary, the resolution favored asking the Legislature to make the change. During floor debate, an amendment was presented to refer the matter to a committee of pharmacists for further study. The amendment was defeated by a vote of 54 No and 35 Yes. After more debate, the original motion passed by a vote of 52 Yes and 35 No. The final approved form of the Uniform Designation for Pharmacists was as follows:

"Whereas pharmacists are licensed rather than registered, the time has come for a uniform designation for pharmacists which is more appropriate than R.Ph.; and Whereas all pharmacists, regardless of the educational degree...are granted equal powers and limitations by the Board of Pharmacy; and Whereas the title Doctor of Pharmacy more correctly identifies the level of expertise associated with the education and experience required of South Dakota licensed pharmacists; Therefore be it resolved that SDPhA endorse and adopt the professional designation, P.D., with the accompanying title Doctor of Pharmacy, and request the Board of Pharmacy to adopt the P.D. designation as the title for all licensed pharmacists in South Dakota and, if necessary seek a legislative amendment which would require South Dakota licensed pharmacists be designated as P.D.'s with accompanying title, Doctor of Pharmacy."[11] .

Attorney Keith Tidball advised that it would be better for the Association to only authorize the designation P.D., rather than seeking Legislative authority. By October 1983, 233 P.D. certificates had been ordered by both in-state and out-state South Dakota registered pharmacists. The P.D. concept soon changed because of the movement to create a six-year Pharm.D. program at SDSU College of Pharmacy in 1987.

Pharmacist Polls and Surveys

A 1981 Gallup Poll rated twenty-four professions in terms of honesty and ethical standards. Pharmacists ranked first with 59%, dentists 50%, and medical doctors 50%. A *Lilly Digest* survey of 2,070 community pharmacies in 1980, listed the following averages per pharmacy: sales $416,161; cost of goods sold $273,390; gross margin $142,771 or 34%; total expenses $126,987 or 31%; net profit $13,784 or 3.3% before taxes. Total income of a self-employed proprietor before taxes was $39,875. Other averages per pharmacy included: 51.2% sales were from prescriptions and 48.8% from other; 49.6% were new prescriptions and 50.4% were refills. The average charge per prescription was $7.85.[12]

In 1984, a survey of in-state pharmacists was conducted by Association Secretary Harold H. Schuler. He used pharmacist renewal information and Board of Pharmacy records. Total male pharmacists registered were 432, and total women pharmacists registered were 163 for a total of 595 in-state pharmacists. The survey showed where pharmacists are working in South Dakota: in retail pharmacy, 84 women and 286 men; in clinic pharmacy, 13 women and 11 men; in hospital pharmacy, 51 women and 72 men; pharmacists unemployed, 4 women and 0 men; doing relief work, 4 women and 9 men; working other than in retail, clinical, or hospital pharmacy, women 4 and men 24; reporting other occupations, women 0 and 4 men; reported as salespersons, women 0 and men 5; and reported as retired; 0 women and 22 men.

A SDSU College of Pharmacy Economic Survey, funded by a SDPhA grant, was conducted in 1987. One hundred and five South Dakota pharmacists completed the survey. The survey showed that the average age was 38; median hourly salary was $12.43; median weekly salary was $553; and median hours worked per week was 40. A news story in the *South Dakota Pharmacist*, September 1987, indicated that the registered pharmacists by gender in the state were 74% men and 26% women.

According to a 1988 Lilly Digest report, the average prescription price was $15.37. It increased by 10% in 1989 to $16.74. Further statistics from the 1988 Lilly Survey showed that prescriptions sales were 66% of total sales, compared to 51.2% in 1980. In 1960, pharmacy hours open per week was 75, which decreased to 60 hours in 1987. Third party prescriptions in 1988 totaled 37% of all prescriptions filled, 7% more than in 1987.[13]

SD Board of Pharmacy, 1980-1989

On June 30, 1981, Glenn Velau, Rapid City, changed from a full-time drug inspector to a part-time inspector in the West River area. Later, the Board hired Les Hetager, Sioux Falls, as the East River inspector. Hetager had been a pharmacist at the VA Center in Sioux Falls. The Board in 1983, approved a new inspection form for use in the inspection of pharmacies. The new form was much more comprehensive and relevant. In July 1985, Glenn Velau and Les Hetager both retired. Both were given special recognition at the 1985 SDPhA convention for a "job well done." New drug inspectors were hired in that same year. Cliff Thomas, former owner of Cliff Thomas Drug, Belle Fourche, was hired for the West River area. James "Jack" Jones, former owner of Jones Drug, Miller, was hired for the East River area. Jones, a 1950 SDSU graduate, had been mayor of Miller. In 1987-1988, he served as a State Representative in the South Dakota House of Representatives.

The Board of Pharmacy continued to be in sound financial shape. On June 30, 1986, the Board had $11,463 in savings, and $41,464 in checking. Its main source of revenue was from licensing: $39,040 from pharmacies; $7,320 from part-time pharmacies; $3,540 from household remedies; $4,932 from patent medicines; and $2,712 from poisons. Adding other fees from grades, exams, interns, certificates, etc., the total revenue for FY 1985-1986 was $65,164. Some of the expenditures were $9,864 secretary's salary; $6,151 administrative assistant salary; and $13,050 for two part-time inspectors. The total expenditures were $61,467.

Board of Pharmacy members between 1980 and 1989 were: Frank Post, Pierre; Shirley Heitland, Brookings; James Hersrud, Keystone; Jack Bailey, Winner; John Nelson, Arlington; Kenneth B. Jones, Yankton; Marlyn Christensen, Mitchell; Dennis M. Jones, Huron; Robert Gregg, Chamberlain; Jack Dady, Mobridge; and Joan Hogan. Board members were appointed by the Governor for a three-year term.

Executive Secretary Galen Jordre made a statistical comparison of the pharmacy profession in South Dakota between 1964 and 1989: [14]

	1964	1989
In-state registered pharmacists	466	605
Women pharmacists	58	191
Sioux Falls pharmacists	65	153
Independent pharmacies	217	172
Chain pharmacies	6	31
Hospital Pharmacies	9	65

When mandatory continuing education became effective October 1, 1980, pharmacists were required to keep their records for the twelve hours they needed to renew their license. The Board of Pharmacy was given authority to ask 5% of the pharmacists each year, to send in verification of the earned hours. A 1983 audit, showed that some pharmacists had inadequate records and were sent letters of reprimand. The board amended the rules in 1989. Pharmacists had to report twelve hours of earned CE time each year, however, the hours could be earned over a twenty-four month period. The regulation is still in force.

In March 1987, Governor George S. Mickelson signed a new law requiring a pharmacy to have any one of the following references on hand: USP-NF; USPDI Drug Information; Facts and Comparisons; or American Hospital Formulary Service. That same year, the Board reminded pharmacists that they cannot accept returned unused drugs. However, in a hospital with a licensed pharmacy, a pharmacist can accept the return of unused drugs of a particular hospital patient. Unit doses unused in a nursing home can be returned for credit if still in the original unopened containers.

Al Pfeifle, Sioux Falls, who was appointed to the NABP Blue Ribbon Committee in 1968, worked with them in the early 1970s developing a national exam called NABPLEX. The South Dakota Board of Pharmacy began using the five-part exam in the spring of 1976. NABP in 1983, presented Pfeifle a certificate of appreciation for his work on the Blue Ribbon Committee. In 1986, the Board gave the NABPLEX exam to fifteen candidates—in two, four-hour sessions.

In 1989 there were 220 full-time pharmacies and 48 part-time pharmacies. That year, the board passed new regulations for computer pharmacy. Some of the highlights were:
- Input of drug information into a computer can only be performed by a pharmacist, or a person under the immediate supervision of a pharmacist. The identity of the pharmacist must show in the record
- Requirements for storing prescription information must meet the following requirements: guarantee confidentiality; produce a hard copy daily of controlled substance transactions; provide for on-line retrieval; carry all dates of refills and initials of pharmacist; maintain a patient profile; and be capable of reconstruction of records in case of a computer malfunction
- A later rule permitted pharmacies to utilize a common electronic data base, as long as there is an audit trail.

SD College of Pharmacy, 1980-1989

Enrollment was 214 for the school year 1980-1981. Pharmacy Board member Shirley Heitland, in May 1981, administered the Pharmacist's Oath to 26 men and 17 women graduates. Enrollment was 193 for the school year 1981-1982. Thirteen men and 13 women graduated in May 1982. The class of 1982 was the first to graduate from the new 1-4 curriculum [one-year pre-training and four years professional]. The change from the 2-3 program was implemented to allow more time in the professional curriculum for clinical experiences. Dr. Kenneth Redman administered the Pharmacist's Oath in the Christy ballroom. All of the 1982 graduates found jobs. There were thirteen on the faculty in 1982: 8 with Ph.D.; 3 with Pharm.D.; 1 with M.S.; and 1 with B.S. All but one were licensed to practice in South Dakota.

Enrollment was 189 in the fall of 1984. Dean Ray Hopponen, in his 1985 SDPhA convention report, stated, "Over the past 10 years [1975-

1985], 89% of South Dakota residents studying pharmacy have enrolled at SDSU. In the past 10 years, of 588 graduates, 29% have stayed in South Dakota. Over the 10 years that the national examination (NABPLEX) for licensure has been utilized, SDSU graduates have averaged two points above the national average on each of the five parts of the examination. The College of Pharmacy has fifteen faculty members. Over 75% of pharmacy faculty nationally are paid more than SDSU pharmacy faculty."[15]

Enrollment in the fall of 1988 was 223, up 17 from 1987. Of the 223 students, 167 were from South Dakota, 11 from Iowa, 11 from Minnesota, and the remainder from other areas. In the school year of 1989-1990, 245 students enrolled and 51 graduated in May 1990.

Outreach

Dean Ray Hopponen in his 1985 SDPhA convention report reminded pharmacists that the College of Pharmacy had a large outreach program of correspondence courses, workshops, and seminars for pharmacists and non-pharmacists. He said, "During the period, 1979-1984, 659 pharmacists were provided correspondence courses for professional education requirements. Another 484 participated in college sponsored workshops or seminars for a total of 1,143. Other health professionals, nurses, optometrists, and dieticians, were also served.

"Off-campus college credit courses were given to 406 non-pharmacists. Workshops and seminars reached another 820 for a total of 1,226. Altogether, 2,369 health professionals were served. On campus, 720 nursing students and 360 others were taught. Between 1975 and 1982, resignations from the [USD] Medical School faculty created problems in teaching pharmacology. During those eight years, [SDSU] pharmacy faculty taught all or part of the pharmacology course to a total of 520 medical students."[16].

In 1986, the College of Pharmacy prepared its first newsletter, *Pharmacy Focus*, and distributed it to alumni, S.D. pharmacists, and parents of students.

Centennial Celebration, 1888-1988

A twenty-eight page, *College of Pharmacy, a Centennial Celebration*, was published in 1988, to celebrate its first 100 years. Dean Bernard E. Hietbrink, in his centennial greeting said, "This is a special week in the life of the College of Pharmacy. It is inviting to reflect upon the accomplishments, changes and progress experienced during the past century. We could follow the evolution of pharmacy from an 'industrial study' to a two-year course, to the Ph.G. degree...to a Department of Pharmacy, a Division of Pharmacy...the initiation of a five-year curriculum in 1960,

A History of Pharmacy in South Dakota

the establishment of the College of Pharmacy in 1964, [and to] the possible adoption of a Pharm.D. program."[17] The booklet contained fifty-four photographs and an excellent summary of the history of the College of Pharmacy.

The week-long celebration during October 17-23, 1988, included a wine and cheese reception for the President of APhA, followed with a banquet and auction. Some of the items auctioned were: Clark T. Eidsmoe's pharmacy calculations workbook; a Guilford C. Gross pipe; set of antique bottles; two porcelain pill tiles from the old dispensing laboratory; and other items dear to the hearts of former 'SDSU Pharmics.'

Student Groups

The *Industrial Collegian* on May 3, 1921, refers to a pharmacy society that met and heard a talk by Captain Walz. Following entertainment, they conducted their business meeting. Historically, however, there have been five active students groups established at SDSU College of Pharmacy. The Whitehead Chapter of SDPhA was established in 1923. It became the S.D. Chapter of Student APhA in 1954 and in 1987 it became the Academy of Students of Pharmacy (ASP). Tau Chapter of Rho Chi was organized in 1931. Kappa Epsilon for women was organized in 1956. Gamma Kappa Chapter of Kappa Psi was created in 1958. In 1991, Phi Lambda Sigma was founded for the purpose of promoting leadership in pharmacy.

Academy of Students of Pharmacy (ASP)

Fourteen members volunteered to help with hypertension screening at the Brookings Mall in March 1981. Lori Lund reported that the "clinic was a fantastic success." The Chapter published an *All Pharmacy Directory* and sold it for $.25. Their magazine *Pharmic Focus* was first published in 1976. The APhA-ASP Chapter Achievement Award was established in 1974 to recognize outstanding activities of the ASP Chapters in the nation's Colleges of Pharmacy. Not only was Brookings Chapter the outstanding chapter in the nation in 1979, it also won for the years 1984 through 1990, 1992, 1998, 1999, 2000, and 2003.

ASP officers elected in 1985 included President Edane M. Goetz; First Vice-President Jamie J Mayer; Second Vice-President Lance R. Calhoon; Recording Secretary Carol A. Dewald; Corresponding Secretary Jody L. Schumacher; and Treasurer Deborah K. Nelson. In 1987, ten members were awarded USP-DI's in the local Patient Counseling Competition. First place winner Nancy Feuerstein went to the national competition, held in Chicago in conjunction with the annual meeting. SDPhA awarded a $250 grant to the Chapter to attend the 1988 annual APhA meeting.

Rho Chi, Tau Chapter

Tau Chapter of Rho Chi, Pharmacy Honor Society, inducted six new members in 1987. The fourth-year students were selected on the basis of academic performance and leadership. They joined the ranks of 41,000 members nationwide. The six members recognized were: John A. Auchampach, Garner, Iowa; Nancy J. Dietz, Norfolk, Nebraska; Tracy G. Greiman, Garner, Iowa; Sandy K. (Ruter) Hartwig, Kanawha, Iowa; Jeff J. Larsen, Madison, South Dakota; and Lisa A. Swenson, Bridgewater, South Dakota.

Kappa Epsilon

In 1981, the fraternity for women, initiated nine new members and celebrated its 60th birthday. [On campus since 1956]. Dr. Joye Ann Billow, was chapter adviser. New officers elected in 1983 included: President Terri Michael; Vice-President Kellie Lapour; Secretary Debbie Hunt; Treasurer Monica Jones; Chaplain Lisa Olson; and Pledge Trainer Ann Kloucek.

The group held the chapter Christmas party in 1987 with forty members attending. The chapter also hosted the annual All-Pharmacy Christmas party at the Alumni Center. Students and faculty enjoyed the food, fun, and door prizes. A food drive, to help the Brookings Food Pantry for families in need, was sponsored by the chapter.

Kappa Psi

New officers elected for 1983 included: President Terry Finck, Tyndall; Vice-President Jon Berkley, Aberdeen; Secretary Tom Koch, Puallina, Iowa; Treasurer Tim Gallager, Yankton; and Chaplain Perry King, Chamberlain. Seven new members were activated in November 1986. The Chapter conducted its third diabetes screening program at the Brookings Mall in December 1986, where over 200 people were screened.

Pharmacy Float

Pharmacy students in 1980 won first place with their float, "A Spoonful of Sugar Helps the Medicine Go Down," at the SDSU Hobo Day Homecoming Parade. All the pharmacy students in 1981, conducted a Heart Fund Sunday Drive in Brookings and raised $1,460. The pharmacy float, "Onward to Education" won first place again in the 1982 Hobo Day Parade. Float chairpersons were Mark Tokach, Greg Madsen, and Jeff Kloss. During the 1988 Centennial Celebration, the pharmacy float was selected first for the best theme and second for the most beautiful. The Centennial float was the joint effort of ASP, Kappa Psi, and Kappa Epsilon.

Scholarship and Dinner Dance

A highlight of the pharmacy social season was the annual Pharmacy Dinner Dance. Pharmacy students and faculty joined for a spring gathering for a dinner and awards night. The annual dinner dance and awards night was held at the Staurolite Inn, Brookings, April 10, 1976. It was held at Lake Benton, Minnesota April 22, 1978.

The 1980 event was held in Brookings, where over 120 persons attended, emceed by Zachary Smith. The highlight of the evening was the presentation of scholarships and awards. The Awards Committee consisted of three faculty members, Dr. Gary Omodt, Dr. Peter Cascella, and Dr. Gary Chappell. By 1980, there were twelve pharmacy scholarships available for pharmacy students. The twelve scholarships presented at the 1980 Pharmacy Dinner Dance were:

- Jean Taylor Nelson Memorial and Carney Nelson Fund, $150 to Bonnie J. Salonen
- E. Keith Edgerton Memorial Fund, $120 to Thomas D. Glatt
- F.O. Butler Scholarship, $400 each to Barry L. Hendrickson, Rhonda L. Fredrickson, and Debra L. Stibral
- Kenneth and Elizabeth Redman Scholarship, $250 to Bryan L. Gregor
- Earl and Daphne Serles Memorial Scholarship, $250 each to Tamara J. Heinzerling, Vertus D. Anderson, and Steven E. Martinson
- SDPhA Scholarship, $300 to Brian L. Temple
- Sandra Grover Memorial Scholarship, $150 to Donna F. Gustad
- Dr. Ted Reichmann Memorial Scholarship, $100 to John M. Lichty
- Druggists' Mutual Insurance Co. Scholarship, $300 to Jeffrey L.Bendt
- Greater State Fund Scholarship, $200 to Monica L. Waltner
- Richard J. Duffner Memorial Scholarship, $300 to Lynn T. Carlson
- Brown Drug Co. Scholarship, $250 to Janet R. Goens

Awards presented at the dinner included the following:
- Lilly Achievement Award, to Melanie Wilkens.
- Ladies' Auxiliary, SDPhA, $65 to Lois F. Kredit.
- Upjohn Achievement Award, $100 to Jeffrey R. Herron
- Merck Award of Merck Index to Steven A. Williams and Dianne M. Habbena

- Bristol Award, plaque and publication to Patricia A. Nelson
- Druggists' Mutual Ins. Co., $35 to Rebecca L. Murphy
- Owen Benthin Scholastic Achievement Award, $500 to Patricia A. Rezek.

Remarks were made by Diane Sturdevant, Rho Chi president; Joel Gaub, Kappa Psi Regent; Patty Rezek, Kappa Epsilon president, and Gary Van Riper, Kappa Psi adviser. SAPhA President Lois Kredit, presented SAPhA awards to Cheryl Hassing and Jeffrey Herron. Elizabeth White was named Kappa Psi sweetheart and the Kappa Psi Award was given to Gene Locken.

The annual pharmacy dinner dance and awards ceremony was held in April 1987, where 280 people attended. Chairperson Julie Breitbach said it was a wonderful dinner and dance and many awards and scholarships presented.

Phonathon

Some scholarship money was raised at the first Pharmacy Phonathon in May 1987. Eighty students volunteered and called alumni and friends for donations to the College of Pharmacy. Each night, for four nights, twenty students gathered at the Alumni Center, and after a brief training period, began calling alumni and friends of the college. They had great success at the first Pharmacy Phonathon, with 671 people pledging $21,000 in cash, and donations of computers, and equipment. The cash was used to purchase books, supplies, research equipment, and five scholarships. The 1989 Phonathon raised $26,000 cash.

A resolution was approved to start and fund a Floyd LeBlanc Scholarship Fund at the 1980 SDPhA convention. They also agreed to close out active solicitation for the Earl R. and Daphne C. Serles Memorial Scholarship Fund because the fund had grown enough to provide three or four annual scholarships. It had grown to $18,189 by June 1982, the interest of which provided three scholarships of $350 each. The LeBlanc Fund had increased to $4,651 by June 1985, and the interest would be large enough to award one scholarship in the spring of 1986. The Serles Fund totaled $19,036 in 1985.

Pharmacy Days

Pharmacy Days were begun by Dean Ray Hopponen. He set the date of December 13, 1983, as the date for prospective employers to interview members of the 1984 graduating pharmacy class. SDPhA President James Stephens, Pierre, and the Executive Committee agreed to sponsor a 5:00 p.m. reception and buffet for the graduating class and faculty the night before in the Student Union. President Stephens and Executive Secretary

Harold H. Schuler attended the event and showed a film, *The South Dakota Pharmacy Story*.

The event was held again in 1984 at the Walder Dining Room of the Student Union. If any pharmacists wanted to meet the graduating seniors, they could pay the $7.56 cost of the dinner and attend. The buffet-social was tied in with pharmacist recruiting days held the next day at SDSU. The two-day event, was called Pharmacy Days.

Sixteen companies conducted 233 interviews with forty-two fifth-year students during the fourth annual Pharmacy Days December 4 and 5, 1986, held on the campus of SDSU. Salary offers ranged from $29,000 to $42,000 with the median at $32,000 to $35,000 per year. Pharmacy Days were a joint effort of the College of Pharmacy and the SDSU Career and Academic Planning Center. SDPhA continued its practice of hosting all the fifth-year students and faculty to a dinner the night before Pharmacy Days. In 1989, twenty-one companies conducted 391 interviews with the second, third, fourth, and fifth year students.

Early Computer Use at the College of Pharmacy

An early use of the computer was created through a joint venture of the College of Pharmacy, State University Extension Service, and Yankton Sacred Heart Hospital in 1974. The joint effort resulted in the establishment of a computer terminal in the Sacred Heart Hospital. It allowed hospital pharmacist Donald Strahl to use the computer to check the effect of drugs on patients. Dean Ray Hopponen said the computer will "check the effects of one drug on a patient when that patient is already on other medication. In addition, it will provide information to the doctors on the effects of several drugs if used in combination."[18] The terminal tied into the SDSU Computer Center.

The South Dakota Board of Pharmacy passed regulations pertaining to the use of computers in pharmacy in 1979. Computer training had been given in Pharmacy Management at the College of Pharmacy. In 1980, an AdHoc Committee to study the use of computers in pharmacy practice was created by the College of Pharmacy. IBM's personal computer was introduced in 1981. In April of that year, the College of Pharmacy and Rho Chi Society sponsored a seminar "Computer Use in Pharmacy—the Future." Faculty member Gary Van Riper reported that over 100 had attended the seminar.

Word processing equipment purchased to furnish the new Guilford C. Gross Pharmacy Building in 1981 included: $6,000 for typewriters; $5,184 for memory typewriters; $7,200 for a word processor; and $11,600 for computer equipment. It was obvious the College of Pharmacy used both manual and electric typewriters as well as the latest computer equipment. The transition from the old methods to the new did not happen overnight. Dr. Kenneth Redman in 1983 predicted that "Pharmacy will continue to be computerized in all aspects of the profession."[19]

Change of Deans

Dean Ray Hopponen, who had ably served as the Dean of the College of Pharmacy since 1966, retired July 1, 1986. The Board of Regents appointed Bernard E. Hietbrink as acting dean. He was appointed Dean of the College of Pharmacy January 1, 1987. Hietbrink had received his B. S. in pharmacy from SDSU in 1958 and his Ph.D. from the University of Chicago in 1961. He started his career at SDSU in 1964 as an assistant professor in the College of Pharmacy. Hietbrink was promoted to associate professor and department head, Pharmacology in 1966 and to professor and department head, Pharmaceutical Sciences in 1983.

Distinguished Alumnus Award

The award was created to honor graduates of the SDSU College of Pharmacy who had served their profession with distinction. The first distinguished alumnus was Clark T. Eidsmoe, presented in 1988. Eidsmoe earned his Ph.G. in pharmacy from SDSU in 1913; his B.S. in 1929; and his M.S. in 1931. After practicing the profession for seventeen years he joined the SDSU College of Pharmacy in 1929, where he served as an instructor and professor until his retirement in 1964. The award has been presented at the scholarship and awards night in the spring of the year. Subsequent distinguished alumnus since that time include:

    1989 Guilford C. Gross
    1990 Richard F. Wojcik
    1991 J. Bruce Laughrey
    1992 Harlan Stai
    1993 Mary Waggoner Kuper
    1994 Donald A. Strahl
    1995 Garrett Gross
    1996 Dwight W. Hustead
    1997 Kay Coffield Pearson
    1998 Merle E. Amundson
    1999 Marian L. Roberts
    2000 Allen A. Pfeifle
    2001 Bernard E. Hietbrink
    2002 Kenneth B. Jones
    2003 Richard A. Smith

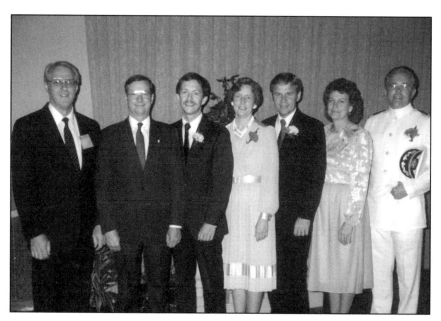

Officers for 1985-1986, from left to right, Past Pres. Al Pfeifle, Pres. Robert Gregg, Pres. Elect Dave Helgeland, 1st V-Pres. Mary Kuper, 2nd V-Pres. Arvid Liebe, 3rd V-Pres. Marilyn Schwans, and Treas. Craig Hostetler.

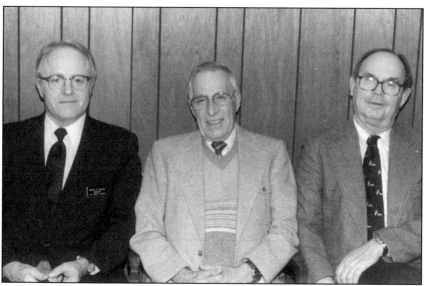

Waiting for a 1983 Board of Pharmacy meeting are left to right, Secretary Harold H. Schuler, and drug inspectors Glenn Velau and Les Hetager.

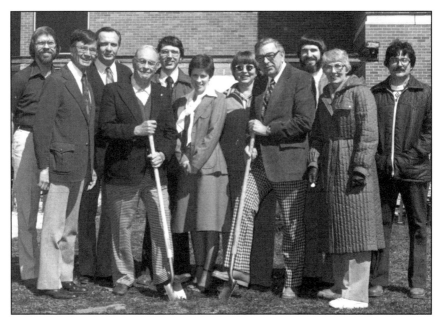

Ground-breaking for the new pharmacy building from left to right include: Gary Omodt, Dean Ray Hopponen, Bernard Hietbrink, Kenneth Redman, Joel Houglum, Colleen Jones, Joye Billow, Guilford Gross, Gary Chappell, Jean Bibby, and Peter Cascella. April 1980.

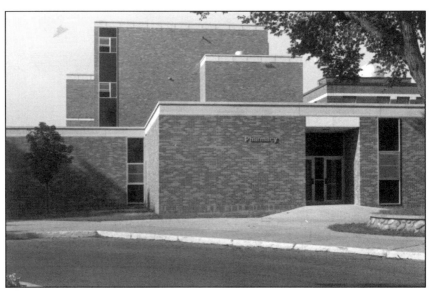

The new Guilford C. Gross Pharmacy Building dedicated 1981.

A History of Pharmacy in South Dakota

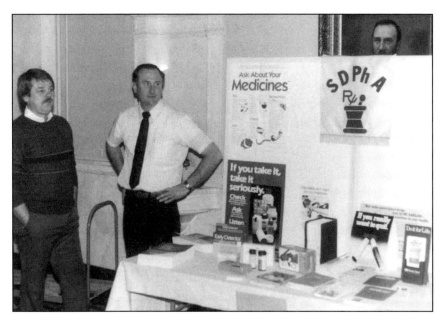

A 1987 Health Fair at the capitol with Lynn Ketelsen and Bob Brost.

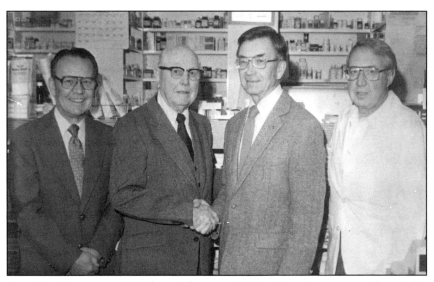

Dean Ray Hopponen, third from left, congratulates Harry Lee, second from left for establishing a pharmacy scholarship. The gathering included three generations of owners of Alcester Pharmacy: Harry Lee original owner, sold to Vere Larsen, left, in the 1940s. Larsen later sold to William "Bud" Peterson, right, in the early 1980s. 1985 photo.

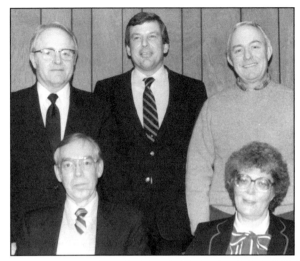

1981-1985 Board of Pharmacy. Top left to right, Secretary Harold H. Schuler, Board Members Frank Post, Ken Jones; bottom left to right, John Nelson, Shirley Heitland.

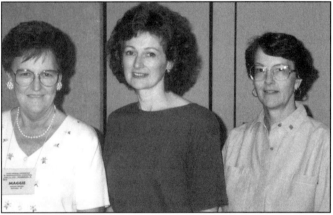

SDPhA Auxiliary presidents: left to right, Maggie Nelson, 1997; Karen Jones, 1998; and Janelle McKinstry, 1999.

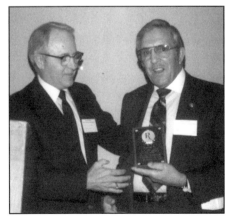

Secretary Harold H. Schuler presents U.S. Senator James Abdnor with a plaque for outstanding support of the objectives of the Association, at the 1985 SDPhA convention in Sioux Falls.

CHAPTER 12
1990-2003

SD Pharmacists Association (SDPhA), 1990-2003

South Dakota Pharmaceutical Association

Historical Background

When the South Dakota Legislature approved a pharmacy law for the new state in 1890, they created a unique administrative feature. The secretary and the treasurer of the Board of Pharmacy were also the secretary and the treasurer of the Pharmaceutical Association. Statutory duties were outlined for each agency. When pharmacists paid their $2.00 license renewal fee to the Board of Pharmacy, they automatically became a member of the Association. The pharmacist license renewals fees, although collected by the Board, were transferred to the Association to finance their operations. The Board financed their operations with other license fees.

The close-connectedness of the Association and the Board was subject to Legislative review, especially in the 1970s and 1980s. For example, between 1975 and 1980, there were seven Legislative bills attempting to separate the Board and Association. All of the bills were defeated in the Legislature by Association lobbyists. Board members and Association officers believed the arrangement was not causing a public problem, and besides, it cost less money to operate the two groups.

Incorporation of South Dakota Pharmacists Association

Separation of the Association and Board of Pharmacy were discussed at the 1994 convention in Pierre. Convention minutes show that some pharmacists were concerned about the increasing workload of the current joint office, such as publishing the *South Dakota Pharmacist*, increased convention and meeting responsibilities, added licensing responsibility, and an increase in distribution of information. Each entity with its own executive secretary, might be in a better position to face the future of the profession. Another concern was that the Association was a quasi-state agency and not incorporated. A separation from the Board of Pharmacy, would allow the Association to better function in a changing health care system, as well as establishing pharmaceutical care as a standard of practice in South Dakota.

In 1995, the SDPhA Executive Committee recommended steps be taken to pass legislation which would permit the Association to become a non-profit corporation. All registered pharmacists would be entitled to its rights and privileges including the right to vote and be an officer. Specifically, the Executive Committee favored deleting the requirement that the secretary of the Association also be secretary of the Board. However, they strongly favored that the Association continue to receive pharmacist license renewal fees to finance its operations.

With the help of the pharmacy profession, the 1996 Legislature, through House Bill 1249, passed a law separating the Board of Pharmacy and the Pharmaceutical Association. The law contained these features:

- Changed name to South Dakota Pharmacists Association
- Provided authority to the Association to create a non-profit organization
- Authorized all registered pharmacists to be members
- Deleted requirement that the Association secretary also be the Board secretary
- License renewal fees collected by the Board go to the Association
- License fees would be raised by Board of Pharmacy regulation rather than by statute.

Following passage of the new law, President Robert Wik, Gregory, and the Executive Committee met in Chamberlain April 28, 1996 and approved a number of procedural steps to incorporate the Association as well as adopt a new Constitution and By-laws.

The first step was the action taken at the annual convention on June 7-9, 1996 at the Radisson Resort Hotel at Cedar Shore, Chamberlain. Convention delegates, by a vote of 47 Yes and 1 No, approved the amendments to the Constitution and By-laws. The amendments would be discussed and voted upon again at special meetings.

At a July 27-28, 1996 meeting, the Executive Committee voted to call a special meeting to be held at the Radisson Resort Hotel at Cedar Shore, Chamberlain, September 22, 1996. They also asked Secretary Galen Jordre to send notice to all pharmacist members, and include the Articles of Incorporation [Constitution] of the South Dakota Pharmacists Association and the final draft of the By-laws.

President Pam Jones, Huron, reminded pharmacists about "The Three R's of Pharmacy" in the plan for the future. She was quoted in the *South Dakota Pharmacist*, July-August 1996 issue: "Reengineering our future through pharmaceutical care is the national focus of our profession. Reorganization of our Association is our state focus so that we will continue to meet the needs of our profession as we reengineer through pharmaceutical care. Refocusing is what each of us needs to do to reengineer and reorganize for our individual practice."[1]

Twenty-nine pharmacists attended that September 22, 1996 special Association meeting. President Pam Jones, Huron, announced that a quorum was present. A motion was made and seconded to ratify the Articles of Incorporation and approve the By-laws. It passed with a unanimous vote, 29 Yes and 0 No.

Following the September 22, 1996 meeting, the new Board of Directors and Incorporators held an organizational meeting by telephone conference on September 26, 1996. The Board of Directors and Incorporators were Pam Jones, Huron; Mark Gerdes, Sioux Falls; Earl McKinstry, Piedmont; James Bregel, Chamberlain; Cheri Kraemer, Parker, and Robert Wik, Gregory. They adopted the By-laws approved September 22, 1996; accepted the transfer of assets and liabilities of the South Dakota Pharmaceutical Association; and agreed to appoint an executive director.

After 106 years, the South Dakota Pharmacists Association replaced the South Dakota Pharmaceutical Association and the close-connectedness with the Board of Pharmacy was dissolved. Pam Jones, Huron, was the last president of the South Dakota Pharmaceutical Association and the first president of the South Dakota Pharmacists Association.

The American Pharmaceutical Association changed its name to American Pharmacists Association in 2002. The National Association of Retail Druggists (NARD), also changed its name to National Community Pharmacists Association (NCPA).

Highlights, By-laws of the South Dakota Pharmacists Association
- Membership consists of active members, associate members, student members, pharmacists emeritus, life members, honorary members, and members of Academies of the Association hereafter created. Only the active members could vote or hold office.
- All registered pharmacists who have secured a current annual certificate from the Board of Pharmacy shall be active members.
- Officers shall be president, president-elect, first vice-president, second vice- president, and secretary/treasurer. At the annual meeting, the president-elect, first vice- president, and second vice-president advance in office. A new second

vice-president and secretary/treasurer shall be elected at the annual meeting.
- The elected officers form a Board of Directors who shall appoint an executive director.
- Standing committees include public affairs, professional affairs, college of pharmacy, pharmacy management, and nominations. Each committee shall consist of at least one member of the Board of Directors and four other members who serve staggered three-year terms.
- A commercial and legislative section shall raise money through voluntary membership fees to finance legislative lobbying.
- The Board of Directors shall establish a network of district organizations to serve South Dakota pharmacists.

Administrative Matters

Executive Directors

Galen Jordre, RPh., who had been executive director since February 1986 resigned January 27, 1997 to become executive director of the North Dakota Pharmaceutical Association. Executive Director Galen Jordre, had skillfully led the Association into the new era of pharmaceutical care, pharmaceutical counseling, patient records, and the pharmacy practice act. He compiled and introduced the Association news journal, The *South Dakota Pharmacist*, in 1986, which is still being published. He handled all of the details pertaining to the separation of the Association and the Board, and the incorporation of the South Dakota Pharmacists Association, in 1996. His wife Ann, also a pharmacist, was awarded the Honorary President Award at the 1999 convention in Rapid City.

On April 29, 1997, the SDPhA Board of Directors hired Terri McEntaffer, RPh., as executive director. McEntaffer was president of the South Dakota Society of Hospital Pharmacists in 1996, and was also president of the SDPhA Mobridge District, 1993-1995. Pam Stotz, administrative assistant in the pharmacy office, resigned February 17, 1999. She had ably served as administrative assistant for both the Board and the Association since 1985. Rogene Dutton, Pierre, served as administrative assistant between November 1, 1999 and February 26, 2003. Terri McEntaffer resigned November 30, 1999 to be executive director of the Illinois Pharmaceutical Association.

Bob Coolidge, RPh, Pierre, was hired May 1, 2000 as executive director. He had served seven years as a consultant pharmacist with the State Department of Health in Pierre. For twelve years previously, he had managed a pharmacy for Lewis Drug. Bob and his wife Kelly have four children. President James Bregel, Chamberlain, said "I feel he brings excellent qualifications to the position. His experience in retail and his experience working for the state should bring a well-rounded individual...to our Association for years to come."[2] Coolidge's grandfather, George Tammen owned a drug store at Yankton in 1901.

Coolidge, interested in the history of the Association, had asked Historian Harold H. Schuler, Pierre, to write a history of the beginning of the Association, between 1886 and 1893, for the *South Dakota Pharmacist*. After completion of that early history, Bob Coolidge; Cliff Thomas, Belle Fourche; and others believed that the entire history should be compiled. After reviewing the matter, the Board of Directors, on January 6, 2002, authorized Harold H. Schuler to write the history. Bob Coolidge resigned in June 30, 2002 and accepted a job as pharmacist consultant at the State Department of Health. President Steve Aamot, Aberdeen, said, "We would like to sincerely thank Bob for his two years of service, dedication, and support that he has given to the Association."[3]

On July 1, 2002, the Executive Board appointed Tobi Lyon as interim executive director. Tobi was raised on the family ranch near Meadow, South Dakota. She attended the School of Mines for three years and then graduated with a degree in Health Service Administration from Mount Mercy College, Cedar Rapids, Iowa. After being named executive director January 1, 2003, she served the Association until May 8, 2003, when she resigned to become Director of Provider Relations with Western Health, a division of Rapid City Regional Hospital. Upon leaving, Tobi Lyon reported that "I have truly enjoyed working for SDPhA and have a real passion for your profession. I thank all of you."[4]

The Board of Directors employed Robert Overturf, Rapid City, as the new executive director August 1, 2003. Bob has a B.S. degree in Political Science and had completed graduate course work toward a Masters Degree, which he plans to continue to pursue. Formerly, Overturf worked with the Drug Enforcement Administration and the South Dakota Division of Criminal Investigation before retiring in 2002 as the DCI Supervisor in Rapid City. During his career he was on the Board of Trustees of the State Retirement System, and often appeared before Legislative Committees. Most recently, Bob worked as a sales representative for a pharmaceutical company, where he met many South Dakota pharmacists.

In April 2003, the Board of Directors hired Jaime Gangelhoff as the communications specialist for SDPhA. Jaime is a graduate of Augsburg College, Minneapolis, where she earned her degree in Fine Arts and a minor in Communications. She has had experience in event planning, graphic design, and sales. She will focus her efforts on improving SDPhA publications and informational material.

Pharmacists

The number of registered pharmacists in South Dakota had increased from 455 in 1891 to 1457 in 2002, a record high. A table showing the number of pharmacists in South Dakota since statehood is as follows:

Year	In-state	Out-state	Total
1891	424	31	455
1908	536	144	680
1915	661	192	853
1924	644	237	881
1932	586	166	752
1942	488	181	669
1950	535	279	814
1971	440	451	891
1978	596	513	1109
1992	-	-	1219
1996	-	-	1377
2000	736	630	1393
2001	757	657	1414
2002	824	633	1457

During the above time frame, license renewal fees were: $2.00 in 1890; $3.00 in 1894; $5.00 in 1921; $10.00 in 1953; raised from $25 to $35 in 1988; $70 in 1996; and $125 in 2001.

Finances

Gross revenue for the Association in 1992 totaled $104,605. Some of the receipts included $42,665 from the $35.00 pharmacist license renewals; $5,724 from advertising in *South Dakota Pharmacist* (6 issues per year); $5,176 from continuing education; and $390 from 78 pharmacy students who paid the $5.00 Association membership. Expenses totaled $108,547, including such items as $20,000 salary for Executive Director (Board paid other part); per diem $10,720; postage $5,108; South Dakota Pharmacist $9,129; and scholarship fund $300.

Revenue in 1999 totaled $185,624. Some of the revenue was from 1345 pharmacists who paid $94,150 for the $70 license renewal fee; excess from the annual convention was $20,485; and $8435 from advertising in *South Dakota Pharmacist/Stat-Gram*. Some of the expenses included $44,813 for executive director salary; $15,400 for administrative assistant salary; $10,819 for expenses for publication of *South Dakota Pharmacist/Stat-Gram*; and cost of annual convention was

A History of Pharmacy in South Dakota

$16,083. Balance on hand June 30, 1999 included checking $3,000 and savings $63,737.

Conventions

Conventions are an important part of the administration of pharmaceutical affairs. The Articles of Incorporation required that the Association meet yearly in convention to conduct business. Conventions can be called, after due notice to the membership, to vote on amendments to the Constitution and By-laws, resolutions from the districts, as well as motions from the floor. A quorum of twenty-five is needed to take official action. Historically, conventions have been a place for action, social gatherings, and improvement of the profession. Sporting events, banquets, social hours, awards, meetings of auxiliary groups, and floor business fill out a convention schedule.

Since the 1980 continuing education (CE) requirement of twelve hours a year, convention planners have included approved CE programs. At the June 1981 convention in the Mitchell Holiday Inn, eleven hours of CE were presented. Twelve hours of CE was presented at the 1993 convention in Sioux Falls, two hours of which were by a panel, including Senator Tom Daschle, discussing "Health Care Reform-The Pharmacy Connection." At the 1993 convention a new Innovative Pharmacy Practice Award was adopted. The award is given to a pharmacist whose work has resulted in improved patient care. The first winner was Yee-Lai Chiu, Sioux Falls.

Planning and producing a convention takes a lot of volunteers and a lot of hard work. Convention Chair Garry Freier of the 1995 convention at the Mitchell Holiday Inn, created eleven committees. Nineteen members served on the committees. Some of the committees included: CE [11 hours], Exhibits, Finance, Food, Hospitality, Golf, Fhun-Run/walk, Registration, Worship, Memorial and Auxiliary. Eleven awards were given at the Saturday night banquet, and three at the Sunday wholesalers luncheon. Margaret Zard, Mitchell, was SDPhA president that year.

The 2000 convention held at the Ramkota Inn Best Western at Sioux Falls September 22-24, included twelve CE programs for a total of nineteen hours of CE. Comparatively, four hours were scheduled for business meetings: two hours Saturday afternoon and two hours Sunday morning. A banquet and awards presentation were held Saturday night. The Memorial Service was held Sunday morning. James Bregel, Chamberlain, was the outgoing president and Cheri Kraemer, Parker, was the incoming president. The usual June convention was moved to September in 2000. The registration fees for the entire convention cost $140 a person, guest $90, technician $70, and student $70. The 2002 convention in Rapid City included twelve hours of CE and the registration fees were similar to those in 2000. Attendance was 100 persons at the 2002 gathering. Steve Aamot, Aberdeen, was president 2001-2002.

Ramkota Hotel in Aberdeen was the site for the June 6-8, 2003 convention. At a business meeting the following officers were installed for 2003-2004: President Monica Jones, Huron; President-Elect Shane Clarambeau, Hermosa; First Vice-President Julie Meintsma, Pierre; Second Vice-President Galen Goeden, Yankton; and Treasurer Robert Reiswig, Spearfish. Past President Karla Overland-Janssen, Rapid City, a SDSU College of Pharmacy student, the president of the South Dakota Pharmacy Technicians Association, and the above officers serve as the Board of Directors of the South Dakota Pharmacists Association.

Memorial Service and Recognition Breakfast
The Veteran Druggists' Association was formed in 1926. Pharmacists who had served twenty-five years were eligible for membership. The veterans met at a convention veterans breakfast. The Association's first Memorial Service was conducted in 1927 at the Mobridge convention. The program opened with a quartette who sang "The Vacant Chair." Secretary W. P. Loesch then read the name of one of the deceased, after which a pharmacist said a few words of tribute as well as a brief biographical sketch. This same procedure was performed for the nine deceased pharmacists. The meeting closed with the quartette singing "Rose of Sharon," and a prayer by one of the local ministers. With a few changes, this format continued for many years. Both events were always held on Sunday morning.

At the 1976 convention, there was a Veterans' Breakfast for those pharmacists who had served twenty-five years or more. Immediately after, a Memorial Service was held with the reading of the names of those deceased that year, followed by music, a message, and a prayer. In 1988, the regular Memorial Service was held followed by a Recognition Breakfast for all pharmacists registered twenty-five years or more. A similar format prevailed until 1994. That year, after the Memorial Service, a Pharmacist Recognition Breakfast was held where all pharmacists attending the convention were recognized.

Murray D. Widdis, Sioux Falls, pharmacist at Lewis Drug for many years, was recognized at the 1997 convention for having been registered as a pharmacist for seventy-five years. Widdis, originally from Chamberlain, passed his exams on October 12, 1922 and held Certificate No. 2233. At the 1999 Recognition Breakfast, pharmacists were recognized as follows: Those who were registered from 10 to 24 years, those from 25 to 34 years, those 35 to 49 years, and those 50 years and over.

The Memorial Service at the 1999 convention in Rapid City included a remembrance of Ted Hustead, Wall, SD. Ted E. Hustead died January 12, 1999 at the age of ninety-six. One of his honors included a Honorary Doctorate for Public Service from SDSU in 1996. The South Dakota Legislature commemorated his memory with a special resolution. Ted and Dorothy founded the internationally famous Wall Drug in 1931. After a slow start during that hot 1931 summer, Dorothy noticed that tourist cars were passing by Wall without stopping. She came up with the idea to offer free ice water at the drug store. Ted made up signs, Free Ice Water at Wall Drug and posted them along Highway 14 and 16. Tourists began to stop in droves. Before the summer was over, they had to hire eight employees to handle the extra work. The business boomed. By 2003, the drug store was serving 20,000 people daily. Its Wall Drug signs are posted around the world. Dorothy passed away in 1995. After their son Bill died in October 1999, Bill's wife Marjorie and their two sons Rick and Ted, and their spouses carry on the business. The drug store now consists of several buildings including a large mall-type structure. Some of the features include a pharmacy, pharmacy museum, traveler's chapel, western art gallery, animated Cowboy Orchestra, thousands of historical photos, a 530-seat dining room and a giant T-Rex in the back yard mall. Ted and Dorothy founded the SDPhA Hustead Award in 1988. Dennis Womeldorf, pharmacist at Wall Drug, was introduced into the Jackrabbit Sports Hall of Fame in 2003, honoring his basketball career while attending SDSU in the late 1960s.

Throughout the years, both the Memorial Service and the Recognition Breakfast [formerly Veterans' Breakfast] were held the first thing Sunday morning. At the 2002 convention in Rapid City, the Recognition, Memorial, and Awards were all held at the Saturday evening banquet. Roger Eastman, Platte, was one of the pharmacists recognized at the Memorial Service. Eastman, a graduate of Creighton College of Pharmacy, owned and operated drug stores at Tripp and Platte. He was eighty-seven years of age when he died February 17, 2002. Eastman, a former President of SDPhA and the Board of Pharmacy, was awarded the Bowl of Hygeia in 1971 and the Hustead Award in 1991.

Public Relations

During National Pharmacy Week, October 20-26, 1991, the Association adopted two themes, Everyone Wins When You Talk, and You and Your Pharmacist Communicate for Good Health. Large posters and smaller pass outs carried that message to the public. The same message was carried in public service radio and newspaper announcements. President Jo Oihus (Prang) said, "We should no longer allow our image to be that of just pill counters. We need to market to the public that the benefit of a patient-pharmacist relationship has much greater value than the discounted price of the prescription. If we can demonstrate benefit to the public, we have proved our worth to the health care system."[5]

Available from the Association office were Patient Medication Kits provided by Lederle Laboratories. The three kits included National Medication Awareness Test; Self-Medication Awareness Test; and Managing Your Medicines. Pharmacists could use these kits for pass outs. In 1992, twenty-two volunteers staffed a SDPhA booth at the State Fair. They passed out packets containing a Personal Medication Record and information about a Medic Alert bracelet. Over 3,500 people, including United States Senator Larry Pressler, registered during the seven-day period.

An APhA sixteen-minute video, Your Medicine, Your Pharmacist and You, was available to pharmacists in 1993. The video, for use at informational meetings, explained the important role pharmacists played as key members of the health care team. Pass outs to over 3,000 people visiting the booth during the 1993 State Fair, included the same type materials as in 1992, plus information on the Kathy's Kids Program. After evaluation of the 1992 and 1993 appearances at the State Fair, the Executive Committee decided not to exhibit at the 1994 State Fair.

The public relations theme for the 1994 National Pharmacy Week was, Talk About Your Prescriptions Month. To help pharmacists present programs, NARD provided a number of speaker assistance kits. The kits provided speeches, promotional ideas, 35 mm slides, and handouts on six pharmacy-related topics: Getting the Best Results from Your Medicine; Patient Compliance, How Important It Really Is; Your Prescription; Saving Money on Prescription Drugs; How to Avoid Drug Interactions; and the Proper Use of Over-the-Counter Drugs. The kits cost $35 each for member pharmacists.

President Earl McKinstry, Piedmont, appointed the following to the Association's Public Affairs Committee for 1998: Chair Steve Aamot, Shirley Guthmiller, Leslie Shoenhard, Mark Kantack, Renee Sutton, and two SDSU ASP members Joan Case and Susan Rosenau. The committee listed their activities during 1998 National Pharmacy Week: letters to the editor and public service announcements were sent to forty-five newspapers; information was sent to all State Representatives and State Senators; public service announcements were provided to thirty-four radio stations; information was also provided to eight television stations of which KBNB-TV of Rapid City interviewed President Earl McKinstry and KEVN-TV of Rapid City interviewed Paula Stotz. Governor William

Janklow proclaimed National Pharmacy Week in South Dakota for October 22-28, 2000. Association newsletters such as *South Dakota Pharmacist* and *Stat-Gram* helped keep pharmacists informed. Advertisement rates for the *South Dakota Pharmacist* in 2001, were one page $350, if run four times it was $330 a page. Classified ads were $15.00 for five-lines per issue.

President Karla Overland-Janssen, Rapid City, said the 2002 Board of Directors developed a mission statement: "To promote, serve and protect the pharmacy profession" as well as a vision statement, "To lead pharmacy into an ever changing future."[6]

Rankings, Surveys, and Practice

Pharmacy service and business has grown throughout the first ninety years of the twentieth century. Secretary Galen Jordre alluded to that at the 1990 convention. He reported that less than thirty years ago there were about 700 prescription drugs on the market which increased to 2,800 in 1990. Consumers spend an estimated $30 billion a year on 1.63 billion prescriptions, an average of six per person. He further said, "The American consumer expects to receive medicines to treat their health problems. The rapidity of new drug development...increases the need for patients to learn how to use their medicines safely."[7]

According to a 1991 *Lilly Digest* survey, the average independent community pharmacy had total sales of $918,318 and a net profit of 2.9% of sales [or $26,631]. Third party pay prescriptions accounted for 40.4% of prescriptions filled. The average prescription cost rose 11%, or $2.02; the average Rx cost was $20.39. The average hospital pharmacy inventory worth increased 22% to over $170,000.[8]

A Gallup Poll in 1994 asked 1,008 adults how they would rate professions and occupations in terms of honesty and ethical standards. Pharmacists ranked the highest with 62%. The next four were clergy 54%, dentists 51%, college teachers 50%, and medical doctors 47%.[9] A similar CNN/USAToday/Gallup Poll in 1998 of the most trusted professionals, ranked pharmacists with 64%, clergy 59%, doctors 57%, and dentists and college professors at 53%.[10]

A SDSU College of Pharmacy survey of salaries for both full-time and part-time pharmacy work was completed in 1998 and in 1999. The 1998 survey of 208 full-time pharmacists, who worked an average of 43.7 hours a week, earned $53,468 per year. A 1999 survey of 76 pharmacists who worked less than forty hours per week, showed that the men earned $21.22 an hour and the women $23.25. The overall salary of the seventy-six pharmacists was $22.81 per hour.[11]

The 2001 report of the Board of Pharmacy listed where pharmacists are practicing in South Dakota. Their study showed that of the 757 in-state pharmacists; 502 are in retail, 156 in hospital, 15 manufacturing/wholesaler, 35 teaching, and 49 other. According to a Board of Pharmacy manpower study in 2002, pharmacy service is lacking in fifteen South Dakota counties. They also reported that a serious problem may develop in eighteen other counties in five years. New regulations may be necessary to permit a pharmacist to make a living and serve these low populated areas.[12]

Legislation

Pharmacist Legislative Days at the state capitol in Pierre, continued with the same format as used in the 1980s. The January 29, 1990 event, began Tuesday evening with a dinner and briefing at the Ramkota Inn, Pierre. The next morning, pharmacists, spouses, and students served a continental breakfast to Legislators in lobbies of the House and the Senate. The menu included bagels, assorted cream cheeses, orange juice and coffee. Afterward, the pharmacists attended committee meetings as well as talking with Legislators. They returned to the Ramkota for a luncheon and legislative debriefing. That year, Attorney Robert Riter, Pierre, was the lobbyist. The 1991 event, when Terry Casey, Chamberlain, was Association president, was similar to the 1990 Legislative Days.

Pharmacist Legislative Days was actually hosted and funded by the Commercial and Legislative (C&L) Section of the Association. In 1993, 211 individuals, 87 businesses, and 5 corporations contributed $15,463 to the fund which was used for lobbying and legislative purposes. The expenditures for the year totaled $13,354 of which $5,662 was paid to Attorneys Robert Riter, Jr. and John Brown for lobbying expense. The fund in 1993 had a surplus on hand of $30,164. In 1999, C&L fees were $35 for individuals, $100 for pharmacies, and $200 for corporations. That year a grand total of $15,288 was voluntarily contributed to the C & L Section.

Each district selected several pharmacists to attend Legislative Days at the capitol. District pharmacists, Association officers, spouses, and students totaled fifty people in 1992. Usually a faculty member or two accompanied the students. Emily Maydew, ASP president said, "ASP took thirty-seven students from pre-pharmacy to P3 to Pierre for [February 2003] Legislative Days sponsored by SDPhA. We performed blood glucose, blood pressure, and cholesterol screening for Legislators and capitol staff. We enjoyed the unique opportunity to experience the Legislature and represent the profession."[13]

A resolution had been introduced at the 2002 convention in Rapid City to have SDPhA host a social and dinner for the members of the South Dakota Legislature [like the format of the 1960s, and 1970s] but it failed. The format of a continental breakfast for members of the Legislature used in the 1980s and 1990s was satisfactory to pharmacists.

Pharmaceutical Care

In 1992, a federal government program mandated that when a prescription is issued to a medicaid patient, the pharmacist must provide counseling to the patient about the drug. This prompted Pharmaceutical Associations, including the South Dakota group, to seek Legislation requiring pharmacists to counsel private patients as well as those in the government medicaid program. The theory is that pharmacists are not only dispensers of drugs but also dispensers of information. Don McGuire, *Pharmacy and the Law*, said, "The trend has been to move from product dispensers to providers of pharmaceutical care."[14]

SDPhA President Jo Prang commented on the direction toward which the Association was heading, "The reality is, the pharmacy profession is moving towards disassociation with the product, and more association with service, communication, and knowledge. We are ready to take our responsibility as part of the health care team for the best therapeutic outcome for the patient. Even if we are not ready, we will all soon be mandated by government to participate in this patient-focused profession of pharmacy. This change in emphasis came about because the government can see the benefits to a health team approach to medicine."[15]

Patient Counseling and Patient Records

The South Dakota Legislature passed a law, effective July 1, 1992 stating that when a pharmacist provides a prescription to a patient that the pharmacist must offer to counsel that patient about the drug. A pharmacist must also maintain a prescription record for each patient. Regulations for the law were issued by the Board of Pharmacy effective December 31, 1992.

The prescription record system for each patient must include: name, address, phone, list of drugs, known allergies, known reactions, and known diseases. Records must be kept one year either on paper or electronically. Patient counseling, according to the Board of Pharmacy, required review of the patient's record before filling a new prescription for that patient. When the filled prescription container is issued to the patient, the pharmacist must offer counseling which could include special directions, proper use, common side effects, storage requirements, and information on refills. If there is no record it signifies that counseling was accepted and provided or that an offer was made.

The Board also reminded pharmacists that only pharmacists can offer and provide counseling. It cannot be performed by technicians or other support personnel in the pharmacy. Board Secretary Dennis M. Jones said, "two very important questions to ask the patient when counseling are 1. Do you have any allergies? and 2. What did your prescriber tell you this medication was to be used for? Many errors have been prevented by asking these two questions."[16]

Association President Linda Pierson, Mitchell, in reviewing the 1992 Legislative Session as to patient counseling said, "Mandated counseling may upset many of you for various reasons, but I believe that 'information transmission' is the pharmacist's function. We are or should be in this profession for the sake of the patient and promoting good drug health care. If we don't meet this challenge there are always others waiting in the wings to take over."[17]

NABP made a national survey in July 1994 on the impact of patient counseling. They found that over forty states passed similar laws to the one passed in South Dakota. The study also showed that 60% of the patients had not been offered counseling on their medications. Only 38% of the patients reported they had been offered counseling. Patients also reported that about two-thirds of the time pharmacists did the counseling and about a third of the time counseling was provided by technicians or clerks in the pharmacy. However, when patients were counseled, they felt that pharmacists had done a fairly good job.[18]

To be sure South Dakota pharmacists were complying with the new law, the Board of Pharmacy in 1995 adopted a new regulation creating a Pharmacy Counseling Score Sheet to be used by their two drug inspectors. Compliance with the new law had varied around the state, so the Board believed the new score sheet would provide uniformity in enforcing the minimum standards of patient counseling.

A number of continuing education programs were available, both in conventions and separate meetings, pertaining to counseling and patient records. President Mark Gerdes, Sioux Falls, said, "we are trying to offer more in the way of [CE] certificate programs. A pharmacist can hang that certificate, thus giving credibility with the patient and other professionals."[19] Executive Director Terri McEntaffer, in 1999 reaffirmed that view, "I would encourage you to take pharmaceutical care courses. At some point you have to jump. You have to say I am going to take the extra time to really talk to this patient about this drug, find out how they are responding, are they having trouble taking it as prescribed. [You have to] say I am going to move beyond dispensing."[20]

Al Pfeifle, Sioux Falls, predicted the profession is changing "from product-oriented to patient oriented. There is nothing more satisfying than helping patients."[21] Pharm.D. Robert D. Gibson, speaking at the 2000 APhA convention told the delegates that the prescription markup and professional fee have dominated the profession for years. Now "pharmacists provide value to the health care system...drugs don't work alone."[22] President Steve Aamot, Aberdeen, said, "We can make it happen. Studies have shown that pharmacists can reduce medication errors, improve patient outcomes, and decrease costs by providing patient-care services in a variety of settings."[23]

There had been a trend in the profession to shift from product dispensers to dispensers of pharmaceutical care. Executive Secretary Dennis M. Jones, in his 2000 report to the SDPhA convention remarked, "The pharmaceutical care message is being heard, and for the first time, newly built or remodeled pharmacies are adding patient counseling areas and restrooms for pharmacists and patients. Pharmacists are asking to use their education, not just fill prescriptions."[24]

Pharmacy Practice Act

Another important law passed in 1993 was the Pharmacy Practice Act. It specifically states that the practice of pharmacy means: interpretation of prescription orders and dispensing in the patient's best interest; responsibility for compounding, labeling, and storage of drugs, and maintaining records for them; and the provision of patient counseling and pharmaceutical care. President David Kuper, Sioux Falls, stated that the new Pharmacy Practice Act, "has expanded the pharmacist's traditional role of compounding, distributing, labeling, and storage of drugs. It now includes the interpretation and evaluation of prescription drug orders and the provisions of patient counseling and pharmaceutical care. These two activities hold promise for new professional opportunities."[25]

Association Executive Secretary Galen Jordre, helped secure passage of the Pharmacy Practice Act of 1993. He said, "The establishment of the Pharmacy Practice Act of 1993 was a major advancement for pharmacy in the state. Prior to that time, the only role for pharmacists outlined in the laws was to fill prescriptions. Representatives of all facets of pharmacy in the state worked together as a committee to develop the practice act language. There were several meetings of the committee and the proposal was previewed to other health care groups in the state. The resultant list of duties for pharmacists broke new ground. The significant advance in the practice act were to allow for collaborative therapy practice to initiate and modify medication regimens. The other significant aspect was the ability of pharmacists to administer medications. There had to be a compromise with the Medical Association that placed some limitations on pharmacists administering injectable medications. The compromise required that rules be established, a process that took several years. When looked at in comparison to other states, South Dakota has one of the more progressive practice acts in the country."[26]

Other Legislative Matters

In 1993 the Legislature repealed the provision requiring two lines on a prescription by which a doctor could authorize a pharmacist to substitute by signing substitution permitted or dispense as written. The new law simply authorized a doctor to avoid substitution by writing on the prescription, 'brand necessary'. A doctor could not preprint this authority on the prescription form.

The old problem of discriminatory pricing by manufacturers was addressed in House Bill 1265 in the 1994 session. It mandated that manufacturers must make available to retail pharmacies the same price as to other pharmacies in government facilities or in hospitals. After a committee hearing, the bill was referred to a summer study. The same language was listed in Senate Bill 3 for the 1995 Legislature which passed the Senate by a vote of 24 Yes and 10 No. But it was defeated in the House of Representatives.

Considering that 20% of a pharmacists time is devoted to handling third party prescriptions, the different kinds of insurance cards used by the patients became a real problem. President James Bregel, Chamberlain, expressed concern about this problem in 1999. He said, "One of the problems with these cards is that there is no uniformity with the information provided on the cards. Each card has it own unique style, and sometimes the information needed to process the claim is not even on the card. What is the solution? Mandate legislation which would require uniform prescription benefit cards."[27] House Bill 1189 was introduced in the 2000 Legislature to create a uniform prescription drug information card, but it was defeated. The measure was introduced again in the 2002 Legislature in Senate Bill 87. It passed and was signed into law by Governor William Janklow, effective July 1, 2002. The law authorized the South Dakota Division of Insurance to pass regulations and implement standards for a uniform prescription ID card in South Dakota.

Association President Monica Jones, Huron, in 2003 summed up the need for participation in the Legislative process: "Involvement in the political process is absolutely necessary in today's environment. With all of the changes we have seen at the state level and with discussions and debates on the national level about Medicare covering prescriptions, we need to be active in letting our Legislators know what we as pharmacists do. We need to be fairly paid for our product, but we also need to let them know what an impact our involvement in patient care can have on the outcomes of that patient. And just as importantly, we need to be paid to do it."[28]

SD Board of Pharmacy, 1990-2003

Board Philosophy

The Board of Pharmacy, consisting of Dennis M. Jones, Huron; Dale Stroschein, Sturgis; Jack Dady, Mobridge; and Lay Person Joan Hogan, Brookings, presented the philosophy of the Board at the 1992 SDPhA convention: "The Board, in acting to protect the public, does not want to be seen only as enacting laws and rules that set procedures for pharmacists to follow or as a disciplinary agency. Through regular inspections of licensed facilities, the Board hopes to raise the level of voluntary compliance to state and federal laws and rules. The provision of pharmacy services cannot be isolated from the rest of the health care services, and the board will work to insure that the health of the public is protected by pharmacists becoming an integral part of total health care system."[29]

South Dakota Statute 36-11-1, also helped define the philosophy of the Board of Pharmacy declaring, "The practice of pharmacy in South Dakota is hereby declared to be a professional practice affecting the public health, safety, and welfare and is subject to regulation in the public interest."

Administrative Changes

Board of Pharmacy Separated From South Dakota Pharmacists Association

The 1996 Legislature passed House Bill 1249 which separated the Board of Pharmacy from the South Dakota Pharmacists Association (SDPhA), that had been an administratively connected operation since 1890. The new law changed the name South Dakota Pharmaceutical Association to South Dakota Pharmacists Association. It deleted the requirement that the Association secretary also be Board of Pharmacy secretary. It also stated that the Board of Pharmacy will continue to issue the pharmacist license renewals, however, the monies so collected must be transferred to the South Dakota Pharmacists Association, which uses the renewal fees for their operation. The Board of Pharmacy will continue to collect and use other license fees to fund their operation. The Board of Pharmacy according to the new law was a separate state agency.

Galen Jordre, who had been executive secretary of both the Board of Pharmacy and the Association since 1986, resigned January 27, 1997 to take a job as executive director of the North Dakota Pharmaceutical Association. In June 1997, the Board of Pharmacy hired Dennis M. Jones, Huron, a former Board of Pharmacy member between 1987-1997, as their executive secretary. Jones, a graduate with a B.S. degree from SDSU, was in charge of the pharmacy at Huron Regional Medical Center. On December 1, 1997, he moved the Board of Pharmacy office from Pierre to Sioux Falls.

Board of Pharmacy members in 1998, consisting of Duncan Murdy, Aberdeen; Mark Graham, Mitchell; Steve Statz, Sioux Falls; Lay Person Nora Hussey, Sturgis; and Executive Secretary Dennis M. Jones, listed a number of Board responsibilities at the SDPhA convention, which included: certification of CE programs; conducting Board examinations for licensure; examining reciprocity candidates from other states; licensing pharmacists, pharmacies, non-resident pharmacies, wholesalers, vendors of non-prescription drugs, vendors of poisons; adopting budgets; administering intern regulations; enforcing laws and regulations; investigating concerns of the public expressed to the Board; holding public hearings; and administering disciplinary actions.[30]

Licensure Changes

Wholesale Drug Distributors

The Legislature in 1991, passed a law authorizing the Board of Pharmacy to license wholesale drug distributors. Wholesale drug distributors included manufacturers, jobbers, brokers, warehouses, wholesalers, and some pharmacies, delivering human prescription drugs into South Dakota. The annual license of $200 is payable to the Board of Pharmacy. The effective date of the law was January 1, 1992. In 1993, the Board issued 234 licenses to wholesalers which increased to 562 in 2003.

Non-Prescription Drugs

Since 1890, pharmacists had the exclusive right to sell all factory-packaged patent medicines as well as prescription drugs. The Legislature in 1933, however, permitted lay persons to sell factory-packaged patent medicines under a $3.00 license purchased from the Board of Pharmacy. In 1934 the board issued 599 Patent Medicine Licenses. The annual license fee was raised to $6.00 in 1964. In 1971, 1,860 Patent Medicine Licenses were issued, compared to 861 in 1996.

Only pharmacists, since 1890, could sell factory-packaged drugs listed in the United States Pharmacopoeia (U.S.P.) and National Formulary (N.F.). However, the Legislature in 1945 authorized lay persons to sell certain U.S.P. and N.F. factory-packaged drugs, called household remedy drugs. The annual $3.00 license permitted lay persons to sell twenty-two of the U.S.P. and N. F. drugs. In 1996, the Board sold 478 Household Remedy Licenses for a fee of $6.00 each.

In 1997, the Legislature repealed both the Household Remedy Law and the Patent Medicine Law and created a new class of drugs called Non-Prescription Drugs, which could be sold without a prescription. The Legislature in 1997, for the protection of public health, believed there must be some state control of the sale of the factory-packaged Non-Prescription Drugs, the same as in 1933 with Patent Medicines and in 1945 with Household Remedies. They again placed that state control with the South Dakota Board of Pharmacy. Lay persons with a $20.00 license issued by the Board, could sell Non-Prescription Drugs in their original packages.

The outside wrapper had to show the following: common name of the Non-Prescription drug, quantity of contents, adequate directions for use, adequate warnings, and name of manufacturer. In 1998, the Board of Pharmacy passed a regulation that required a lay person dealer to maintain a segregated display of the Non-Prescription Drugs. A licensed pharmacy was also required to maintain a segregated display of the Non-Prescription Drugs outside of the prescription department. In 1999 the Board issued 777 of the Non-Prescription Drug Licenses, which increased to 869 in 2003.

Nonresident Pharmacies

The South Dakota Legislature in 1997, passed a law giving authority to the Board of Pharmacy to license nonresident pharmacies. A nonresident pharmacy is one that mails or delivers any dispensed drug to a person in South Dakota, pursuant to a legally issued prescription. The license fee was set at $200 and the Board was authorized to pass rules governing nonresident pharmacies. In 1999, the Board issued 109 of the nonresident pharmacy licenses which increased to 264 in 2003.

Other Licenses Issued by the Board of Pharmacy

In 1991, the Board issued 225 full-time pharmacy licenses. Seven pharmacies had closed. Ten new pharmacies were licensed: 5 in Wal-Mart, 1 in K-Mart, 2 in Hy-Vee Food and Drug, 1 in a hospital, and 1 in a nursing home. In 1992, the Board issued 228 full-time pharmacy licenses. That year, four pharmacies had closed, and eight new pharmacies were licensed: 3 in K-Mart, 1 in Wal-Mart, 1 in Medicine Shoppe, and 3 others.

In 1993, the Board issued 230 full-time pharmacy licenses which was twenty more than the 210 issued in 2002. Presently, the fee is $200. In 1993, the Board issued 41 part-time pharmacy licenses which is similar to 42 in 2002. The fee is $160. The number of Poison Licenses issued in 1993 was 325 which had decreased to 288 in 2003.

The Board of Pharmacy also administers the yearly personal pharmacist license renewal. The fee was raised to $125 in 2001. In 2002, the board issued 1,406 personal license renewals to both in-state and out-state pharmacists. Although the license renewal fee is collected by the Board of Pharmacy, the proceeds by law, are transferred to the South Dakota Pharmacists Association.

The Board of Pharmacy finances its affairs by license and administrative fees. Their budget was $177,597 in 2000 which grew to $208,679 in 2003. The principal source of revenue for the South Dakota Pharmacists Association is from pharmacist renewal fees. The total amount from pharmacist renewal fees collected by the Board and transferred to the Association in 2002 was $168,375.

Pharmacists Licensed Since 1890
On October 1, 1890 the South Dakota Board of Pharmacy issued the first pharmacist License No. 1 to W. S. Branch, Parker, S.D. Since that time and up to October 15, 2003, 113 years, the Board has registered and licensed 5,308 pharmacists.

Patient Counseling, Patient Records, and Pharmacy Practice Act
In 1992, the Legislature passed a law requiring pharmacists, when providing a prescription to a patient, to offer counseling as to the proper use of the drug. Counseling could include information about incorrect dosage, side effects, storage, proper use, and numbers of refill.

The same law required the pharmacist to maintain a patient record system for each patient. The record must maintain the name of the drug dispensed, name and address of patient, phone, age, list of drugs used by patient, known allergies, known reactions to drugs, etc. It is required that the pharmacist consult that record before filling a patient's prescription.

In 1993, the Legislature passed the Pharmacy Practice Act listing many new standards for the practice of pharmacy. According to the statute, the practice of pharmacy means:
- interpretation and evaluation of prescription drug orders and dispensing in the patient's best interest
- provision of patient counseling and pharmaceutical care, and
- the responsibility for compounding, distributing, labeling and storage of drugs and for maintaining proper records for them.

The Legislature granted authority to the Board of Pharmacy to pass regulations pertaining to patient counseling, patient records, and practice of pharmacy and to enforce both the laws and the regulations.

Compliance with Laws and Regulations

It states in the application for a pharmacy license, "the provisions of law, and the Board of Pharmacy Rules and Regulations relative to conducting a pharmacy in the state of South Dakota, will be faithfully observed." It is incumbent upon the pharmacist applicant as well as the pharmacists employed in the licensed pharmacy to know and understand the pharmacy laws and regulations. To help pharmacists know the law and regulations, the South Dakota Pharmacists Association published *South Dakota Pharmacy Law and Information*. The eighty-page booklet can be purchased for a small fee. Pharmacy Law and Board of Pharmacy Regulations are also provided by the South Dakota Board of Pharmacy or the Legislative Research Office.

To help with compliance, the Board of Pharmacy employs two Drug Inspectors, Jack Jones of Miller, and Cliff Thomas of Belle Fourche, both hired in 1985. They are charged with inspecting pharmacies, pharmacists, wholesalers, pharmacy practices, and other Board of Pharmacy license holders. State reimbursement rates for their expenses in 2003 included $.29 a mile for private car use, $23 a day for meals, and $40 for lodging.

In 1995, the Board updated inspection forms used by the inspectors. After a pharmacy inspection, a copy of the inspection report is sent to the pharmacist owner, or if a corporation, to the corporate officer. All inspection reports are carefully reviewed by the executive secretary. The Board approved a Patient Counseling Score Sheet for use by the inspectors. These steps resulted in greater uniformity of inspections throughout the state. Drug Inspector Jack Jones, in a 1997 report to the Board, reported that many computer systems need updating to comply with Board regulations. He also reported that patient counseling is improving, but it is very limited.

In a 1999 Board report, Executive Secretary Dennis M. Jones said, "The area of greatest concern during inspections has centered on the lack of patient counseling, perpetual inventory control [of controlled substances and drugs], and resistance to development of pharmaceutical care programs. However, progress is occurring."[31] In 2001, twelve formal complaints were filed with the Board. Most of the complaints were handled by Board follow up, a letter of reprimand or corrections, or, in a few cases, hearings for pharmacists have been held to resolve reported complaints or violations found during inspections.

Some of the most frequent deficiencies found on inspection reports in 2002 included: license not displayed; incomplete prescription records; failure to provide last inventory for controlled drugs; outdated medication on shelf; computer not capable of carrying initials of a pharmacist;

incomplete patient profiles; no record of counseling the patient when issued a new prescription; and failure to document request not to use child resistant closures.[32]

Board Examinations for Licensure

Background

The first South Dakota Board of Pharmacy examinations were given in 1890-1891. They consisted of three parts: 20 questions on chemistry, 10 questions on pharmacy, and 19 questions on materia medica. The exams lasted one day starting at 9:00 a.m., and after the three main exams, the Board members united for an examination in manipulation, oral, and identification and finished by 6:00 p.m. Board members corrected the hand written exams at their homes, usually in six to eight days. A candidate was required to answer correctly not less than 65% of the questions and not less than 50% in any of the three main branches. Assistant pharmacists needed to answer correctly not less than 50% of the questions and not less than 40% in any of the three main branches. Thirty candidates qualified to take the exams that first year, 11 were registered as pharmacists, 6 were registered as assistant pharmacists, and 13 failed.

When Executive Secretary Harold H. Schuler started with the Board of Pharmacy in 1964, the exam procedure was very similar, except for more subjects, longer exams, laboratory work, and orals. Each Board member prepared their own mimeographed examinations and corrected the handwritten answers at home. Sometimes it took two to three weeks to obtain the results. Similar procedures continued until 1976 when the Board began using the NABP exam called NABPLEX.

NABPLEX AND NAPLEX

National Association Boards of Pharmacy Licensure Examination (NABPLEX) was prepared by NABP. Candidates using paper exams, used a No. 2 pencil to fill in one of the circles following the question. The five-part national exams were easy to correct, and results were available in a short time. Candidates also had to pass a paper jurisprudence examination which was prepared by members of the South Dakota Board of Pharmacy. In 1986, NABP introduced the integrated NABPLEX which had all the testing materials in one section.

NABP in 1981, also developed a Score Transfer Program whereby a candidate could transfer their score to another state in which they may wish to also be licensed. If a candidate met all the requirements of that state, their score transfer can be used as the exam requirement for registration as a pharmacist. The score transfer fee is $75 per state.

During 1992, sixty-four new pharmacists were licensed: 30 by passing NABPLEX; 18 by score transfer; and 26 by reciprocity. Seventy were newly licensed in 1993: 29 by passing NABPLEX; 27 by score transfer; and 14 by reciprocity. Although many of the pharmacists did not practice in the state, they transferred their score should they want to practice in South Dakota at a later time. Sixty-four graduates took the NABPLEX in 1995 and 96.7% passed the examination on the first try.

NABP introduced a new process whereby pharmacists can transfer their licenses between states by electronic transfer. It is a computerized program called Electronic Licensure Transfer Program (ELTP). It can be used by state boards when processing reciprocal transfers. The fee is $250 for the first state and $50 for each additional state. ELTP eliminated a lot of paperwork for NABP, Boards of Pharmacy, and pharmacists.

Because of a switch to an all Pharm.D. program, there wasn't a graduation class in 1997. However, NABPLEX was given and 17 candidates were licensed by examination and another 14 by reciprocity. A student needed a passing grade of 75%.

In 1997, NABP introduced a new examination, North American Pharmacy Licensure Examination (NAPLEX). The exam is based on the Pharm.D. six-year curriculum, testing a pharmacist's education and knowledge to provide pharmaceutical care to patients. This computer adaptive examination is given at Prometric Testing Centers, one of which is located in Sioux Falls. Candidates desiring to take the test and who meet South Dakota requirements apply to the Board of Pharmacy. The Board notifies NABP of eligible candidates. The Chauncey Group International Ltd. issues an Authorization to Test (ATT) to the candidate who then goes to the testing center to take the examination, which takes four hours and fifteen minutes. Candidates use a provided computer and can use its on-screen calculator during the test. NABP sends the test score to the Board. A grade of 75% is needed to pass. The exam fee is $250 plus a $110 vendor fee for a total of $360. NABP also provides a Multistate Pharmacy Jurisprudence Examination (MPJE) for a fee of $135. It is a two-hour computer adaptive exam. A grade of 75% is needed to pass.[33]

In 2001, forty-four candidates took the NAPLEX and all passed. Twenty-six of the candidates listed South Dakota as their home state. The South Dakota Board does not use MPJE, but administers their own law examination; however, thirty-eight states do use the MPJE exam.

Intern Rule Changes

The Board passed new regulations effective in 1996, which required interns to earn 1,500 hours of practical experience under the sanction of the College of Pharmacy's experiential [experience] program, generally through its extern and clinical pharmacy programs. However, 880 hours had to be earned in a licensed pharmacy under the supervision of a registered pharmacist.

Pharmacy students are eligible to register as an intern if they have completed one week of classes or have graduated from a college of pharmacy. The fee is $40 and is good for the entire intern period. In 2001, 134 interns were registered with the Board of Pharmacy. An intern must wear an intern badge during their practical training experience.

Board Activities

In 1995, the State Personnel Office reclassified Secretary Galen Jordre from a medical secretary to Board of Pharmacy executive secretary. The change placed the position within the same salary range as other consultant pharmacists working for the state.

The Board certified CE programs for various sponsors as follows: 102 in 1998, 126 in 1999, and 118 in 2001. The Board accepted NABP's offer in 2000 to join with them in a state newsletter. The inside sheets of the four-page newsletter, contains National Pharmacy Compliance News compiled by NABP. Outside sheets contain South Dakota Board of Pharmacy News compiled by the executive secretary. It costs the Board $523 for an issue of 1,400 copies, which includes production, printing, and mailing to in-state and out-state South Dakota pharmacists. Board members, President Steve Statz, Sioux Falls, Arvid Liebe, Milbank, and Executive Secretary Dennis M. Jones, attended the national ninety-sixth NABP meeting in Nashville, Tennessee, May 2000.

District 5 of the National Boards of Pharmacy (NABP) was created in 1937, and included representatives from Boards and Colleges of Pharmacy from four or five states including South Dakota, who met to review common problems. The group in 2001, consisted of Boards of Pharmacy from Iowa, Minnesota, Nebraska, North Dakota, South Dakota, and Manitoba, Canada. It also included the College of Pharmacy faculties from Drake, University of Iowa, University of Minnesota, Creighton University, University of Nebraska, North Dakota State University, University of Manitoba, and South Dakota State University. Board members Arvid Liebe, Milbank; Steve Statz, Sioux Falls; Duncan Murdy, Aberdeen; Nora W. Hussey, Sturgis; and Executive Secretary Dennis M. Jones, hosted representatives from District 5 in the Rushmore Plaza, at Rapid City, August 2001. The three-day meeting included CE programs; separate and joint meetings; discussions about manpower, automation, telepharmacy, and legislative issues. A trip to Mount Rushmore was also enjoyed.

A History of Pharmacy in South Dakota

Following the passage of a 1996 South Dakota law, the Board of Pharmacy, Board of Nursing, Board of Medical and Osteopathy, and Veterinary Board joined forces and established the Health Professional Assistance Program (HPAP). The program is designed to help practitioners in the four professions who have problems with depression, liquor, drug abuse, or mental impairment. During 2002, HPAP spent $57,545 to help 70 participants with impairment problems. Each board is assessed a share of the expenses depending upon the number of participants in the program from that board.

In 2000, the South Dakota Board of Pharmacy joined the Health Integrity and Protection Data Bank (HIPDB). Each health care profession, through its regulatory agency, provides information to HIPDB about health care providers whose license has been reprimanded, suspended, or revoked. Names of the pharmacists who have had their license reprimanded, suspended, or revoked are sent to NABP who in turn transmits the names to HIPDB. NABP acts as the agent for the South Dakota Board of Pharmacy. In 2000, the South Dakota Board of Pharmacy submitted the names of six pharmacists who were reprimanded or had their licenses suspended or revoked. In 2002, the national organization was called National Practitioner Data Bank-Healthcare Integrity and Protection Data Bank (NPDB-HIPDB). Data bank information is available to state and federal agencies in the United States.

In 2001, the Legislature passed a law authorizing pharmacists to give influenza immunizations. The Board of Pharmacy passed regulations in 2002 stating that a pharmacist may administer flu shots to eligible patients eighteen years of age and older, if the pharmacist has completed an approved training program for the administration of influenza immunizations. Those pharmacists that do administer flu shots must keep records in their pharmacy for five years. Some of the required information which must be documented for the record include: name, birth date, and address of patient; date of the immunization and site; name, dose, lot number and expiration date of vaccine; name of pharmacist administering vaccine; and name of health provider.

SD College of Pharmacy, 1990-2003

Administration

New Deans

Dr. Bernard E. Hietbrink, who had served as Dean of the College of Pharmacy since January 1, 1987, announced his retirement as of August 31, 1994. Dr. Gary S. Chappell was appointed acting dean while a search committee, including Mary Kuper, Sioux Falls, representing SDPhA, began the task of finding a new dean. Dr. Hietbrink had earned his B. S. degree in pharmacy from SDSU in 1958 and his Ph.D. at the University of Chicago in 1961. He began as an assistant professor in the College of Pharmacy and in thirty years worked his way up to dean. SDPhA Secretary Galen Jordre complimented Dr. Hietbrink for his excellent work as Dean College of Pharmacy, "In seven years as dean, the number of faculty has doubled, the Masters Degree in Pharmaceutical Sciences has been reinstated, and the Pharm.D. program began with the first class."[34]

During Hietbrink's time as Dean of the College of Pharmacy, the faculty grew from 14 in 1984 to 21 in 1995. The budget grew from $575,000 in 1986 to $1,627,000 in 1995. The South Dakota Pharmaceutical Association honored Dr. Hietbrink by awarding him the Honorary President's Award at the 1994 convention. Dean Hietbrink and his wife Elaine retired at Bella Vista in northwest Arkansas.

Dr. Danny L. Lattin began as the new dean July 1, 1995. He had earned his B.S. degree in pharmacy from the University of Kansas in 1965 and his Ph.D. from the University of Minnesota in 1970. Dean Lattin, who had effectively guided a growing College of Pharmacy and the new Pharm.D. program for seven years, announced his retirement effective September 30, 2002. According to a story in *The College of Pharmacy*, Lattin had, "overseen the expansion of the doctor of pharmacy degree program, made sure the college received its full accreditation from ACPE...and elevated the College to new heights, mainly due to the effective way Lattin has connected with constituents, alumni, and friends."[35] ASP Chapter President Kris Lulewicz, said, "Dean Lattin is a kind, compassionate, and caring man. We will greatly miss him."[36] Dean Lattin and his wife Ferrol, returned to Lawrence, Kansas to spend their retirement.

In the meantime, the campus learned more about two earlier deans of the College of Pharmacy. Dr.Guilford C. Gross, Bowdle, died March 21, 1997. Gross had taught at the College for over thirty years including two years as dean 1964-1965. The new pharmacy building was named after him in 1981. Former Dean Raymond E. Hopponen was awarded the title of professor and dean of pharmacy emeritus by the Board of Regents in December 1999. Hopponen had served as dean from February 1, 1966 until his retirement on June 30, 1986. During his term as dean, "more than 1,000 students earned pharmacy degrees, the Guilford C. Gross Pharmacy Building was constructed, the faculty more than doubled, and SDSU became a national pioneer in placing pharmacy students in a workplace setting as a part of the required curriculum."[37]

Dr. Brian L. Kaatz, was appointed acting dean of the College of Pharmacy on October 1, 2002. In November, 2002 a thirteen-member search committee announced three finalists for the deanship, one of whom was Dr. Brian Kaatz. The search committee consisted of members from SDPhA, Board of Pharmacy, SDSU faculty, and College of Pharmacy faculty. Later, the committee recommended Dr. Brian Kaatz for the position. On March 13, 2003, the Board of Regents named Dr. Kaatz, Dean of SDSU College of Pharmacy. Kaatz earned his B.S. degree in pharmacy from SDSU in 1974, and his Doctor of Pharmacy degree from the University of Minnesota in 1977. He had worked as a clinical pharmacist in a South Dakota hospital pharmacy and was professor and head of the Department of Clinical Pharmacy, at SDSU College of Pharmacy.

Dr. Kaatz was honored by his SDPhA colleagues when they presented him with the Hustead Award at the 2001 convention in Pierre. The honor recognized his thirteen years of service to SDSU and the Association. In 2003, he received the APhA Good Government Pharmacist-of-the-Year Award. The award recognized his work, during a July-December 2000 sabbatical, as a Senior Health Care Policy Fellow for United States Senator Tim Johnson. Kaatz helped educate the senator and his staff about the impact pharmacists can have on improved health outcomes for patients. Consequently, Senator Johnson introduced Senate Bill 974, the Medicare Pharmacist Services Coverage Act. Medicare only pays pharmacists to fill prescriptions, however, Johnson's bill would have expanded that to paying for pharmacists' patient care services. Brian and his wife Joyce, have two grown children, David and Julie.

Faculty
Between 1924 and 1935 the average enrollment in the College of Pharmacy was 73, and the average number of faculty for the same period was between three and four. Of course, the number of students enrolled in the professional school, as well as available monies, helped determine the number of faculty needed for instruction. However, here are some representative years showing the number of faculty on duty in the College of Pharmacy: 6 in 1954; 8 in 1968; 14 in 1984; 21 in 1995; and 31 in 2002.

In 1990, Dean Hietbrink began a program to recognize outstanding faculty in the College of Pharmacy. Those recognized in 1995 were: David Helgeland, MBA, for Service to Students; Mustapha Beleh, Ph.D. for Classroom Teaching; Paul Price, Pharm. D. for Individual Teaching; Kalpana Kamath, Ph.D. for Research and Scholarship; and Brian Kaatz, Pharm.D. for Service to the Profession.

Those faculty who were recognized in 2001 were: Dr. Thomas J. Johnson, Classroom Teaching; Dr. James R. Clem, Individual Teaching;

Dr. Janet R. Fischer, Innovative Teaching; Dr. Rajender R. Aparasu, Research and Scholarship; Mr. Gary C. Van Riper, Service to the Profession; Dr. Chandradhar Dwivedi, Service to Students (Dwivedi had been named Teacher of the Year in 2000); and Dr. Debra K. Farver, Special Service.

Further recognition of faculty in 2001 included Dr. David Helgeland who was promoted to associate professor of Pharmaceutical Sciences and awarded tenure; Dr. Wendy Bender was promoted to associate professor of Clinical Pharmacy; associate professors Dr. Rajender Aparasu and Dr. Xiangming Guan were both awarded tenure. Dr. Debra K. Farver was promoted to professor Clinical Pharmacy; and Dr. Kim Messerschmidt was promoted to associate professor in Clinical Pharmacy. Dr. Bruce Currie on July 1, 2001 was named Head of the Department of Pharmaceutical Sciences. Dean Emeritus Bernard Hietbrink was named Distinguished Alumnus in 2001.

Two faculty members were elected to offices in 2001: Shelly Pulscher, Department of Clinical Pharmacy, was elected secretary-treasurer of the South Dakota Pharmacists Association; and Gary Van Riper, Department of Pharmaceutical Sciences, was elected secretary of the South Dakota Society of Health-System Pharmacists.

The 2002 organizational chart lists Dean Danny Lattin in charge of two main divisions: Pharmaceutical Sciences, with Dr. Bruce Currie as Head; and Clinical Pharmacy, with Dr. Brian Kaatz as Head. One area of faculty growth was in the field of Clinical Pharmacy. That growth began when the Board of Pharmacy passed regulations in 1972 permitting intern students to earn up to 400 hours concurrent with attendance in the College of Pharmacy. Former Dean Ray Hopponen said, "until this innovation in 1972, the pharmacy curriculum didn't extend beyond the campus. This change had students spend one semester of their five-year program off campus...between working with the clinical pharmacist, the hospital pharmacist, and the community pharmacist."[38] By 1996, students could earn all of their 1,500 hours of intern time under the sanction of the College of Pharmacy, however, 800 of those hours had to be earned in licensed pharmacies.

Recruiting and retaining faculty has always been a challenging problem at the College of Pharmacy. Dean Danny L. Lattin reported in 2002, that to maintain an "adequate numbers of highly qualified pharmacy faculty, the College of Pharmacy must have the resources to retain current and in attracting new faculty [for] the numbers of students presently being admitted to the professional program. A very serious differential...exists currently between salaries at our College of Pharmacy and those in the practice sector, as well as for salaries at other colleges and schools of pharmacy. The amount of the gap has increased dramatically since 1998. Furthermore, five colleges of pharmacy have opened since 1995. All of these new academic institutions are competing for an inadequate national supply of pharmaceutical science and clinical pharmacy faculty."[39]

Gary Van Riper, editor of *The College of Pharmacy* reported, "The pharmacy graduation class of May 2001 showed an average starting salary of $71,000 in the private sector. By comparison, the College recently hired a new professor with two years of post-graduate training for $62,000."[40] A campaign was started in January 2002 to provide additional funds to keep and attract quality faculty. The fund drive was formulated by Dean Lattin and the Pharmacy Advisory Council. Later, a ten-member development committee directed a campaign to raise a three-million dollar endowment to keep and attract faculty.

A Dean's Club was started in 1989 to strengthen programs and provide scholarships. Those contributing from $250 to $499 received a brass desk plaque inscribed with their name. Fifty-six contributed to the club in 1994. Another important and active group is the fifteen-member College of Pharmacy Advisory Council. Membership includes five each from the following groups: SDPhA, SDSHP, and Alumni. Recent chairpersons of the Advisory Council include Ron Johnson, Mitchell; Pam Jones, Huron; and David Kruger, Lake Bluff, Ill.

A 1969 SDSU College of Pharmacy graduate, Dennis Ludwig, Boulder, Colorado, was elected president of the National Community Pharmacists Association (NCPA) [formerly NARD] at the 1997 convention in New Orleans.

Pharm.D. Program

The degree programs offered at the College of Pharmacy have passed through various stages throughout the years: two-year Ph.G. 1893-1924; three-year Ph.C. 1918-1930; four-year B. S. 1931-1959; and five-year B.S. 1960-1994. Sixty-one students graduated with the five-year B. S. in Pharmacy May 1994.

A movement was growing around the country to establish a six-year Pharm. D. program. Delegates at the American Association of Colleges of Pharmacy gathering in 1992, voted 92 Yes to 57 No to adopt the Doctor of Pharmacy as the entry level degree to the profession. Pharmacists at the 1992 SDPhA convention, endorsed the Pharm.D. program. The members of SDSHP unanimously supported the Pharm. D. program at their 1992 convention. Representatives from SDPhA and the Board of Pharmacy appeared before the Board of Regents registering their support for the new program. The Board of Regents agreed to ask a consultant team to visit the SDSU College of Pharmacy to determine if a Pharm.D. program could be established.

SDPhA Executive Secretary Galen Jordre said there is a need for the six-year Pharm.D. program because, "Society is demanding more from pharmacists, and pharmacists must be prepared to meet the challenge. The pharmacy profession is embracing the concept of 'pharmaceutical care'— improving therapeutic outcomes and helping patients make the best use of their medications. Pharmacists must be equipped to deliver pharmaceutical care in both community and institutional settings."[41]

The consultant team of three College of Pharmacy Deans, from University of Kentucky, University of Illinois at Chicago, and Idaho State University, visited the campus and clinical sites April 21 and 22, 1992. Later, they strongly recommended the Doctor of Pharmacy program at the College of Pharmacy. On March 19, 1993, the Regents approved the six-year Pharm.D. as the entry level degree to be offered in the fall of 1994.

The College of Pharmacy started a program between 1994-1998, whereby former B. S. degree graduates could return to school and take course work to complete the Pharm.D. degree. The first ten, following a hooding ceremony, graduated with a post B.S. Pharm.D. degree May 6, 1995. The graduates were: Del Mandl, Wendy Jensen, John Theobald, Stacie Tomkins, Kathy Lynch, Mary Tom, Becky Baer, Telene Bettcher, Kim Messerschmidt, and Mary Tasler. The last group with post B.S. Pharm.D. degrees would graduate in May 1998. During the period, thirty-one pharmacists obtained their Pharm.D. degree. There was no graduating class in 1997. The first six-year all Pharm.D. class would graduate in May 1998.

An entry level Pharm.D. class of fifty students had been selected from 163 applicants in the fall of 1994. The class, with a 3.54 GPA, consisted of 42 SDSU students and 8 transfers. It included 31 women and 19 men. A M. S. in Pharmaceutical Sciences program also began in the fall of 1994. The graduating 1998 Pharm.D. class consisted of 45 students, 28 women and 17 men. In the 2001 graduating class, there were 45 who graduated at the May 4 hooding ceremony. Eighteen accepted positions in South Dakota: 14 in community practice and 4 in hospital practice. The class consisted of 12 men and 33 women.

Twenty-six women and 16 men graduated with their Pharm.D. in the spring of 2000. That fall, the College of Pharmacy accepted 60 in the professional school instead of 50. The curriculum consisted of a two-year pre-pharmacy and a four-year professional school. In May 2003, 47 graduated: 8 of whom continued their education. Of the remaining 39, 85%

A History of Pharmacy in South Dakota

entered community practice, 10% hospital practice, and 5% were undecided. Forty percent of the 39, began their careers in South Dakota. Dean Kaatz said, "For the fifth time, each graduate that took the licensure exam passed on the first try. We have a 100% rate going for the fifth year in a row. We are in the very highest tier of average scores, as compared to the other eighty-three schools of pharmacy."[42]

Dean Brian Kaatz reported in 2003, that the ACPE accreditation team visited the College of Pharmacy in September 2002. He said, "The accreditation term granted for the Doctor of Pharmacy program extends until July 2009, a full six-year cycle. They recognized the high quality of our program. They also pointed out we need to begin thinking about future improvements in our classroom, laboratory, and office spaces."[43]

Externship and Clinical Pharmacy Intern Program

In 1996, the Board of Pharmacy further expanded the role of the College of Pharmacy in the intern training program. Their regulation stated that all of the required 1,500 hours of practical experience could be acquired as part of the college-based experiential program, if the intern is enrolled as a student in the College of Pharmacy. However, 800 of those hours had to be earned working in a licensed pharmacy where the primary work involved interpreting prescription orders; dispensing prescription orders; reviewing patient medication profiles; communicating with the patients; and managing a pharmacy. There were 134 interns registered with the Board of Pharmacy in 2001 and 160 in 2002. Dr. Dennis Hedge, Associate Professor of Clinical Pharmacy, was selected as the 1998 Teacher of the Year by the pharmacy student body.

The Clinical Pharmacy faculty of the College of Pharmacy implements both an intern training program at the College of Pharmacy and at community and institutional pharmacies around the state. According to the SDSU College of Pharmacy Web-Site, "the Department of Clinical Pharmacy provides classroom and clerkship instruction for the last two years of the (Pharm.D.) degree program. Faculty are located at various practice sites which provides students the opportunity for diverse learning experiences. The Department of Pharmaceutical Sciences provides a firm foundation in the pharmaceutical sciences leading to the Doctor of Pharmacy (Pharm.D.) degree."

The P4 (senior year) program for fifty-eight students in 2003 is representative of the intern training program at the College of Pharmacy. Bernard Hendricks, Clinical Pharmacy Instructor and Continuing Education Coordinator, supervises a student rotation program that acquaints the students with all aspects of pharmacy. Hendricks, who started with the College of Pharmacy in 1982, states that the rotation program, running from May to May, for a period of forty-four weeks, requires each student to complete ten different rotations. The rotation program, which had been an elective, became a requirement in May 2002.

The twenty members of the Clinical Pharmacy Department faculty at SDSU serve as preceptors at community and institutional pharmacies for the following required four week rotations:

Internal Medicine I (4 weeks)

Community Pharmacy Care (4 weeks)

Ambulatory Care (4 weeks) or Internal Medicine II (4 weeks)

Three of the following—(each 4 weeks) Pediatrics, Psychiatry, Critical Care, Infectious Disease, Geriatrics, Directed Studies

Two of the following electives—(each 4 weeks) Oncology, Home Health, Pharmacy Administration, IHS, Cardiology, Nephrology, Pharmacokinetics, Managed Care, Nuclear Pharmacy, or Directed Studies.

Licensed pharmacists (non-SDSU faculty) also serve as preceptors for the six-week rotation in community pharmacies. Some of the community pharmacy sites are: Walgreen's and K-Mart in Sioux Falls; Thrifty White in Brookings; Wal-Mart in Pierre; Medicine Shoppe in Yankton; Pioneer Drug in Elk Point; and Liebe Drug in Milbank.

Licensed pharmacists (non-SDSU faculty) serve as preceptors for the six-week rotation in institutional pharmacies. Some of the institutional pharmacy sites are: McKennan Hospital in Sioux Falls; Rapid City Regional Hospital; and Sacred Heart Hospital in Yankton.[44]

Generally the rotation program meets the 1500 hour practical experience requirement to take the Board of Pharmacy examinations. Some fourth-year professional (P4) students, depending on their electives, may need to earn some intern time during the summer, to meet the required 800 hours of the intern time earned in licensed community or hospital pharmacies.

Each year the members of the College of Pharmacy Externship Program select one of the voluntary pharmacist preceptors, at either the community or institutional six-week rotations, as the Preceptor of the Year.

Preceptors of the Year

1983 Ron Nelson, St. Joseph's Hospital, Mitchell

1984 William Ladwig, Lewis Westgate, Sioux Falls

1985 Brian McFarland, Snyder Clinic, Brookings

1986 Paul Sinclair, Liebe Drug, Milbank

1987 Dennis M. Jones, Huron Regional Medical Center, Huron
1988 Ken Main, Kendall's Drug, Brookings
1989 Don Munce, Lewis Eastgate, Sioux Falls
1990 Thomas Carlson, Ray's Snyder Drug, Brookings
1991 Margaret Zard, Shopko, Mitchell
1992 Dana Darger, St. Mary's Hospital, Pierre
1993 Elizabeth Pettersen, VA Hospital, Sioux Falls
1994 Tim Gallagher, Yankton Rexall Drug, Sioux Falls
1995 Elizabeth Lechner, VA Hospital Pharmacy, Sioux Falls
1996 Elizabeth Lechner, VA Hospital Pharmacy, Sioux Falls
1997—
1998 Laurie Garry, Queen of Peace Hospital Pharmacy, Mitchell
1999 Mike Talley, Rapid City Regional Hospital Pharmacy, Rapid City
2000 Julie Lindgren, Osco Pharmacy, Sioux Falls
2001 Tom Iverson, Safeway Pharmacy, Rapid City
2002 Christopher Sonnenschein, Lewis Drug, Sioux Falls
2003 Shelly Pulscher, Hot Springs VA Medical Center, Hot Springs

College of Pharmacy Publications

A March 16, 1920 issue *Industrial Collegian* carried a 'Pharmic Special' that five pharmics were on the 1919 SDSU football team. Recent publications of the College of Pharmacy included *Focus on Pharmacy*, started in 1986. The eight-page newsletter-style format reviewed activities about the College of Pharmacy, its students, and its alumni. Gary C. Van Riper was the editor. Over 3,500 copies were distributed to friends of pharmacy. Its publication costs were supported by pharmacy friends and alumni.

In 1997, the College of Pharmacy Advisory Council, Dean Danny L. Lattin, and Editor Gary C. Van Riper changed the publication to a magazine-style format. The first issue of the new magazine, *The College of Pharmacy*, was printed in the Spring of 1997. It contained a color cover, table of contents, feature stories with color, lists of alumni contributors, names of graduates, and pharmacy news in general. Over 3,500 copies of the well-written and well- prepared magazine were printed by the College of Pharmacy with the financial support of alumni and friends. The 1997 title page shows the following persons responsible for its publication: Dean Danny L. Lattin; Head of Clinical Pharmacy, Brian L. Kaatz; Head of Pharmaceutical Sciences, Gary S. Chappell; Coordinator for Alumni

Affairs, James E. Powers; Editor, Gary C. Van Riper; Co-editor, Nan Steinley; Graphics, Virginia Coudron; Writers/Photographers, Kate Gundvaldson, Jennifer Widman, and Brent McCown; and Publications Editor, Dan Tupa.

The College of Pharmacy began a weekly column in 1992 in the *South Dakota Medical Journal* called "Pharmacology Focus". Contributors are from the Department of Clinical Pharmacy faculty.

Student Activities

Campus Pharmacy Organizations
Alpha Kappa Chapter of Phi Lambda Sigma was formed on the campus on October 28, 1991. The society, promoting leadership in pharmacy, placed third in Phi Lambda Sigma Leadership Challenge competition at the APhA convention in Los Angeles, March 1997. Eight new members were initiated in September 1998. More than $500 was contributed for the Cystic Fibrosis Foundation from the proceeds of a bowl-a-thon in March 1999. In January 2002, the chapter submitted a leadership challenge application and gave a poster presentation on it at the national meeting in March at San Francisco. They won the Leadership Challenge plaque and $500. According to their President Teresa Seefeldt, the challenge for 2003 is to develop a leadership workshop emphasizing stress management and task delegation for pharmacy students. Dr. David Helgeland is the Phi Lambda Sigma adviser.

Dr. Gary Chappell was elected Outstanding Chapter Adviser for the Academy of Students of Pharmacy (ASP) in 1989. He began advising the group in 1975 and continued through 1993. During that time the chapter won the national Outstanding Chapter Award ten times: 1979, 1983-89, and 1991-1992. ASP Chapter was awarded the Chapter Achievement Award in 2000. Dr. Chappell, former Head of the Pharmaceutical Sciences Department, retired at the end of the 1999-2000 school year. The Chapter in 2001 had 170 members. In the spring of 2002, ASP members attended the annual Legislative Days in Pierre where they performed diabetes, blood pressure, and cholesterol screenings for Legislators and staff. President Erin Koopman that same year reported the group held the annual charity auction to benefit Berakhah House and Children's Inn at Sioux Falls. In October 2003, President Kris Lulewicz and twenty-three members made the trip to an ASP Region V midyear meeting in Omaha. They won the Traveling Trophy for most students in attendance from a chapter. Present ASP advisers are: Dr. Rebecca Baer, Dr. Kelley Keller, and Dr. James Clem.

Tau Chapter received the Award for Sustained Contribution from the National Rho Chi Society in 1995. They were also awarded first place for

Academic Excellence by SDSU and the South Dakota Board of Regents. In April 1999, Tau Chapter of Rho Chi inducted eleven new members at an initiation banquet in Walder Room, University Student Union. The new members were: Krista Beastrom, Joan Case, David Gums, Cassi Houska, Jacqulene Howley, Cathy Koch, Emily LaBay, Jodi Meerbeek, Mary Quenzer, Susan Rosenau, and Carla Schwensohn. The chapter in 2000-2001 offered free tutoring services to all interested students in the College of Pharmacy. Tau Chapter in 2002, again received the Board of Regents Award for Academic Excellence. Only students in the top 20% of their class in the spring of their second professional year (P2) are eligible for membership in the academic honor society. Present Rho Chi advisers are: Dr. Chandradhar Dwivedi and Dr. Brian Kaatz.

In 1995, Kappa Psi members participated in two blood drives in Brookings, decorated the pharmacy float for Hobo Days, and raised money for the Make-A-Wish Foundation. The Gamma Kappa Chapter of Kappa Psi voted in 1999 to pledge women as members. They also participated in an Adopt-A-Highway Program for a section of U. S. Highway 14. Regent Scott Bergman reported that the chapter in 2002 made Valentine's Day and Halloween door decorations for the Ronald McDonald House. The group held its first annual Kappa Psi/College of Pharmacy Scholarship Golf Tournament. In November, the chapter sponsored a campus blood drive to help relieve the blood shortage. Vicki Riemer, Owatonna, MN, a P2 student, won $1,000 Kappa Psi scholarship for leadership capabilities and academic success. Vice Regent Thomas K. Chiu, attended Legislative Days in Pierre and joined with other students to conduct blood glucose, blood cholesterol, and blood-pressure checks on Legislators. In September 2003, the chapter hosted a GVR Fest, a three-day celebration in honor of their distinguished Grand Council Deputy, Gary Van Riper, chapter adviser.

During 1995, Kappa Epsilon teamed up with ASP to host a Wellness Fair booth explaining what questions patients should ask their pharmacists. During the fall and spring rush, 32 new members were initiated. The pledges visited the elderly, sold raffle tickets, held a bake sale, and met for pizza. Members of Kappa Epsilon, a pharmacy fraternity for women, delivered ten painted pumpkins to the residents of local nursing homes in 1999. In 2002, President Angie Fouts and several members attended Kappa Epsilon national convention where they received the Outstanding Collegiate Chapter Award for Chi Chapter. Members that same year, promoted breast-cancer awareness, volunteered for Habitat for Humanity, and picked up litter for the Adopt-A-Highway program. In the spring of 2003, the College of Pharmacy held a retirement party for Chi Chapter

Kappa Epsilon adviser Dr. Joye Ann Billow. A number of the Chi sisters attended to show their appreciation for her twenty-nine years serving as Chi Chapter adviser and for her contributions to the College of Pharmacy. Dr. Billow, although retired, continued as Chi Chapter adviser. She began her service with them in 1973. Membership then was five which grew to sixty-three in 2002.

Scholarship and Awards Night

One of the outstanding College of Pharmacy events had been the Annual Pharmacy Dinner Dance where scholarships and awards were presented. During an event, held in March 1992, $29,000 in scholarships and awards were presented to worthy students. Dean Hietbrink noted an 80% increase in the value of the scholarships in the past five years. Over $35,000 was awarded in 1993. The Dean Hietbrink Scholarship Fund was created upon his retirement in 1994. By 1995, the fund had grown to $14,164, large enough to provide one scholarship at the 1995 awards banquet. At the 1995 event, the name Annual Pharmacy Dinner Dance was changed to Annual Scholarship and Awards Banquet. Seven awards and thirty-eight scholarships were given at the 1998 event.

The College of Pharmacy distributed over $60,000 in scholarships and awards in 2002, including $10,800 raised by the phonathon. The distribution included nine new scholarships, one of which was the Jack M. Bailey endowed scholarship. Bailey served on the Board of Pharmacy 1976-1981 and was awarded the Bowl of Hygeia in 1982.

Mrs. Marilyn Eighmy, administrative assistant to the dean, was presented the Distinguished Service Award by the South Dakota Pharmaceutical Association in 1999. Marilyn started in her position on July 1, 1969 and retired in 2003. Betty Behrends was appointed administrative assistant to the dean that same year.

Phonathon

The first phonathon was held in 1987 where 671 friends of pharmacy pledged $21,000. Proceeds from the annual phonathon had grown to $50,000 in 1994 and to $60,000 in 1996. Funds raised in 1998 were distributed as follows: $7,400 scholarships; $4,900 grants to student organizations; $35,964 for faculty development; $5,987 for the magazine *The College of Pharmacy*; and $4,877 to Pharmacy Advisory Council and activity support. In 2002, seventy-five students worked the phones and raised $70,329.

Pharmacy Days and Opportunities Night

Pharmacy Days began in 1983. Dean Ray Hopponen set a December date for employers to interview members of the 1984 graduating class. It was held in two rooms of the Career and Academic Planning Center. Because of extra space needs, it was moved to the Student Union in 1990. It continued throughout the years and in November 1992, twenty employers interviewed students at Pharmacy Days held on the campus. Pharmacy Days organizer Gary C. Van Riper explained the procedure for the 2001 event: "There are three aspects to Pharmacy Days. The first night is for students who are seeking internships. Virtually all of the school's 110 third and fourth-year students spent time with some of the twenty-seven employers on hand November 1. An internship, which is required for licensure, also can be attractive financially, with some firms offering $20 per hour for summer internships. The second night is a time for the sixth-year students to get acquainted with prospective employers. Interviews are held the following day. Emily Ingalls of Baltic had interviews with eight firms. Classmate Cassi Houska of Pukwana had six. Each are pursuing retail opportunities."[45]

Pharmacy Days Career Fair was held October 30-31, 2003 in the Student Union Ballroom. A number of employers, including Bill Ladwig, vice president of professional services at Lewis Drug, Sioux Falls, interviewed students. Ladwig said, "For me, this (Pharmacy Days) is a social exchange with the students. It's a networking. You get to know a couple good students."[46]

Another night for students to meet employers is at South Dakota Pharmacy Opportunities Night, which was started in 2002. This time, however, the program is organized to provide pharmacy students with information about career opportunities in South Dakota. It is held ahead of Pharmacy Days so that South Dakota employers get first chance to meet with the pharmacy graduates. The agenda for October 6, 2002 in the Volstorff Ballroom, University Student Union, included opening remarks at 4:00 p.m.; presentation of employers at 4:30 p.m.; buffet at 5:30 p.m.; and small groups for personal interviews at 6:15 p.m. Sixteen in-state employers and forty students from the first through the fourth year of the professional school were present. The event is hosted by the College of Pharmacy, SDPhA, SD Society of Health-System Pharmacists, and Jewett Drug, Aberdeen.

Pharmacy Class Makes History at SDSU

Fifty-seven pharmacy students made history Jan. 8 when they participated in the first annual College of Pharmacy White Coat Ceremony at South Dakota State University.

"We are making history together," said Brian Kaatz, dean of the SDSU College of Pharmacy, adding that this is the first in what will hopefully become an annual tradition at State.

"The white coat ceremony symbolizes the student's transition from being a regular student into being a professional," said Dr. Jane Mort, chairperson of the committee that organized the event.

Mort, professor of clinical pharmacy at SDSU, said that recognizing professionalism among students is a rising trend in colleges of pharmacy throughout the nation.

"It is very important to acknowledge and honor the students' transition into a professional. It's a step that we want to make sure all students recognize they are taking," she said. Because of this emphasis on professionalism, Mort said more colleges are hosting ceremonies like the white coat.

Students receive their white coats during their first year in the professional pharmacy program, after completing at least two years of pre-pharmacy coursework.

Mort said that some colleges award students their white coats at the beginning of their first year of pharmacy school. However, students at SDSU received their coats in January, in the middle of their first year, to allow them a "better sense" of what they are committing to.

Around 200 people attended the event. Planning for the ceremony began in September. A committee of four faculty members and one student, along with pharmacy department staff members, organized the event. Walgreens sponsored the ceremony. The sponsorship included the provision of funds for the white coats, which featured the Campanile logo as well as the words "SDSU College of Pharmacy."

At the ceremony, Kaatz explained that the white coat, a symbol of a student's journey into professionalism, is an "outward expression of aspirations" as well as a "visual attempt" to represent bigger ideas, such as altruism and responsibility.

"While wearing these coats, you will get more and more responsibilities over the next three and a half years," said Kaatz. "While wearing these coats, you will find yourselves in some tough spots. You will be nervous, challenged and even a little afraid from time to time. But, importantly, while wearing these white coats, you will be looked upon by many people for answers, for guidance and for help."

Keynote speaker Victoria Roche, associate dean for administration at the Creighton University School of Pharmacy and Health Professions, said "White coat ceremonies are all about a public commitment to professionalism."

A professor of pharmaceutical sciences, Roche compared professionalism to a tapestry, stating that, as a tapestry is a thing of beauty that is proudly displayed, students should display the visible signs of a professional. Roche encouraged students to "take the high road" in actions, words, deeds and language. She compared the backing of a tapestry to the attitudes, beliefs and values, such as honesty, accountability and respect, which support and make possible what the public sees in a pharmacy professional.

In addition, Roche told students to learn from faculty and other pharmacy professionals.

"Watch them. Emulate them. Talk with them. Challenge them. And make them proud to recognize you as a deserving fellow in the great community of pharmacy," she said.

"Keep the magic and the passion of this white coat ceremony alive for as long as you practice."

Tiffany Hoffman of Platte, a representative for the class, worked as a technician prior to receiving her white coat. Now, she said, "You actually do get more respect from the customers. They realize that you are an authority."

Hoffman said the general consensus from the class was that the students appreciated the ceremony and were glad they participated. The first semester was difficult for many, she said, and the event provided some helpful recognition from parents, pharmacists and fellow classmates.

"You start to feel a little bit of that respect as soon as you wear the coat," said fellow class representative John Kappes of Sioux Falls. "It's a symbol of the profession and, without that, you're just another person working."

Kappes said that the students are still getting to know one another and the ceremony helped promote class unity.

"We had fun," said Kappes. "Getting the class together is always a good time." Both Hoffman and Kappes said that parents appreciated the ceremony as well.

"I hope that they continue to do it for future years," Hoffman said.

Students who participated in the ceremony were:

Alcester: Carrie Larsen.
Arlington: Sara Spilde.
Bridgewater: Rachel Paweltzki.
Brookings: Rebecca Bitter, Tyler Bryant, Tamara Burt, Jerri Cox, Kate
Englin, Jess Haensel, Angela Livingston, Andrea Schmidt, Daniel Sneeden,

Angela Taylor, Thomas Thorne and Crystal Todd.
Chamberlain: Danielle Dykes.
Elk Point: Angela Curry.
Estelline: Rebecca Meyer.
Mitchell: Leah Bartscher, Tara Jones and Tara Miiller.
Pierre: Jocqueline Herman and Krista Schmidt.
Platte: Tiffany Hoffman.
Rowena: Amanda Funke.
Sioux Falls: Misti Albers, Myla Anderson, Craig Beers, Craig Brodie, Joseph Buren, Kallie Dunlap, Steffanie Gramlick, Karin Jacobson, John Kappes and Daniel Pratt.
Valley Springs: Robyn Dump.
Watertown: Scott Roby.
White: Jacob Hoefler.
Wolsey: Jenilee Johnson.
Yankton: Beth Goeden and Gregory Kotschegarow.

Alta, Iowa: Jessica Loehr.
Buffalo Center, Iowa: Carmen Garst.
Sioux City, Iowa: Krasen Boshnakov.
Storm Lake, Iowa: Lori Sorensen.

Buffalo Lake, Minn.: Heather DeRock.
Fairmont, Minn.: Sara Fowler.
Mankato, Minn.: Jessica Johns and Sarah Rothi.
Minneota, Minn.: Melissa Gorecki and Danielle Hennen.
New Hope, Minn.: Manisha Besterwitch.
Perham, Minn.: Gregory Delaney.
St. Cloud, Minn.: Jeffrey Jonas.

Crofton, Neb.: Michael Kuchta and Gregory Peitz.
Lincoln, Neb.: Heidi Hejl.
Ponca, Neb.: Jamie Keller.

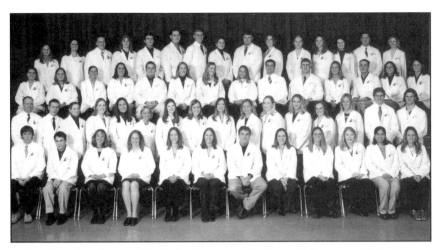

The first class to participate in the annual College of Pharmacy White Coat Ceremony at South Dakota State University on Jan. 8, 2004.

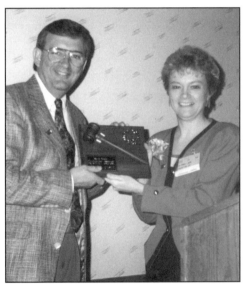

SDPhA Past President Terry Casey receives his gavel from President Jocelyn Prang at the 1991 Chamberlain convention.

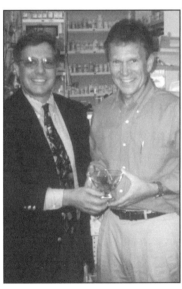

NARD representative John Rector, met with U. S. Senator Tom Daschle at the 2001 Sioux Falls SDPhA convention

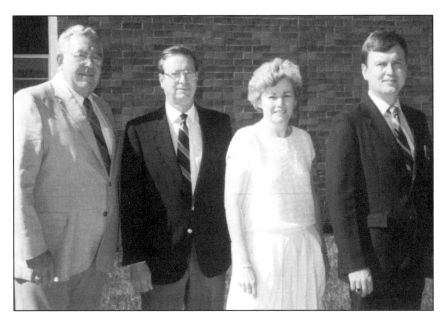

Board of Pharmacy members left to right, Jack Dady, Robert Gregg, Joan Hogan, and Dennis M. Jones prepare for a 1991 meeting at the College of Pharmacy. Jones was named executive secretary of the Board in 1997.

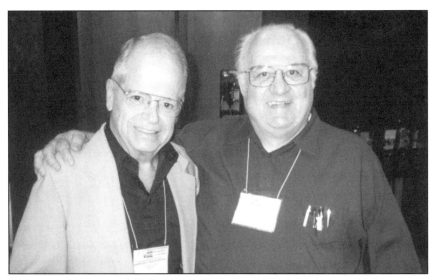

Jack Jones and Cliff Thomas, have served as Drug Inspectors for the Board of Pharmacy since 1985.

A History of Pharmacy in South Dakota

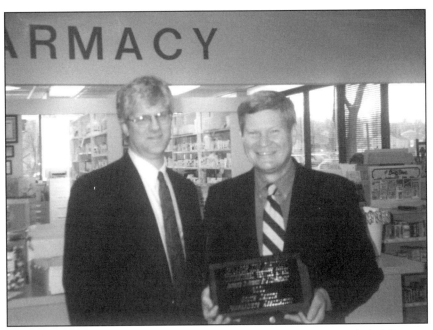

Dr. Brian Kaatz, left, and U. S. Senator Tim Johnson. The senator is holding an award he received from SDPhA in November 2001. Dr. Kaatz was named Dean SDSU College of Pharmacy in 2003.

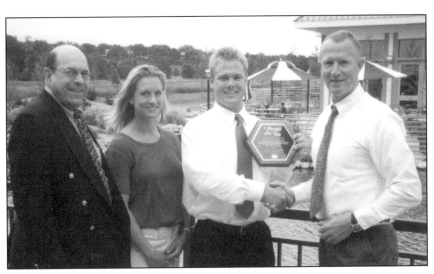

SDSU College of Pharmacy Externship Coordinator Bernard Hendricks, right, congratulates Pharm.D. Chris Sonnenschein upon being named Preceptor of the Year for 2002. Chris is with Lewis Drug, Sioux Falls. Dean Danny Lattin, and Mrs. Chris Sonnenschein are observers of the proceedings.

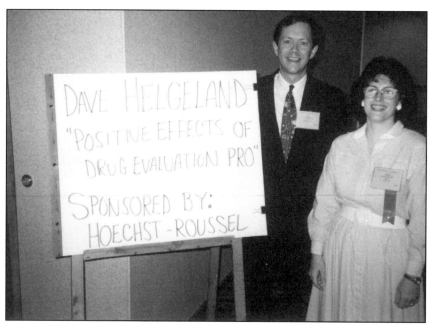

Dave Helgeland, SDSU College of Pharmacy, ready to speak at the 1994 convention. Standing at his right is Terri McEntaffer, who later served as Executive Director of SDPhA in 1997-1999.

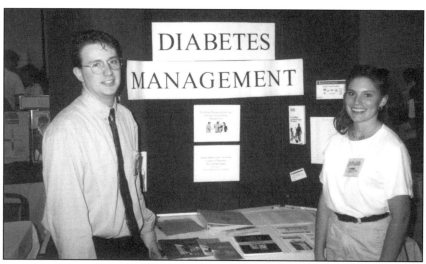

Scott Stizman and Jenna Fleeger, students at SDSU College of Pharmacy, display information on a diabetes care plan as part of Phi Lambda Sigma Leadership Challenge. 1996 photo.

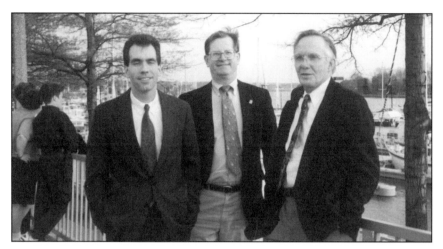

SDPhA officer Tim Gallagher, Executive Secretary Galen Jordre, and Dean Bernard Hietbrink, enjoying the scenery at a May 1993 national pharmaceutical meeting.

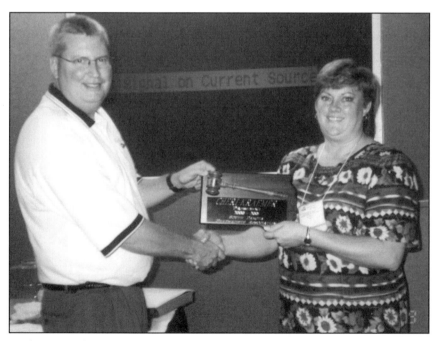

SDPhA Executive Director Robert Coolidge, 2000-2002, presents a gavel to retiring President Cheri Kraemer at the 2001 convention.

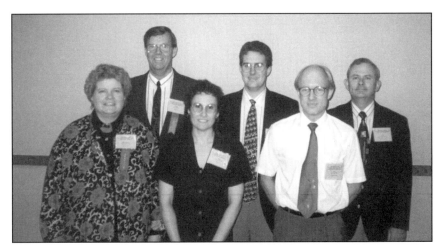

1995 SDPhA officers, left to right, Past President Margaret Zard, President Robert Wik, Pam Jones, Mark Gerdes, James Bregel, and Earl McKinstry. All were involved in incorporation of South Dakota Pharmacists Association.

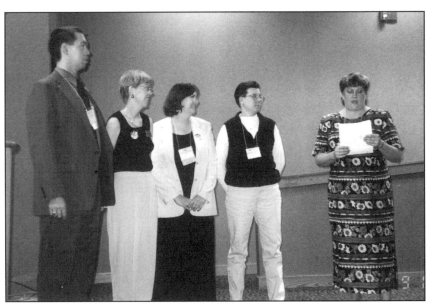

2001 SDPhA officers, left to right, President Steve Aamot, President-elect Karla Overland-Janssen, First Vice President Monica Jones, Treasurer Julie Meintsma, and Past President Cheri Kraemer. Second Vice President Shane Clarambeau not available when picture taken.

A History of Pharmacy in South Dakota

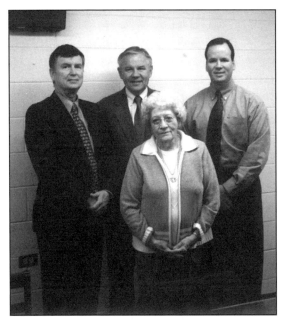

2003-2004 Board of Pharmacy, left to right, Dennis M. Jones, Executive Secretary; Arvid Liebe; Nora Hussey; and Stephen Statz. Duncan Murdy not available when picutre taken.

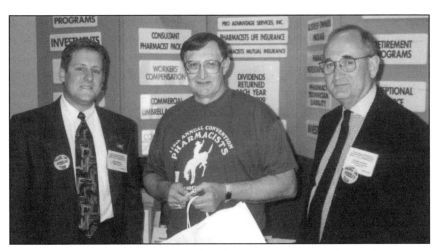

Pharmacists Mutual booth at 1996 Chamberlain convention. Pharmacist Everett Randall, Redfield, center. Representatives of Pharmacists Mutual, on left, Todd Westby, on right, Dan Carter.

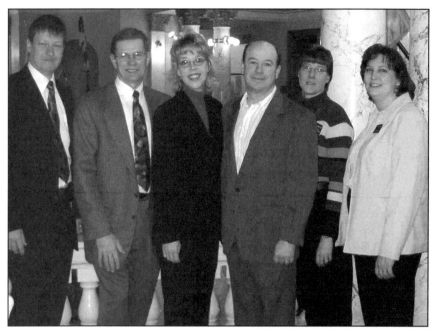

2003-2004 SDPhA officers. From Left: Treasurer Robert Reiswig, 2nd Vice President Galen Goeden, Past President Karla Overland-Janssen, President Elect Shane Clarambeau, 1st Vice President Julie Meintsma, President Monica Jones.

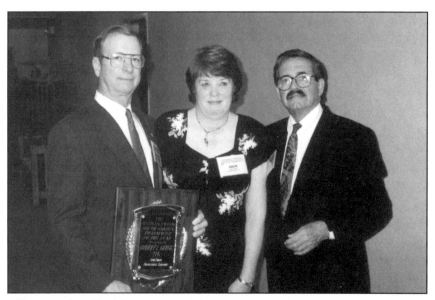

Bill Hustead, Wall, right, presented the 1996 Hustead Award to Robert Gregg, Chamberlain, left. Mrs. Julie Gregg is in the center.

A History of Pharmacy in South Dakota

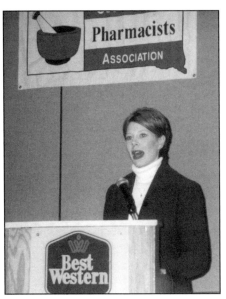

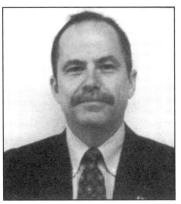

Robert Overturf, SDPhA
Executive Director, 2003-present

Tobi Lyon, SDPhA Executive Director,
2002-2003

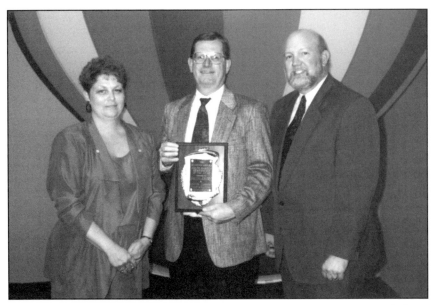

Galen Jordre, center, SDPhA Executive Director, 1986-1997 was presented the
Hustead Award in 1993. President Linda Pierson, left, and President-Elect
David Kuper, right.

CHAPTER 13
South Dakota Society of Health-System Pharmacists (SDSHP), 1976-2003

The South Dakota Society of Hospital Pharmacists was founded in 1976 to enhance the practice of hospital pharmacy and provide the professional needs of an increasing number of pharmacists practicing in hospital pharmacies.

In 1962, there were nine licensed hospital pharmacies in the state. The hospitals and pharmacist managers were: St. Luke's Hospital Pharmacy, Aberdeen, Lyle E. Anderson; St. John's Hospital Pharmacy, Huron, Sr. Mary Grace Kujawa; Bennett-Clarkson Memorial Hospital Pharmacy, Rapid City, Gwen V. Miller; St. John's McNamara Hospital Pharmacy, Rapid City, J. Toomey and M. Frances Beecham; McKennan Hospital Pharmacy, Sioux Falls, Ella Vogelsang; Sioux Valley Hospital Pharmacy, Sioux Falls, Linus C. Werner; Memorial Hospital Pharmacy, Watertown, Derald Hughes; Sacred Heart Hospital, Yankton, Annette L. Smith; and State Hospital Pharmacy, Yankton, Daniel Gackle.

There were sixty-one hospitals in South Dakota in 1967: 11 with licensed pharmacies and two with part-time pharmacies. At the time, the Department of Health and the Board of Pharmacy were working on regulations for the handling of medications in nursing homes and homes for the aged. The federal government was also working on regulations that would have required nursing homes to have either a full or part-time pharmacy. To meet the growing need, the Board of Pharmacy and SDPhA in 1967, supported the part-time pharmacy concept in the recodification of South Dakota's Pharmacy Law.

A part of the 1967 law authorized nursing homes, as well as hospitals, to obtain a part-time limited pharmacy license for in-patients only. The first to obtain a part-time pharmacy license under the new law was St. Joseph Hospital in Mitchell, and Memorial Hospital in Sturgis. Merle Walker, Walker Pharmacy, acted as part-time pharmacist in the Memorial Hospital pharmacy, and continued as a pharmacist in his business. By 1969, the Board of Pharmacy issued forty-three part-time pharmacy licenses. The license fee was $25.

In 1972, there were ten full-time licensed hospital pharmacies and forty-six part-time licenses in hospitals and nursing homes. The number of pharmacists practicing in institutional pharmacy was growing rapidly in the state and nation. Nationally, Cohen and Helfand found that in 1947 only 3% of the pharmacy graduates were entering hospital pharmacy. That figure grew to 25.1% in 1988. They also found that 90% of the pharmacy graduates were entering practice in community pharmacies in 1947. The figure dropped to 57.1% in 1988.[1]

SDPhA in 1976, created an Institutional Pharmacy Committee. The committee reviewed problems of pharmacy practice in institutions and reported them to the Association. That same year, there were 35 full-time pharmacists and 55 part-time pharmacists working in hospitals. There were also many pharmacists working part-time in nursing homes. Pharmacists practicing in hospitals believed they should have a Society of Hospital Pharmacists to promote their professional interests. Hospital pharmacists, meeting at Sioux Falls in 1976, organized the South Dakota Society of Hospital Pharmacists. It would be separate from the South Dakota Pharmaceutical Association, however, its members would also continue with the Association.

Its first convention was held in 1977, where they elected Galen Jordre as president. The mission statement of the Society according to its Membership Brochure was "to provide leadership and education to support its members in helping people make the best use of medications." The society also aspired "to be a highly effective professional organization devoted to ensuring its members are valued members of the health-care team." The purpose of the society is also outlined in its Web-site, "To advance the public health by promoting the professional interest of pharmacists practicing in health systems." In 1981, the Society became an ASHP chapter affiliate.

At SDSHP's March 1983 convention in the Airport Holiday Inn, at Sioux Falls, eight hours of continuing education was on the program. Some of the CE subjects were "Ethical Dilemmas in Medicine" by Pharm.D. Brian Kaatz, Sioux Valley Hospital; "Update on Respiratory Therapy" by Dr. Lowell Hyland, Sioux Valley Hospital; and "Cancer—Statistics and Treatment" by Dr. David Elson, US School of Medicine. Delegates elected Ron Nelson president, and presented the Pharmacist of the Year Award to Ron Huether. Registration fees were $30.00, $20 for members.

With the growing number of support personnel [pharmacy technicians] assisting registered pharmacists in hospital pharmacies, the American Society of Hospital Pharmacists (ASHP), as early as 1975, created training guidelines for technicians. Those guides were used by SDSHP to train technicians in hospital pharmacies. In 1984, the Society began certifying technicians. The following year, the South Dakota Board of Pharmacy passed regulations defining the duties of support persons [pharmacy technicians] working in licensed pharmacies. A technician, under the immediate and personal supervision of a registered pharmacist, could assist a pharmacist in a pharmacy.

In 1986, SDSHP certified ten pharmacy technicians. The 1987 SDSHP convention was held in Brookings. The three-day event included continuing education for the twenty-three pharmacists who had paid the registration fee. Twelve pharmacy technicians also attended some of the CE programs. Twenty-one pharmaceutical companies, located in the exhibit area, had displays on new drugs, delivery systems, and computer systems. At the time, the membership of SDSHP had grown to 90 members and 2 associates. Society committees included: Public Relations, Membership, Education, Nominations, Convention, Technician Certification, Task Force on Student Involvement, and Constitutional Revision.

The Society met at Aberdeen in April 1988. Fifty-five registered for the convention. Membership at the time was 101, plus 2 associates and 5 students. At a business meeting, the delegates voted to raise annual dues to $20 by a vote of 11 Yes and 6 No. They also agreed to continue publishing Society news in SDPhA's *South Dakota Pharmacist*. The Constitution was changed in 1988 affecting the following committees: Public and Professional Affairs, College of Pharmacy, Peer Review, Third Party Programs, Nominations, and Discriminatory Pricing. Each committee had one Executive Committee member and four other members. The Technician Certification Committee held its exam October 21, at Sioux Valley Hospital. A third annual Society dinner meeting was held in Sioux Falls November 1988.

The 1989 meeting was guided by the following theme, "Pharmacy as a Clinical Profession." Membership totaled 103, plus 6 associates and 4 students. President Brian Kaatz reported on SDSHP activities during the year:

- Published directory of hospital services
- Established line of communications between SDPhA and SDSHP
- Sixty-eight registered for the annual meeting, but only 26 members attended the business meeting
- An approved position paper stated the Society believes, "except under unusual circumstances (emergencies in rural

areas), that it is not in the patient's best interest for physicians to dispense drugs."

• Convention profit was $2300 [2]

Governor George S. Mickelson was the banquet speaker at the April 1990 convention in the King's Inn at Pierre. Jerome Kappes was elected president and Laurie Garry was named Pharmacist Of The Year. President Kappes' message, printed in the *South Dakota Pharmacist*, presented an excellent statement about the role of hospital pharmacists. He said, "I would like to share with you a portion of our pharmacy department's mission statement. We want to be known as drug information specialists within the institution for the benefit of patients, physicians, nurses, and allied health professionals. Our goal in providing medications is to relieve pain and suffering and restore the health of our patients and prevent future medical problems."[3]

In 1991, the Society of Hospital Pharmacists created a lending library of references for its members in institutional practice. Some of the Video Tapes available from the library included: *Medication Errors: A Closer Look*; *Drug Theft by Health Care Personnel*; and *Cost Benefits of Contemporary Pharmacy Services*. Some of the demonstration software available were: Medteach Demo, Data Kinetics Demo, Triage Demo, and IV-Ease Demo. Items could be obtained from Secretary Gary Van Riper, University Station, Brookings. Fifteen different books were also available, such as: *Handbook for Injectable Drugs*, *Medication Teaching Manual*, *1990-1991 ASHP Practice Standards*, *Criteria for Drug Use Evaluation*, and *1991 Residence Directory*. The lending library was discontinued in 1995. Useful items were donated to the College of Pharmacy.

With the help of Doug Smith and Terri McEntaffer of the local Convention Committee, a successful convention was held at the Crossroads Hotel in Huron April 24-26, 1992. The theme for the convention was "Therapeutic Advances-Accent on Biotechnology." One event which drew many interested pharmacists was an open hearing on the proposed Pharmacy Practice Act. It was introduced as a bill in the 1993 Legislative Session, and passed into law. Over ninety members, spouses, and exhibitors registered for the convention. President-elect Michael Duncan became president.

One of the projects in 1992 was to review proposed ASHP Guidelines for Pharmacy Prepared Sterile Products. President Mike Duncan said, "These guidelines, when approved will undoubtedly be the quality standards for pharmacy prepared sterile products in all settings (hospital, community pharmacy, home health care etc.)"[4] Duncan appointed a task force to review the proposed guidelines and draft a response from the Society. Some other proposed projects supported by the Society that year were: Pharmacy Practice Act, mandatory patient counseling, and the Pharm.D. program at the College of Pharmacy. Galen Jordre was presented the Upjohn Excellence in Research Award at the convention.

The Society in 1994 consisted of 144 members. Its Board of Directors, headed by President Kari Shanard-Koenders, consisted of the past president, president-elect, secretary, treasurer, and two board members. The Board met three times during the year. That year the Society funded two $500 scholarships, one to Kim Messerschmidt and one to Stacie Tomkins, to further their Pharm.D. degrees at SDSU. Dave Meyer and Deb Dees were selected as delegates to the ASHP House of Delegates.

In 1995, APhA and ASHP created the Pharmacy Technician Certification Board (PTCB). The purpose of the new group was to create more uniformity as to the qualifications of Pharmacy Technicians. That same year, SDSHP and SDPhA entered into a joint agreement to sponsor the National Technician Certification Exam. The Society of Hospital Pharmacists had been certifying pharmacy technicians since 1984. With the advent of PTCB, SDSHP dissolved its Technician Certification Committee in 1996. With the passage of the Pharmacy Practice Act, SDSHP and the College of Pharmacy, on April 22, 1995, co-sponsored a teleconference on the implementation of pharmaceutical care on the state television network, RDTN. A grant from ASHP helped fund the teleconference.

In 1994, the American Society of Hospital Pharmacists changed its name to American Society of Health-System Pharmacists. At the March 1995 convention, where President-elect Terri McEntaffer became president, the Society directed its Board of Directors to prepare the materials to change its name to South Dakota Society of Health-System Pharmacists. SDSHP met in convention at Aberdeen in 1996. By a unanimous vote the members changed its name from South Dakota Society of Hospital Pharmacists to South Dakota Society of Health-System Pharmacists. The new name "more accurately described the Society in a time of rapid change and reform in the health care system."[5] New standing committees included: Continuing Education, Education, Promotion, Nominations, and Annual Meeting. The new committees would provide, "More interaction from the Board of Directors and more involvement from the membership to drive and chair these committees."[6] Also in 1996, the Board of Pharmacy passed a new regulation permitting two technicians to assist one pharmacist in the pharmacy area.

At an August 1997 meeting of the Board of Directors, President James Clem announced that Linnea Putnam, Wendy Jensen, and Earl McKinstry would be coordinators for the 1998 annual meeting. Ron Johnson was selected to represent SDSHP on the SDSU College of Pharmacy Advisory Committee. Glenn Voss and Carol Breitkruetz were appointed to the Pharmacy Outreach Steering Committee. At an October meeting, plans were made for the annual officers retreat. Janet Fischer, professor of Clinical Pharmacy, was named as the Pharmacist of the Year at the 1997 April convention held in Pierre. Fischer had worked for SDSU since 1986, when she graduated with a Pharm.D. from Creighton University. She divided her time between the College of Pharmacy and Sioux Valley Hospital. She taught in the classroom of the College of Pharmacy as well as at the hospital.

The Board of Directors from SDSHP and SDPhA met jointly at the June 6, 1998 convention. It was agreed that the two organizations will have their first joint convention on September 2000 in the Ramkota Inn at Sioux Falls. The next joint convention was set for Pierre in September 2001. Many details needed to be coordinated in order to meet jointly, but both groups looked forward to the challenge and opportunities.

ASHP announced its first annual National Health-System Pharmacy week, February 8-12, 1999. The theme for the event was "Helping Patients Make Their Medications Work." This helped Health-System Pharmacists throughout the nation to show the valuable role pharmacists play in patient care. Activities included: media outreach and interviews, open houses, and speaking engagements. Treasurer Kimberley J. Cogley, in her 1999 report listed 121 active members, 20 student members and 1 associate member. Her records also showed $14,221 income and $11,374 expenses. December 31, 1999 checking balance was $7229 plus a $4600 certificate of deposit.

The program for the joint three-day September 2000 meeting of SDSHP and SDPhA at Sioux Falls included twelve hours of CE over a three-day period. Also scheduled was a Friday afternoon golf tournament. The evening began with a tailgate party buffet, after which golf and sales persons of the year awards were presented. Next day's meeting consisted of several business and resolution meetings and an awards banquet in the evening. A Memorial Service was held Sunday morning followed with a two-hour business meeting and election of officers.

Although the joint meetings in 2000 and 2001 were successful, it was agreed by both groups to have separate conventions in the future. Membership of the Society in 2001 was 128 active members, 59 students, and 1 associate. The SDSHP convention was set for March 2002 in the

Holiday Inn Downtown, at Sioux Falls. Over 100 attended the convention which featured 15 CE speakers, 20 vendor displays, and 12 scientific posters. Bruce Scott, past president of ASHP spoke. Awards presented at the banquet included Technician of the Year Award to Ann Hilson, Yankton, and Pharmacist of the Year Award to Dennis Hedge, Sioux Falls.

President Tom Johnson reported the Society has added a second pharmacy student to the Board of Directors. In 2002, Sarah Pochop, a P3 student was appointed. In 2003, Annie Hegg, a P1 student was also appointed. Johnson said the students "provide insight and directions to the Board regarding student issues."[7] In 2003, the Board of Directors also appointed Pharmacy Technician Deborah Cummings to the Board. Cummings is pharmacy technician supervisor at Sioux Valley Hospital and at USD Medical Center. The post was created because of the increased technician membership in the Society. Both the students and technician are non-voting Board members.

President Tom Johnson attended the ASHP midyear clinical meeting in Atlanta. The SDSU College of Pharmacy clinical skills team of Brianna Hoffman and Teresa Mathwig tied for first place in ASHP's clinical skills competition. There were sixty-eight competing teams from around the country. Misty Jensen, a clinical pharmacist at Avera McKennan in Sioux Falls, became president of the Society during its convention in the spring of 2003. Events scheduled for 2003-2004 included the second annual Society open golf tournament at Spring Creek Country Club July 18th. The midyear education meeting will be held at Cedar Shore Resort September 13. The 28th annual SDSHP meeting will take place April 16-17, 2004 in Rapid City.

New officers elected at the 2003 spring convention were: President Misty J. Jensen, Sioux Falls; Past President Tom Johnson, Sioux Falls; President-elect Anne Morstad, Sioux Falls; Secretary Gary Van Riper, Brookings; Treasurer Annette M. Johnson, Sioux Falls; and Board Members Vince Reilly, Sioux Falls, and Mike Lemon, Rapid City.

See Appendix F for list of SDSHP presidents, 1977-2003, and SDSHP Pharmacist of the Year Awards.

A History of Pharmacy in South Dakota

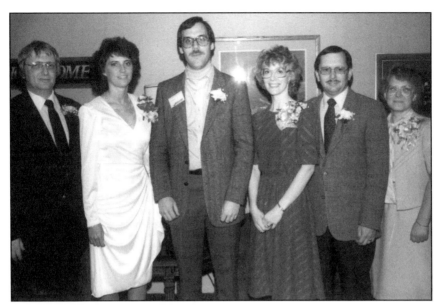

SDSHP 1985 officers, from left to right: Gary Van Riper, Rosemary Hooten, Mark Zwaska, Laurie Garry, Ron Huether and Janet Goens

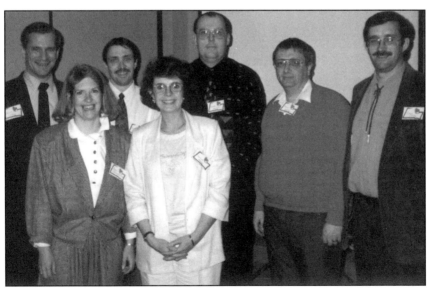

Top left, Brian Meyer-ASHP. Next 1992 SDSHP officers, from left to right: Kari Shanard-Koenders, Mike Duncan, Connie Atkins, Don Nettleton, Gary Van Riper, and Dana Darger.

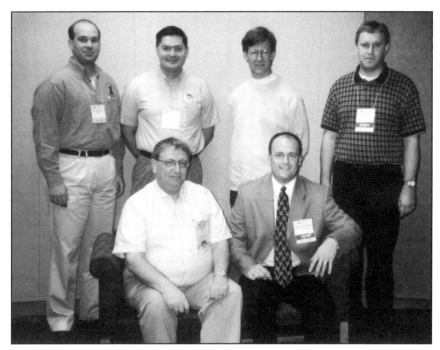

SDSHP 2001 officers top row left to right: Dennis Hedge, Vince Reilly, Tim Page, and Paul Price. Bottom row left to right: Gary Van Riper and Tom Johnson.

A History of Pharmacy in South Dakota

CHAPTER 14
South Dakota Association of Pharmacy Technicians (SDAPT), 1988-2003

The role of support persons [pharmacy technicians] assisting registered pharmacists advanced rapidly following World War II. As early as 1969 the American Society of Hospital Pharmacists (ASHP), in one of their workshops noted: "The establishment of nationally recognized educational standards for pharmacy technicians would be of value...without such standards, there would [be] hospital pharmacy personnel with various levels of training and capabilities."[1] That same year, an APhA task force listed duties that pharmacists and technicians may perform and stated that "nearly without exception these supporting personnel have been trained on the job by the pharmacist."[2]

At first, pharmacy technicians in South Dakota played a larger role in hospital pharmacies than in community pharmacies. At that time, pharmacy technicians received most of their training from pharmacists practicing in the hospital. That was the case of Jeanine Icenogle who was trained as a pharmacy technician after she started work in McKennan Hospital Pharmacy at Sioux Falls in 1973. Training of technicians within a hospital pharmacy was given a boost in 1975 when ASHP created a set of training guidelines for hospital technicians.

In 1977, ASHP also created competency standards for pharmacy technicians and defined qualifications of entry-level hospital pharmacy technicians.[3] The South Dakota Society of Hospital Pharmacists, organized in 1976, following ASHP guidelines, took a leading role in training pharmacy technicians. By 1984, the Society was certifying trained hospital pharmacy technicians. Ten were certified in 1986. At the Society's convention in 1987, several continuing education programs were available for twelve pharmacy technicians who had attended the convention.

The concept for a state pharmacy technician organization originated at McKennan Hospital, Sioux Falls, in 1986. Jeanine Icenogle, at the time was a pharmacy technician working for pharmacist Jerome Kappes in the hospital pharmacy. They believed there was a need for a state organization of pharmacy technicians. In 1987, Icenogle organized the east river with eight technicians present. Pat Skancke from Rapid City Regional organized the west river. It was agreed to hold an organizational meeting on February 6, 1988 at the Black Watch Restaurant in Sioux Falls. At that meeting, seventeen pharmacy technicians organized the South Dakota Association of Pharmacy Technicians (SDAPT), and adopted a Constitution and By-laws.[4]

Judy Rennich, one of the charter members at that meeting said, "SDAPT is an organization of certified and non-certified pharmacy technicians, pharmacists and anyone else that supports the profession of pharmacy technicians. Our goals when we were first organized were to increase membership, provide continuing education, plan meetings, and help with state conventions. Our objectives were to establish and promote a group of qualified pharmacy technicians, to promote a closer liaison between pharmacy technicians and other organizations, to promote and provide educational programs and to participate in activities for the advancement of pharmacy."[5]

The South Dakota Board of Pharmacy in 1986, passed regulations defining what duties support persons [pharmacy technicians] could perform in the pharmacy. This was the first time duties were defined for non-professional support persons working under the personal and immediate supervision of a registered pharmacist.

Western Dakota Technical Institute, Rapid City, had been educating pharmacy technicians since 1989. The course was greatly expanded in 1993, when Pharmacist Earl McKinstry, Piedmont, as pharmacy technology instructor, led an educational program for pharmacy technicians at the Institute. The nine-month program consisted of general education courses as well as pharmacology, medical terminology, pharmacy calculation, pharmacy operations, pharmacy law, and computer literacy. Twenty-four students enrolled that fall. Each student would also need to complete 320 hours of practical experience training in Black Hills hospitals and retail pharmacies.[6]

A 1993 resolution from the SDPhA Black Hills District urged the Board of Pharmacy to determine the number of support personnel per pharmacist in a retail/hospital setting, and define the specific tasks they can perform. The Board in August 1994, passed new regulations which only allowed two support persons to assist each pharmacist in the pharmacy area. The Board referred to support persons rather than to pharmacy technicians. Some of the ways a technician may assist a pharmacist, under the immediate and personal supervision of a pharmacist, are enumerated in 20:51:22:03 of Board regulations:

- Accept a written prescription from a patient and present it to pharmacist
- Accept a refill prescription number over the phone and present it to pharmacist
- Retrieve prescription data from the computer file
- Obtain original containers of drugs from stock and return them
- Count tablets after they have been selected by the pharmacist
- After review by the pharmacist, package the dispensed prescription container for delivery
- Handle or deliver completed prescription to the patient or patient's agent
- Place tablets in unit-dose containers as selected and directed by the pharmacist.

Earl McKinstry, pharmacy technician instructor at Western Dakota Technical Institute, also listed some duties technicians can do when working under the personal and immediate supervision of a pharmacist in a retail pharmacy and in a hospital pharmacy:

Retail pharmacy—
- stock and inventory prescription and OTC medication
- maintain written or computerized patient medication records
- type labels for containers
- prepare insurance claim forms
- manage cash register
- count or pour medications into dispensing container.

Hospital pharmacy—can do all of the above plus:
- assemble 24 hour supply of medications for each patient
- repackage medications
- maintain nursing station medications
- deliver medications to patient rooms
- operating computerized dispensing and/or robotic machinery
- and duties assigned by the pharmacist.[7]

Generally, technicians can perform many duties working under the immediate and personal supervision of a pharmacist, except those which are considered a practice of pharmacy.

In 1995, ASHP, APhA, Michigan Pharmacists Association, and Illinois Council of Health-System Pharmacists created a national Pharmacy Technician Certification Board (PTCB). Technicians would be certified through a voluntary national examination process. The objective was to "enable pharmacy technicians to work more effectively with pharmacists to offer safe and effective patient care service." Up to this time in the state, SDSHP had been certifying hospital pharmacy technicians. That same year, SDSHP and SDPhA agreed to sponsor and use the PTCB examination to certify technicians. In 1996, SDSHP discontinued certifying hospital pharmacy technicians and dissolved its Technician Certification Committee.

To be eligible to take the PTCB exam, a person must have graduated from high school and pay the fee of $95. Candidates for the exam were given a Candidate Handbook which included the content outline for the exam. Candidates could also review technician training texts and other references. Later, SDPhA offered a 300-page training manual, at a cost of $22.50. It included information on terminology, abbreviations, calculations, pharmacology, unit dose, and aseptic technique. A PCTB calculations workbook was also available at a cost of $20. In 1995, exams were given at 120 test centers around the nation, where 6,000 pharmacy technicians passed the exams. Individuals who passed the PTCB examinations were permitted to use the initials CPhT after their names. Certification was valid for two years.

To be recertified, a technician needed to have completed twenty hours of continuing education. Ten hours could be earned at the pharmacy where they practiced, under the supervision of a registered pharmacist. Appropriate CE programs included those on medication distribution, inventory control systems, pharmacy operations, calculations, pharmacy law, pharmacology/drug therapy, and programs specific to pharmacy technicians.

A 1992 South Dakota Law required pharmacists to provide patient counseling when transferring the dispensed medication to a patient. The 1993 Pharmacy Practice Act also called for patient counseling and pharmaceutical care. Past SDPhA President Al Pfeifle, Sioux Falls, predicted the profession would be changing "from a product-oriented to a patient-oriented." SDPhA President David Kuper, Sioux Falls, said the Practice Act "has expanded the pharmacists traditional role of compounding, labeling...and now includes the interpretation and evaluation of prescription drug orders and the provisions of patient counseling and pharmaceutical care."[8]

Pharmacist Stan Schmiedt in 1996, placed an ad in the *Centerville Journal* congratulating LaVonne Isaak for becoming a Certified Pharmacy Technician. A front-page story told about her accomplishment and the role she played in delivering pharmaceutical care at Schmiedt Drug. Schmiedt said, "Because of new directions in pharmaceutical care in South Dakota...more use of pharmacy technicians is the wave of the future. Pharmacists will no longer focus on counting and pouring and manual record keeping, but will instead focus on pharmaceutical care and patient counseling. We at Schmiedt Drug will be incorporating these changes to better serve our customers' needs and managed pharmaceutical care."[9]

In 1996, the Board of Directors, American Society of Health-System Pharmacists, awarded a certificate of accreditation to Western Dakota Technical Institute in Rapid City. The certificate stated that the Institute meets the conditions required for Pharmacy Technician training programs. Earl McKinstry is the instructor and helped write the PT National Certification Examination administered by the Pharmacy Technician Certification Board. Also in 1996, McKinstry was presented a Honorary Member Award by SDAPT.

The exams are given three times a year at 120 sites nationwide. There was an 82% passing rate in 1998. In 1999, twenty-one South Dakota candidates took the Pharmacy Technician National Certification Examination in Sioux Falls. Sixteen passed the exam, increasing the total of South Dakota Certified Pharmacy Technicians to 113. Overall, 93% of the South Dakota candidates passed the exam, which is higher than the national average. A 1999 National Association of Chain Drug Stores/Arthur Andersen study of Chain Drug Store pharmacy showed how pharmacy technicians spent their time while working in their pharmacies: 75% helped with dispensing; 11% in inventory management; 3% in pharmacy administration; 1% in disease management; and 10% in miscellaneous work including insurance related inquiries. Studies conducted by PTCB showed similar results.[10]

The National Community Pharmacists Association (NCPA) [formerly NARD], informed NABP "that NCPA's first priority is consumer safety, and that NCPA supports technological or pharmacy personnel initiatives that enhance the quality of pharmacy practice; however, the pharmacist's physical presence and personal oversight of all dispensing activities, whether they be automated, centrally filled, or handled by a technician is essential to public safety and quality pharmaceutical care. NCPA also supports uniform technician ratios for all practice settings."[11]

In 2000, the Board of Pharmacy proposed a Legislative Bill to regulate and license technicians. The bill had the support of SDAPT, SDPhA, and SDSHP. Senate Bill 89 was introduced in the 2001 Legislature, but it was not favored by the administration, consequently it was tabled in Senate Committee.

In 1999, forty-three pharmacy technicians were members of SDAPT, 12% increase over 1998. Judy Rennich, White, SD was president. She and the Board of Directors made arrangements to affiliate with the South Dakota Pharmacists Association. Affiliation meant benefits for the membership: receive issues of *South Dakota Pharmacist*, and *Stat-Gram*; half price for convention registration; attend all SDSHP educational, social, and business meetings; two pages in *South Dakota Pharmacist* for SDAPT news; and a 50% reduction of fees for CE programs.

Faculty members Gary Van Riper and Rajender Aparasu, and P4 student Joe Strain of the College of Pharmacy made an Economic Survey of Pharmacy Technicians in South Dakota. The 2000 study of 119 usable responses showed: 63 were pharmacy technicians, and 56 were certified pharmacy technicians. The average wage was $9.33 per hour. There were 112 women and 7 men who participated in the study. Forty-five pharmacy technicians had only graduated from high school, 40 from vocational technical, and 34 were college graduates. Pharmacy technicians practiced in the following settings: 38 in hospitals; 31 in independent retail; 30 other; and 20 in chain retail.[12] As of June 16, 2000, 153 pharmacy technicians from South Dakota had passed the PTCB examination.

A 2001 report by Schering showed that nine out of ten community pharmacies employed pharmacy technicians who assisted with dispensing of prescriptions.[13] The National Boards of Pharmacy in 2002 joined with PTCB and endorsed its examination as the nationwide standard for technician exams. NABP President Mick Markuson said, "The role of the pharmacy technician is an important part of the pharmacy team in the protection of public health. NABP is pleased to be a part of PTCB as it focuses on the national certification program for pharmacy technicians."[14] NABP, ASHP, and APhA support registration of pharmacy technicians but generally oppose licensing. The PTCB exam is based upon the following: knowledge required to assist pharmacists serving patients 64%; knowledge on medication distribution and inventory control 25%; and knowledge about the administration and management of pharmacy practice 11%."[15]

As of July 31, 2003, there were 368 certified pharmacy technicians (CPhTs) in South Dakota.[16] The South Dakota Society of Health-System Pharmacists awarded Technician of the Year Awards to: June Neises,

1997; Kathy Pike, 1999; Katie Timm, 2001; Ann Hilson, 2002; and Karla Schaaf, 2003. In 1992, SDPhA presented Jeanine Icenogle, Sioux Falls, the Outstanding Lay Person of the Year Award. SDAPT has awarded Honorary Memberships to Dave Kuper, Jerome Kappes, Terri McEntaffer, Earl McKinstry, Margaret Zard, Bob Coolidge, and Gary Van Riper.

Charter Members of SDAPT, 1988

McKennan Hospital, Sioux Falls—J.J. Icenogle, Bev Wieking, Kristi Schulte, Donna Hulsey and Kim Maroon.

St. Joseph Hospital, Mitchell—Paula Nielsen

Lewis Southgate, Sioux Falls— Betty Reese

Brookings Hospital, Brookings—Judy Rennich, Sandy Olson

Sioux Valley Hospital, Sioux Falls—Sherrie Fodness, Lynn Rieger, Corrine Hauser

V.A. Hospital, Sioux Falls—Betty Monday, Sally Westphal

Sacred Heart Hospital, Yankton—Jean Pinkelman, Ann Skovly

Scotts Pharmacy, Sioux Falls—Cheryl Wyant.[17]

Presidents, South Dakota Pharmacy Technician Association, 1988-2003

J. J. Icenogle-McKennan—1987 before officially organized, 1988, 1992, 1999

Tammy Sidle—1990, 1991

Lisa Wilson—Indian Health—1992-1993

Kelly Schroer—VA Medical Center—1993-1994

Jenice Casey—Intramed Infusion Therapy—1995-1996

Ann Barlow—VA Medical Center—1996,1997,1998

Judy Rennich—Brookings Hospital—1998,1999,2000

Tawny Erickson—Tel Drug—2000,2001,2002

Tammie Hammer—Family Pharmacy—2002

Melanie Angelos—Tel Drug—2003.[18]

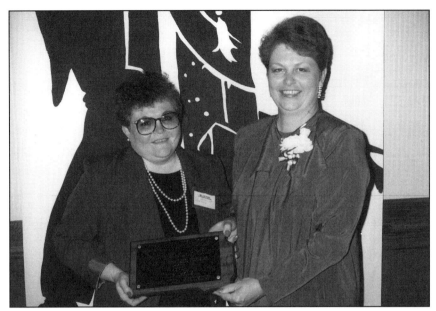

SDPhA President Linda Pierson presents the Association's Distinguished Service Award to Jeanine Icenogle, Sioux Falls, in 1992. Jeanine was one of the original organizers of the South Dakota Association of Pharmacy Technicians in 1988.

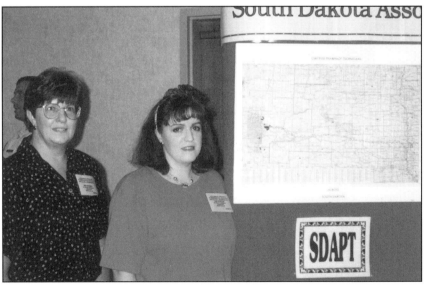

President-elect Judy Rennich and President Ann Barlow standing before their SDAPT exhibit at the 1996 SDPhA convention in Chamberlain.

A History of Pharmacy in South Dakota

Endnotes

Chapter 1, pages 1-10

[1] South Dakota Pharmaceutical Association Annual Proceedings 1908, p.31. (Hereafter cited as SDPhA.)

[2] SDPhA 1909, p. 26.

[3] SDPhA 1901, p. 52.

[4] Ibid.

[5] Eidsmoe, Clark T. *A History of Pharmacy at South Dakota State University, 1877-1974*. Brookings SD:1974, p.8. (Hereafter cited as Clark T. Eidsmoe.)

[6] SDPhA 1921, p. 122-123.

[7] SDPhA 1907, p. 93.

[8] Schuler, Harold H. *A Bridge Apart, History of Early Pierre and Fort Pierre*. Pierre:1987, p.107.

Chapter 2, pages 11-29

[1] SDPhA 1898, p. 22.

[2] Ibid.

[3] SDPhA 1898, p. 37.

[4] Ibid.

[5] SDPhA 1898, p. 50.

[6] SDPhA 1898, p. 45.

[7] SDPhA 1898, p. 47-51.

[8] Ibid.

[9] Pharmacy, *An Illustrated History*. David L. Cowen and William Helfand. New York:Harry N. Abrams, Inc., 1990, p. 162.

[10] Ibid. p. 186.

[11] SDPhA 1891, p. 62-74.

[12] SDPhA 1896, p. 6.

[13] Ibid. p. 13-28.

[14] Ibid. p. 6.

[15] Ibid.

[16] Clark T. Eidsmoe, p. 1.

[17] Ibid. p. 5.

[18] Ibid. p.10.

[19] Kenneth Redman, *History of the South Dakota State University College of Pharmacy 1975-1982*. Brookings, S.D.:Kenneth Redman, 1983. (Hereafter cited as Kenneth Redman.)

Chapter 3, pages 30-51

[1] South Dakota Pharmaceutical Association Annual Proceedings, 1905, p. 48 (Hereafter cited as SDPhA.)

[2] SDPhA 1909, p. 7-8.
[3] SDPhA 1904, p. 25.
[4] SDPhA 1909, p. 83.
[5] Ibid.
[6] Ibid. p. 82.
[7] Ibid. p. 88.
[8] Ibid. p. 42.
[9] SDPhA 1901, p. 30.
[10] SDPhA 1907, p. 82.
[11] SDPhA 1909, p. 25.
[12] SDPhA 1903, p. 85-86.
[13] Ibid. p.132.
[14] Ibid.
[15] Ibid. p.17.
[16] SDPhA 1917, p. 202.
[17] SDPhA 1905, p. 76.
[18] Ibid. p. 33.
[19] SDPhA 1904, p. 3.
[20] SDPhA 1906, p. 102.
[21] SDPhA 1909, p. 39-41.
[22] SDPhA 1901, p. 37.
[23] SDPhA 1903, p. 30.
[24] SDPhA 1905, p. 24.
[25] SDPhA 1906, p. 37.
[26] SDPhA 1907, p. 68.
[27] Ibid. p. 69.
[28] SDPhA 1908, p. 60.
[29] SDPhA 1909, p. 69-71.
[30] Ibid. p. 93.

Chapter 4, pages 52-69

[1] South Dakota Pharmaceutical Association Annual Proceedings 1915, p.63 (Hereafter cited as SDPHA.)

[2] SDPhA 1915, p.57.
[3] Ibid.
[4] Ibid.
[5] SDPhA 1904, p. 95.
[6] SDPhA 1915, p.65.
[7] Ibid. p. 46.
[8] SDPhA 1915, p. 36.
[9] SDPhA 1917, p.109.
[10] Ibid. p.154.
[11] Ibid. p. 84-91.
[12] Ibid. p. 111.

[13] SDPhA 1915, p. 37.
[14] Ibid. p. 37.
[15] SDPhA 1917, p. 103-104.
[16] Ibid. p.59.

Chapter 5, pages 70-85

[1] South Dakota Pharmaceutical Association Annual Proceedings 1917, p. 162. (Hereafter cited as SDPhA.)
[2] SDPhA 1919, p. 97-98.
[3] SDPhA 1931, p. 58.
[4] SDPhA 1924, p. 16.
[5] SDPhA 1929, p.16-18.
[6] SDPhA 1924, p. 87.
[7] SDPhA 1927, p. 89-90.

Chapter 6, pages 86-103

[1] South Dakota Pharmaceutical Association Annual Proceedings 1931, p. 109. (Hereafter cited as SDPhA.)
[2] SDPhA 1932, p. 54-59.
[3] SDPhA 1934, p. 72.
[4] SDPhA 1937, p. 79.
[5] SDPhA 1933, p. 13.
[6] SDPhA 1936, p.57.
[7] SDPhA 1937, p. 12.
[8] Ibid. p. 49.
[9] SDPhA 1927, p. 66.
[10] SDPhA 1931, p. 35-37.
[11] Ibid. p. 97.
[12] SDPhA 1932, p. 12-16.
[13] Ibid. p. 76-77.
[14] Ibid.
[15] Ibid. p. 20-21.
[16] SDPhA 1936, p. 52-53.
[17] SDPhA 1935, p. 75.
[18] Kenneth Redman, p. 34.
[19] Ibid. p.34.
[20] SDPhA 1936, p. 49.
[21] Clark T. Eidsmoe, p. 12.

Chapter 7, pages 104-117

[1] SDPhA 1940, p. 55.
[2] SDPhA 1941, p. 9.
[3] SDPhA 1945, p. 44.
[4] Ibid. p. 13-14.
[5] SDPhA 1942, p. 13-14.

6 SDPhA 1946, p. 29.
7 John Nelson, Letter to author, March 28, 2003.

Chapter Eight, pages 118-132

1 SDPhA 1958, p. 130.
2 SDPhA 1953, p. 55.
3 SDPhA 1954, p. 41.
4 SDPhA 1952, p. 46.
5 SDPhA Minutes, November 7, 1954.
6 SDPhA 1955, p. 75.
7 SDPhA 1954, p. 20.
8 Clark T. Eidsmoe, p.16.
9 Wiley Vogt, Letter to author, November 1, 2003.
10 Terry Casey, Letter to author, March 26, 2003.
11 Kenneth Redman, p. 35.

Chapter 9, pages 133-150

1 Executive Committee Minutes, February 10, 1963.
2 SDPhA 1961, p. 9.
3 Ibid. p. 83-84.
4 SDPhA 1962, p. 19.
5 SDPhA 1964, p. 45.
6 SDPhA 1969, p. 11.
7 Ibid. p. 4.
8 Carveth Thompson, Letter to author, June 14, 2002.
9 SDPhA 1962, p. 65.
10 SDPhA 1961, p. 44.
11 SDPhA 1965, p. 12.
12 SDPhA 1961, p. 8.
13 SDPhA 1962, p. 107.
14 SD Pharmacy Newsletter, November 8, 1967.
15 Clark T. Eidsmoe, p. 15.
16 Ibid. P. 25.
17 Kenneth Redman, P. 36.

Chapter 10, pages 151-177

1 SDPhA 1970, p. 5.
2 SDPhA 1972, p. 5.
3 SDPhA 1973, p. 4.
4 Ed Swanson, Letter to author, April 19, 2003.
5 SDPhA 1969, p. 4.
6 Willis Hodson, Phone conversation with author, April 21, 2003.
7 Executive Committee Minutes, October 10, 1976.
8 Board of Pharmacy, 1973 Manpower Survey.
9 *Lilly Digest*, 1979 Survey.
10 SDPhA 1973, p. 13-14.

[11] Terry Casey, Letter to author, March 26, 2003.

[12] SDPhA 1973, p. 13.

[13] Carveth Thompson, Letter to author, June 14, 2003.

[14] Kenneth Redman, p. 25.

[15] Ibid.

[16] Ibid. p. 27-28.

[17] Clark T. Eidsmoe, p. 28.

[18] SDPhA 1931, p. 83-84.

[19] Clark T. Eidsmoe, p. 19.

[20] Ibid.

[21] Kenneth Redman, p. 44-45.

[22] Ibid.

Chapter 11, pages 178-202

[1] *SD Pharmacy Newsletter*, February 4, 1986.

[2] *South Dakota Pharmacist*, January 1989.

[3] Ed Swanson, Letter to author, April 19, 2003.

[4] Terry Casey, Letter to author, March 26, 2003.

[5] *South Dakota Pharmacist,* July-August 1994.

[6] *SD Pharmacy Newsletter*, April 1980.

[7] *South Dakota Pharmacist,* November 1986.

[8] *South Dakota Pharmacist*, January-February 1989.

[9] *South Dakota Pharmacist*, May-June 1988.

[10] *SD Pharmacy Newsletter*, December 1980.

[11] SDPhA Minutes, June 4, 1982.

[12] *Lilly Digest* Survey of Community Pharmacies, 1981.

[13] *Lilly Digest* Survey of Community Pharmacies, 1987,1988.

[14] *South Dakota Pharmacist*, July 1989.

[15] Dean Ray Hopponen, 1985 SDPhA Convention Report.

[16] Dean Ray Hopponen, 1985 College of Pharmacy Report.

[17] *College of Pharmacy, A Centennial Celebration, 1988.*

[18] *SD Pharmacy Newsletter*, June 28, 1974.

[19] Kenneth Redman, p. 54.

Chapter 12, pages 203-251

[1] *South Dakota Pharmacist*, July-August 1996.

[2] *South Dakota Pharmacist*, Second Quarter 2000.

[3] SDPhA *Stat-Gram*, June 2002.

[4] SDPhA *Stat-Gram*, May 2003.

[5] *South Dakota Pharmacist*, September-October 1991.

[6] *South Dakota Pharmacist*, Third and Fourth Quarter 2002.

[7] *South Dakota Pharmacist*, September-October 1990.

[8] *South Dakota Pharmacist*, March-April 1992.

[9] *South Dakota Pharmacist*, November-December 1994.

[10] *South Dakota Pharmacist*, January 1999.

[11] SDSU College of Pharmacy, *Economic Survey of South Dakota Pharmacists,* 1998, 1999.

¹² Board of Pharmacy Minutes, June 21, 2002.

¹³ *South Dakota Pharmacist*, Second Quarter 2003.

¹⁴ Don McGuire, *South Dakota Pharmacist*, January 2000.

¹⁵ *South Dakota Pharmacist*, May-June 1992.

¹⁶ *National Compliance News*, NABP, October 2001.

¹⁷ *South Dakota Pharmacist*, July-August 1992.

¹⁸ *South Dakota Pharmacist*, November-December 1994.

¹⁹ *South Dakota Pharmacist*, March-April 1998.

²⁰ *South Dakota Pharmacist*, January 1999.

²¹ *The College of Pharmacy*, Spring 2000.

²² *South Dakota Pharmacist*, Second Quarter 2000.

²³ *South Dakota Pharmacist*, First Quarter 2002.

²⁴ Board of Pharmacy Report, 2000.

²⁵ *South Dakota Pharmacist*, May-June 1994.

²⁶ Galen Jordre, Letter to author, October 30, 2003.

²⁷ *South Dakota Pharmacist*, Fourth Quarter 1999.

²⁸ *South Dakota Pharmacist*, Third Quarter 2003.

²⁹ Board of Pharmacy Report, *South Dakota Pharmacist*, July-August 1992.

³⁰ Board of Pharmacy Report, 1998.

³¹ Dennis M. Jones, Board of Pharmacy Report, 1999.

³² Dennis M. Jones, *National Compliance News*, NABP, April 2002.

³³ NAPLEX/MPJE Registration Bulletin 2002, NABP, Park Ridge, Illinois.

³⁴ *South Dakota Pharmacist*, March-April,1994.

³⁵ *The College of Pharmacy*, Summer 2000.

³⁶ *South Dakota Pharmacist*, Second Quarter 2002.

³⁷ *The College of Pharmacy*, Spring 2000.

³⁸ *The College of Pharmacy*, Spring 2002.

³⁹ *South Dakota Pharmacist*, Second Quarter 2002.

⁴⁰ *The College of Pharmacy*, Summer 2002.

⁴¹ Galen Jordre, *South Dakota Pharmacist*, September-October 1992.

⁴² *South Dakota Pharmacist*, First Quarter 2003.

⁴³ Dean Brian Kaatz, *The College of Pharmacy*, Summer 2003.

⁴⁴ Bernard Hendricks, Letter to author, September 17, 2003.

⁴⁵ *The College of Pharmacy*, Winter 2001.

⁴⁶ *The College of Pharmacy*, Winter 2003.

Chapter 13, pages 252-260

¹ David L. Cowen and William H. Helfand. *Pharmacy, An Illustrated History*. New York: Harry N. Abrams, Inc., 1990.

² *South Dakota Pharmacist*, May 1989.

³ *South Dakota Pharmacist*, May-June 1990.

⁴ *South Dakota Pharmacist*, May-June 1992.

⁵ Annual Report, SDSHP 1995-1996.

⁶ Ibid.

⁷ *South Dakota Pharmacist*, First Quarter 2003.

Chapter 14, pages 261-268

[1] Summit Two, Sesquicentennial Stepping Stone Summits, Pharmacy Technicians, May 9-10-2002, Baltimore, Maryland.

[2] Ibid.

[3] Ibid.

[4] Judy Rennich, Letter to author, December 4, 2003.

[5] Ibid.

[6] *South Dakota Pharmacist*, November-December 1993.

[7] Earl McKinstry, RPh, Pharmacy Technician Program, Western Dakota Technical Institute, Rapid City, SD, September 18, 2000.

[8] *South Dakota Pharmacist*, May-June 1994.

[9] *South Dakota Pharmacist*, March 1996.

[10] 2002 White Paper on Pharmacy Technicians.

[11] Board of Pharmacy Minutes, February 25, 2000.

[12] *South Dakota Pharmacist*, Second Quarter 2000.

[13] Shering Report XXIII, Kenilworth, NJ:2001.

[14] *South Dakota Pharmacist*, Second Quarter, 2002.

[15] 2002 White Paper on Pharmacy Technicians.

[16] Judy Rennich, Letter to author, December 4, 2003.

[17] Ibid.

[18] Ibid.

Chronology

1852 APhA was organized in Zane Street Building at Philadelphia College of Pharmacy.

1861 Congress created Dakota Territory (D.T.) including present-day North and South Dakota. Yankton was named capital.

1862 Charley Bramble, New York, opened first drug store in D.T. at Yankton.

1868 All land west of Missouri River in South Dakota part of D.T., designated as Great Sioux Reservation, as stipulated in Laramie Treaty.

1876 Kirk G. Phillips and Dr. A.M. McKinney opened first drug store in Black Hills at Deadwood.

1877 Act of Congress opened Black Hills for settlement, many new pharmacies created.

1881 D.T. Legislature at Yankton, created State College of Agriculture at Brookings.

1884 State College opened at Brookings.

1886 Thirty-eight pharmacists met at Mitchell and organized the Southern District Pharmaceutical Association. Elected Daniel S. White, Flandreau, president and W. S. Branch, Parker, secretary.

1887 D. T. Pharmacy Law passed by Legislature at Bismarck. Created Dakota Pharmaceutical Association north of 7th parallel and Southern District Pharmaceutical Association south of 7th parallel. Established Board of Pharmacy and restricted the sale of drugs and medicines to registered pharmacists.

1888 Pharmacy school established by Board of Regents at State College June 19, 1888.

1889 Statehood approved for South Dakota and voters selected Pierre as temporary capital and Arthur Mellette as Governor.

1890 • Voters selected Pierre as permanent capital.
• Legislature meeting in Pierre January 7, 1890, passed new S.D. Pharmacy Law. Created S. D. Pharmaceutical Association and Board of Pharmacy, both managed by one Executive Secretary.
• After setting land aside for Indian Reservations, remaining land west of the river opened for settlement. Many new pharmacies opened between Pierre and Black Hills.
• At first meeting of S.D. Board of Pharmacy on October 1, 1890, 424 pharmacists were registered, most of whom were registered Territorial pharmacists.

1894 Mrs. Nettie C. Hall, pharmacist at Wessington Springs, was elected second vice-president of SDPhA at the Huron convention, the first woman officer.

1895 Five graduates in pharmacy completed two-year course and were award-
     ed a Ph.G. degree. Recognized as first graduating class in pharmacy from
     State College.
1898 Kirk G. Phillips, Deadwood pharmacist, loses general election race for
     Governor to incumbent Andrew E. Lee.
1899 National Association of Retail Druggists (NARD) formed.
1902 Ladies' Auxiliary organized at Flandreau. Mrs. W. A. Simpson, Flandreau
     was first president.
1903 Legislature required licensing of all peddler medicine wagons.
1904 National Association of Boards of Pharmacy (NABP) organized in
     Kansas City, and perfected in Atlanta in 1905.
1905 •Commercial Travelers' organized at Aberdeen.
     •I. A. Keith, Lake Preston, elected president of NABP.
1907 •U.S. Pure Food and Drug Act effective.
     •West of the river more accessible for new pharmacies with new railroad
     bridges over the Missouri River at Pierre, Chamberlain, and Mobridge.
1908 Department of Pharmacy at State College approved for membership in
     American Association of Colleges of Pharmacy (AACP).
1909 •S.D. Pure Food and Drug Act approved by Legislature.
     •First SDPhA convention held west of the river, at Lead.
1910 New stone capitol in Pierre opened for business.
1914 Congress passed Harrison Narcotic Act.
1917 •Drug Garden planted at State College, north of old college stores build-
     ing. It was discontinued in 1984.
     •During WWI, SDPhA members donated a Motor Army Ambulance to
     the S.D. National Guard. Governor Peter Norbeck accepted it at
     Watertown convention.
1918 Three-year Pharmaceutical Chemist (Ph.C.) degree offered that fall.
     Ended in 1930.
1921 Commercial Travelers changed name to Allied Drug Travelers.
1923 Whitehead Chapter of SDPhA established at State College in 1923.
1924 •Department of Pharmacy at State College changed to Division of
     Pharmacy. Earl R.Serles named dean.
     •Lay persons authorized to sell packaged poisons with a license from
     state.
1925 Ph. G. [Pharmacy Graduate] degree ended with graduating class.
1926 Veteran Druggists' Association formed for those who had been registered
     twenty-five years. Recognized at Veteran Druggists' breakfast at conven-
     tion.
1927 First Memorial Hour conducted at a convention.
1929 APhA convention held in Rapid City. Its president was David F. Jones,
     Watertown.
1931 •New Pharmacy Law required licensure of drug stores; four-year B.S.
     degree needed to take Board examinations; & non-pharmacists couldn't
     own drug stores.
     •Rho Chi Society established at State College.

1932 American College of Pharmaceutical Education (ACPE) approved.

1933 Lay persons authorized to sell packaged patent medicines with a license from state.

1934 American Institute of Pharmacy marble building completed on Constitution Avenue in Washington, D.C.

1937 District 5 of NABP created for South Dakota and four other surrounding states.

1938 Dean Earl Serles, while at State College, was elected president of AACP.

1943 U. S. Army Air Force opened Administration School on campus for 800 enlisted men and 50 officers. Used school's classrooms and dormitories.

1945 Lay persons authorized to sell list of packaged U.S.P. and N.F. household remedies with state license.

1946 Dean Earl Serles, while at University of Illinois, served as president of APhA.

1947 *S.D. Journal of Medicine and Pharmacy* named as official publication of SDPhA. Ended in 1964 with SDPhA publishing *S.D. Pharmacy Newsletter*.

1949 U.S. Supreme Court ruled that limiting ownership of pharmacies to pharmacists only was unconstitutional, but permitted ownership by non-pharmacists if active   management was granted to the pharmacist in charge.

1952 Congress passed Durham-Humphrey Law—any drug bearing prescription legend can only be dispensed and sold by pharmacist, and cannot be sold over-the-counter.

1954 Whitehead Chapter SDPhA affiliated as Student Branch of APhA.

1956 Chi Chapter Kappa Epsilon organized on State College Campus.

1958 •Honorary President's Award approved by Executive Committee.
•Gamma Kappa Chapter of Kappa Psi installed on State College Campus.

1959 Bowl of Hygeia Award, A. H. Robbins Co. approved by Executive Committee.

1960 The first five-year pharmacy B.S. degree program began with the fall class.

1963 Bliss C. Wilson elected president of NABP.

1964 •S.D. State College name changed to S.D. State University.
•Division of Pharmacy name changed to College of Pharmacy.
•State divided into twelve SDPhA districts with required two meetings per year.
•*S.D. Pharmacy Newsletter* started, Secretary Harold H. Schuler, editor.
•Hubert H. Humphrey, Jr., S.D. registered pharmacist, holding certificate 2652, elected Vice-President of the United States. Lyndon Johnson elected president.

1965 Board of Pharmacy passed regulation "Free choice of pharmacy."

1966 George Bender, 1923 Division of Pharmacy graduate, and executive with Parke-Davis, along with artist Robert A. Thom, published original oil paintings *Great Moments in Pharmacy* and *Great Moments in Medicine*.

1967 Complete recodification of S.D. Pharmacy Law: pharmacy declared professional practice; defined dispensing; listed who can prescribe drugs; authorized part-time pharmacies in hospitals and nursing homes.

1968 NABP Blue-Ribbon Committee, including Al Pfeifle, Sioux Falls, began preparing National Board Examination, called NABPLEX.

1969 S.D. Legislature tabled a bill in committee calling for a new College of Pharmacy building.

1972 Carveth Thompson, Faith pharmacist, loses general election race for Governor to incumbent Richard Kneip.

1973 •S.D. Board of Pharmacy transferred to Department of Commerce and Consumer Affairs, and under the Division of Professional & Occupational Licensing.
•Lay person added to the Board of Pharmacy.
•Board approves for first time, 400 hours of intern time to be earned concurrent with attending College of Pharmacy.

1974 •Title 19 Drug Program approved by Legislature.
•Legislature created authority for Health Maintenance Organization (HMO).

1976 •Executive Committee approved Lay Person of the Year Award. [Now Distinguished Service Award.]
•SDSHP founded.
•Board of Pharmacy used NABPLEX for first time.

1977 Mandatory Continuing Education required for pharmacists.

1978 Drug Product Selection [substitution] approved by Legislature.

1980 Auxiliary of SDPhA formed, replacing Ladies' Auxiliary.

1981 •New Guilford C. Gross Pharmacy Building dedicated.
•IBM introduced personal computer.
•NABP began NABPLEX score transfer program.
•SDSHP became ASHP affiliate.

1982 •New law requiring code imprint be placed on all solid dosage drugs, identifying drug and manufacturer.
•First class graduated from 1-4 curriculum, had changed from 2-3 curriculum.

1983 •College of Pharmacy Externship Program began Preceptor of the Year Award.

1984 SDSHP began certifying pharmacy technicians.

1986 •SDPhA changed Constitution calling for two vice-presidents instead of three.
•Pharm-Assist Program established to aid pharmacists/pharmacy students in event of drug/alcohol misuse.
•*South Dakota Pharmacist* journal introduced, Secretary Galen Jordre, editor.
•*Focus on Pharmacy* newsletter started at College of Pharmacy, Gary C. Van Riper, editor.

1987 •Student Branch of APhA became Academy of Students of Pharmacy (ASP).

•First pharmacy Phonathon to raise funds from alumni and friends.

•S.D. Association of Pharmacy Technicians organized.

1988 •Ted and Dorothy Hustead Pharmacist of the Year Award approved.

•College of Pharmacy celebrates Centennial Celebration, 1888-1988.

•Distinguished Alumnus Award began at College of Pharmacy. Clark T. Eidsmoe first recipient.

1989 •Dean's Club started to raise funds to strengthen College of Pharmacy programs.

•Western Dakota Technical Institute began educating pharmacy technicians. Role expanded in 1993, under Earl McKinstry.

1991 •Phi Lambda Sigma founded on SDSU campus.

•Licensure of wholesale drug distributors began.

1992 S.D. law passed requiring pharmacists to offer patient counseling and keep patient prescription record.

1993 •Pharmacy Practice Act passed Legislature, expanding pharmacist's role to evaluate prescription drug orders and provide patient counseling and pharmaceutical care.

•Innovative Pharmacy Practice Award introduced.

•Regents approved six-year Pharm.D. as entry level degree. Offered fall of 1994.

1994 ASHP changed name to American Society of Health-System Pharmacists.

1995 •Annual Pharmacy Dinner Dance now called Annual Scholarship and Awards Banquet.

•National Pharmacy Technician Certification Board (PTCB) created.

•SDSHP and SDPhA agreed to use PTCB examination to certify pharmacy technicians.

1996 •Name South Dakota Pharmaceutical Association changed to South Dakota Pharmacists Association.

•SDSHP changed name to S.D. Society of Health-System Pharmacists.

•SDPhA separated from S.D. Board of Pharmacy with separate executive directors. Board of Pharmacy office moved to Sioux Falls, and Association office remained in Pierre.

•Board joined four other state professional boards and established Health Professional Assistance Program (HPAP). Help professionals who have trouble with drugs, liquor, or mental impairment.

•Board of Pharmacy passed regulations permitting two pharmacy technicians to assist one pharmacist in pharmacy area.

•Board permits 1,500 hours of practical experience to be earned as part of college-based experiential program.

1997 •Patent Medicine and Household Remedy Laws repealed by Legislature. Established new class of Non-Prescription Drugs which can be sold in original packages by licensee.

•Board of Pharmacy given authority to license nonresident pharmacies.

•NAPLEX introduced by NABP, based on Pharm.D. six-year program.

A History of Pharmacy in South Dakota

•Dennis Ludwig, Boulder, CO, and 1969 College of Pharmacy graduate, elected president of National Community Pharmacists Assoc. (NCPA) [Formerly NARD].

Focus on Pharmacy revamped into *The College of Pharmacy* magazine, Gary C. Van Riper, editor.

2000 Board of Pharmacy joined NABP's *National Compliance News*, which provides four pages for S.D.Board of Pharmacy news.

2001 •Legislature authorized pharmacists to give influenza immunizations, pursuant to Board regulations.

•SDPhA (formerly Ladies' Auxiliary) Auxiliary ended.

2002 Pharmacy Opportunities Night affords pharmacy students chance to meet with S.D. employers first.

2003 Dr. Brian Kaatz awarded APhA's Good Government Pharmacist of the Year Award.

Appendix A
Presidents of the
South Dakota Pharmaceutical Association

(South Dakota Pharmacists Association Since 1996)

1886-1887	D. S. White, Flandreau
1887-1888	W. S. Branch, Parker
1888-1889	W. S. Branch, Parker
1889-1890	R. A. Mills, Aberdeen
1890-1891	W. A. Burnham, Groton
1891-1892	Z. A. Crain, Redfield
1892-1893	R. M. Cotton, Tyndall
1893-1894	John McClain, Tripp
1894-1895	James Lewis, Canton
1895-1896	W. S. Branch, Parker
1896-1897	L. T. Dunning, Sioux Falls
1897-1898	C. H. Lohr, Estelline
1898-1899	C. H. Lohr, Estelline
1899-1900	D. F. Jones, Watertown
1900-1901	N. R. Gilchrist, Wakonda
1901-1902	C. M. Serles, Salem
1902-1903	C. W. Peaslee, Redfield
1903-1904	F. G. Stickels, Mellette
1904-1905	Isaac M. Helmey, Canton
1905-1906	W. F. Michel, Willow Lake
1906-1907	G. C. Sabin, Redfield
1907-1908	S. H. Scallin, Mitchell
1908-1909	H. A. Sasse, Henry
1909-1910	Julius Deetken, Deadwood
1910-1911	F. D. Kriebs, Beresford
1911-1912	J. F. Wagner, Garden City
1912-1913	L. E. Highley, Hot Springs
1913-1914	H. J. Schnaidt, Parkston
1914-1915	R. O. Grover, Huron
1915-1916	H. A. Keith, Lake Preston
1916-1917	J. A. Pool, Redfield
1917-1918	Fred L. Vilas, Pierre
1918-1919	Fred L. Vilas, Pierre
1919-1920	Perry Clute, Big Stone City
1920-1921	Selmer Solem, Kadoka

A History of Pharmacy in South Dakota

1921-1922	C. C. Maxwell, Arlington
1922-1923	J. Chris Schutz, Madison
1923-1924	W. E. Bissell, Plankinton
1924-1925	W. L. Buttz, Aberdeen
1925-1926	George Sherman, Huron
1926-1927	C. B. Warne, Redfield
1927-1928	G. F. Swartz, Mobridge
1928-1929	F. W. Brown, Lead
1929-1930	J. J. McKay, Pierre
1930-1931	C.L. "Roy" Doherty, Rapid City
1931-1932	O. J. Tommeraason, Madison
1932-1933	A. C. Thompson, Colton
1933-1934	Bliss C. Wilson, Letcher
1934-1935	George W. Lloyd, Spencer
1935-1936	L. A. Daniels, Aberdeen
1936-1937	Floyd M. Cornwell, Webster
1937-1938	Tom K. Haggar, Sioux Falls
1938-1939	C. A. Locke, Brookings
1939-1940	Herbert S. Crissman, Ipswich
1940-1941	J. A. Clute, Murdo
1941-1942	H. L. Lewis, Hartford
1942-1943	Carl Anderson, Sioux Falls
1943-1944	O. J. Jones, Redfield
1944-1945	A. A. Jarratt, Colman
1945-1946	James Warrell, White Lake
1946-1947	Theodore E. Hustead, Wall
1947-1948	Richard W. Kendall, Brookings
1948-1949	Roger Eastman, Tripp
1949-1950	John H. Sidle, Alexandria
1950-1951	LaVerne J. Mowell, Murdo
1951-1952	Albert O. Bittner, Aberdeen
1952-1953	J. C. Shirley, Brookings
1953-1954	Neil E. Fuller, Chamberlain
1954-1955	Charles F.VanDeWalle,Sioux Falls
1955-1956	Edward W. Peterson, ElkPoint
1956-1957	Alger D. Knutson, Clark
1957-1958	George A. Lehr, Rapid City
1958-1959	Vere A. Larsen, Alcester
1959-1960	Willis C. Hodson, Aberdeen
1960-1961	Albert H. Zarecky, Pierre
1961-1962	Philip E. Case, Parker
1962-1963	L. B.Urton, Sturgis
1963-1964	Wayne C. Shanholtz, Mitchell
1964-1965	Melvin C. Holm, Redfield
1965-1966	Nina D. Lund, Rapid City
1966-1967	Earle T. Crissman, Ipswich

1967-1968	Lloyd E. Wagner, Marion
1968-1969	Robert Ehrke, Rapid City
1969-1970	Clayton Scott, Sioux Falls
1970-1971	James Rogers, Watertown
1971-1972	George Tibbs, Rapid City
1972-1973	Wiley Vogt, Mitchell
1973-1974	M. Lloyd Jones, Aberdeen
1974-1975	Phil VonFischer, Sioux Falls
1975-1976	Clifford Thomas, Belle Fourche
1976-1977	John Nelson, Arlington
1977-1978	Jack Dady, Mobridge
1978-1979	Ed Swanson, Madison
1979-1980	Ron Schwans, Hoven
1980-1981	Ron Huether, Sioux Falls
1981-1982	Dale Stroschein, Sturgis
1982-1983	John F. Halbkat, Jr., Webster
1983-1984	James Stephens, Pierre
1984-1985	Al Pfeifle, Sioux Falls
1985-1986	Robert Gregg, Chamberlain
1986-1987	Dave Helgeland, Yankton
1987-1988	Mary Kuper, Sioux Falls
1988-1989	Arvid Liebe, Milbank
1989-1990	Marilyn Schwans, Belle Fourche
1990-1991	Terry Casey, Chamberlain
1991-1992	Jocelyn Prang, Rapid City
1992-1993	Linda Pierson, Sioux Falls
1993-1994	David Kuper, Sioux Falls
1994-1995	Margaret Zard, Mitchell
1995-1996	Robert Wik, Gregory
1996-1997	Pam Jones, Huron
1997-1998	Mark Gerdes, Renner
1998-1999	Earl McKinstry, Piedmont
1999-2000	James Bregel, Chamberlain
2000-2001	Cheri Kraemer, Parker
2001-2002	Steve Aamot, Aberdeen
2002-2003	Karla Overland-Janssen, RapidCity
2003-2004	Monica Jones, Huron

A History of Pharmacy in South Dakota

Appendix B
South Dakota Board of Pharmacy Members

1890-2003

1890-1891	D.K. Bryant	A.H. Stites	O.H. Tarbell
1891-1892	C.F. Ayer	A.H. Stites	O.H. Tarbell
1892-1893	C.F. Ayer	A.H. Stites	O.H. Tarbell
1893-1894	C.F. Ayer	A.H. Stites	O.H. Tarbell
1894-1895	C.F.Ayer	A.H. Stites	O.H. Tarbell
1895-1896	C.F. Ayer	A.H. Stites	N.J. Bleser
1896-1897	C.F. Ayer	J. Lewis	N.J. Bleser
1897-1898	I.A. Keith	J. Lewis	N.J. Bleser
1898-1899	I.A. Keith	J. Lewis	N.J. Bleser
1899-1900	I.A. Keith	W.J. Hull	N.J. Bleser (res.)
			D.F. Jones
1900-1901	F.C. Smith	W.J. Hull	D.F. Jones
1901-1902	F.C. Smith (res.)	W.J. Hull	D.F. Jones
	I.A. Keith		
1902-1903	I.A. Keith	L.C. Ramsdell	D.F. Jones
1903-1904	I.A. Keith	L.C. Ramsdell	D.F. Jones
1904-1905	I.A. Keith	L.C. Ramsdell	D.F. Jones
1905-1906	I.A. Keith	O.A. Griffis	D.F. Jones
1906-1907	J. Lewis	O.A. Griffis	D.F. Jones
1907-1908	J. Lewis	O.A. Griffis	D.F. Jones
1908-1909	J. Lewis	G.F. Swartz	D.F. Jones
1909-1910	F.W. Brown	G.F. Swartz	D.J. Jones
1910-1911	F.W. Brown	G.F. Swartz	D.F. Jones
1911-1912	F.W. Brown	G.F. Swartz	D.F. Jones
1912-1913	F.W. Brown	G.F. Swartz	D.F. Jones
1913-1914	F.W. Brown	G.F. Swartz	F.W. Halbkat
1914-1915	F.W. Brown	H.J. Schnaidt	F.W. Halbkat
1915-1916	F.W. Brown	H.J. Schnaidt	F.W. Halbkat
1916-1917	F.W. Brown (res.)	H.J. Schnaidt	F.W. Halbkat
	C.B. Baldwin		
1917-1918	C.B. Baldwin	H.J. Schnaidt	F.W. Halbkat
1918-1919	C.B. Baldwin	H.J. Schnaidt	F.W. Halbkat
1919-1920	C.B. Baldwin	H.J. Schnaidt	J.A. Pool
1920-1921	C.B. Baldwin	D.F. Dexter	J.A. Pool
1921-1922	C.B. Baldwin	D.F. Dexter	J.A. Pool
1922-1923	C.B. Baldwin	D.F. Dexter	J.A. Pool
1923-1924	C.B. Baldwin	B.H. Neumayr	J.A. Pool
1924-1925	L.E. Highley	B.H. Neumayr	J.A. Pool
1925-1926	L.E. Highley	B.H. Neumayr	A.R. Williams

1926-1927	L.E. Highley	B.H. Neumayr (d)	A.R. Williams
		H.J. Schnaidt	
1927-1928	L.E. Highley	H.J. Schnaidt	A.R. Williams
1928-1929	L.E. Highley (res.)	H.J. Schnaidt	G. Sherman
	F.L. Vilas		
1929-1930	F.L. Vilas	H.J. Schnaidt	G. Sherman
1930-1931	F.L. Vilas (res.)	H.J. Schnaidt	G. Sherman
1931-1932	H.A. Sasse	H.J. Schnaidt	G. Sherman (d)
1932-1933	H.A. Sasse	H.J. Schnaidt	F.L. Vilas
1933-1934	H.A. Sasse	H.J. Schnaidt	F.L. Vilas (res.)
			E.C. Severin
1934-1935	H.A. Sasse	H.J. Schnaidt	E.C. Severin
1935-1936	H.A. Sasse	G.W. Lloyd	E.C. Severin
1936-1937	H.A. Sasse	G.W. Lloyd	E.C. Severin
1937-1938	S.A. Amunson	G.W. Lloyd	E.C. Severin
1938-1939	S.A. Amunson	G.W. Lloyd	E.C. Severin
1939-1940	S.A. Amunson	G.W. Lloyd (res.)	E.C. Severin
		J.H. Sidle	
1940-1941	E.C. Severin (res.)	J.H. Sidle	S.A. Amunson
	M.C. Beckers		
1941-1942	M.C. Beckers	Floyd Cornwell	S.A. Amunson
1942-1943	M.C. Beckers	Floyd Cornwell	S.A. Amunson
1943-1944	M.C. Beckers	Floyd Cornwell	T.K. Haggar
1944-1945	M.C. Beckers	Floyd Cornwell	T.K. Haggar
1945-1946	M.C. Beckers	Floyd Cornwell	T.K. Haggar
1946-1947	M.C. Beckers	Floyd Cornwell	Harold Tisher
1947-1948	M.C. Beckers	Floyd Cornwell	Harold Tisher
1948-1949	M.C. Beckers	Floyd Cornwell	Harold Tisher
1949-1950	M.C. Beckers	Floyd Cornwell	Harold Tisher
1950-1951	M.C. Beckers	Floyd Cornwell	Harold Tisher
1951-1952	H.W. Mills	Floyd Cornwell	Harold Tisher
1952-1953	H.W. Mills	Floyd Cornwell	Harold Tisher
1953-1954	H.W. Mills	M.L. Schwartz	Harold Tisher
1954-1955	H.W. Mills	M.L. Schwartz	Harold Tisher
1955-1956	H.W. Mills	M.L. Schwartz	Harold Tisher
1956-1957	H.W. Mills	M.I. Schwartz (d)	Harold Tisher
		T.K. Haggar	
1957-1958	H.W. Mills	T.K. Haggar	Harold Tisher
1958-1959	H.W. Mills	T.K. Haggar	Roger Eastman
1959-1960	A.O. Bittner	H.W. Mills	Roger Eastman
1960-1961	A.O. Bittner	Ted Hustead	Roger Eastman
1961-1962	A.O. Bittner	Ted Hustead	Roger Eastman
1962-1963	T.K. Haggar	Ted Hustead	Roger Eastman
1963-1964	Carveth Thompson	T.K. Haggar	Roger Eastman
1964-1965	Carveth Thompson	T.K. Haggar	Roger Eastman
1965-1966	Carveth Thompson	M. Holm	Roger Eastman
1966-1967	Carveth Thompson	M. Holm	Roger Eastman
1967-1968	Carveth Thompson	M. Holm	Allen Pfeifle
1968-1969	Carveth Thompson	M. Holm	Allen Pfeifle
1969-1970	R. Ehrke	M. Holm	Allen Pfiefle
1970-1971	R. Ehrke	M. Holm	Allen Pfeifle

1971-1972	R. Ehrke	T.C. Rutherford	Allen Pfeifle	
1972-1973	Joseph Cholik	T.C. Rutherford	Allen Pfeifle	
1973-1974	Joseph Cholik	Terry Casey	J. Bailey	D. Burns*
1974-1975	Joseph Cholik	Terry Casey	J. Bailey	D. Burns
1975-1976	Joseph Cholik	Terry Casey	J. Bailey	D. Burns
1976-1977	Joseph Cholik	Terry Casey	J. Bailey	S. Heitland*
1977-1978	Joseph Cholik	Terry Casey	J. Bailey	S. Heitland
1978-1979	J. Hersrud	Terry Casey	J. Bailey	S. Heitland
1979-1980	J. Hersrud	Frank Post	J. Bailey	S. Heitland
1980-1981	J. Hersrud	Frank Post	J. Bailey	S. Heitland
1981-1982	Frank Post	K.B. Jones	John Nelson	S. Heitland
1982-1983	Frank Post	K.B. Jones	John Nelson	S. Heitland
1983-1984	Frank Post	K.B. Jones	John Nelson	S. Heitland
1984-1985	Frank Post	K.B. Jones	John Nelson	S. Heitland
1985-1986	Frank Post	M. Christensen	John Nelson	S. Heitland
1986-1987	Frank Post	M. Christensen	John Nelson	S. Heitland
1987-1988	Dennis M. Jones	M. Christensen	Jack Dady	S. Heitland
1988-1989	Dennis M. Jones	Robert Gregg	Jack Dady	Joan Hogan*
1989-1990	Dennis M. Jones	Robert Gregg	Jack Dady	Joan Hogan
1990-1991	Dennis M. Jones	Robert Gregg	Jack Dady	Joan Hogan
1991-1992	Dennis M. Jones	Robert Gregg	Jack Dady	Joan Hogan
1992-1993	Dennis M. Jones	Dale Stroschein	Jack Dady	Joan Hogan
1993-1994	Dennis M. Jones	Dale Stroschein	Jack Dady	Joan Hogan
1994-1995	Dennis M. Jones	Dale Stroschein	Jack Dady (d)	Joan Hogan
1995-1996	Dennis M. Jones	Steve Statz	Duncan Murdy	Joan Hogan
1996-1997	Dennis M. Jones (res.) Mark Graham	Steve Statz	Duncan Murdy	Joan Hogan
1997-1998	Mark Graham	Steve Statz	Duncan Murdy	Nora W. Hussey*
1998-1999	Mark Graham	Steve Statz	Duncan Murdy	Nora W. Hussey
1999-2000	Arvid Liebe	Steve Statz	Duncan Murdy	Nora W. Hussey
2000-2001	Arvid Liebe	Steve Statz	Duncan Murdy	Nora W. Hussey
2001-2002	Arvid Liebe	Steve Statz	Duncan Murdy	Nora W. Hussey
2002-2003	Arvid Liebe	Steve Statz	Duncan Murdy	Nora W. Hussey

(Res.) Resigned
(d) Died in Office
(*) Layperson

Appendix C
College of Pharmacy Faculty

	Year Came to SDSU	Year Left SDSU
Abler, Conald	1950	1951
Ahlquist, Raymond P.	1940	1944
Aparasu, Rajender	1995	current
Baer, Rebecca	1998	current
Bailey, Harold	1951	1961
Beleh, Mustapha	1992	1995
Bender, Wendy Jensen	1996	current
Benton, Byrl	1939	1940
Berg, Thomas	1996	1999
Berg, Warren	1946	1948
Bhavnagri, Vispi	1970	1973
Billow, Joye	1972	2002
Blackwell, Willis	1947	1951
Bloedow, Duane	1974	1976
Bradshaw, Robin	1987	1989
Brenner, George	1971	1976
Bruno, Gerald	1963	1964
Caliendo, Theresa	1988	1993
Cascella, Peter	1976	1989
Chappell, Gary	1973	2000
Clem, James	1992	current
Creekmore, Freddy	1998	2001
Currie, Bruce	2000	2004
Dees, Debra	1991	1992
Dvorak, Sonya	1999	2002
Dwivedi, Chandradhar	1987	current
Edwards, Gary	1980	1983
Eidsmoe, Clark	1929	1964
Engineer, Ferzaan	1990	1992
Farnsworth, Terry	1995	1997
Farver, Debra	1983	1986
Farver, Debra	1989	current
Fiechtner, Helen	1991	current
Fischer, Janet	1986	current
Gaston, Dorothy	1925	1927

Gholami, Kheirollah	1989	1991
Gilbertson, Terry	1968	1972
Gross, Guilford	1940	1980
Guan, Xiangming	1995	current
Gurney, Mary	2003	current
Halbert, Michael	1982	1988
Harris, Wayne	1965	1967
Hedge, Dennis	1992	current
Heins, Jodi	1994	current
Helgeland, David	1976	1979
Helgeland, David	1989	current
Hendricks, Bernard	1982	current
Hietbrink, Bernard	1964	1994
Hikal, Ahmed	1969	1970
Hiner, L. David	1932	1940
Hogstad, Jr.,Anton	1917	1925
Hopkins, Cyril	1893	1894
Hopponen, Raymond	1966	1986
Houglum, Joel	1979	current
Hutton, Sarah	2002	current
Jarat, Mildred	1944	1949
Joens, Colleen	1979	1982
Johnson, Annette Brand	2001	current
Johnson, Thomas	1998	current
Jones, David Franklin	1895	1896
Kaatz, Brian	1977	1978
Kaatz, Brian	1989	current
Kamath, Kalpana	1993	1996
Keller, Kelley	2002	current
Knott, Robert	1963	1965
Koestner, James	1982	1987
Kruse, Heather	2003	current
Kutscher, Eric	2002	current
Lange, Winthrop	1955	1958
Larsen, Ronald	1979	1987
Lattin, Danny	1995	2002
LeBlanc, Floyd	1922	1964
Lee, Steven	2001	current
Leicht, Maya	1998	2000
Lemon, Michael	1997	current
Locke, Charles	1918	1919
Locke, Charles	1940	1946
Marchiando, Rodney	1996	1999
McCoy, Randy	1994	1996
McFadden, G. H.	1936	1937
Menke, Jennifer	1993	2001

Messerschmidt, Kimberly	1995	current
Morrison, Sherman	1922	1924
Mort, Jane	1986	current
Moss, Jeffrey	1979	1982
Mukherjee, Suman	1999	current
Omodt, Gary	1958	1992
Palakurthi, Srinath	2003	current
Parry, Edgar	1949	1951
Pathak, Yashwant	1990	1993
Patterson, Larry	1975	1976
Powers, James	1983	1999
Preuss, Charles	1997	1998
Price, Paul	1993	2000
Pulscher, Shelly	2000	2001
Rang, Karl	1927	1932
Rao, B. K.	1966	1970
Redman, Kenneth	1951	1973
Repschlaeger, Barbara Mason	1983	1986
Sathe, Rajendra	1993	1996
Scherrer, James	1979	1982
Serles, Earl	1917	1940
Shepard, James	1888	1895
Shlanta, Stephen	1970	1972
Singh, Yadhu	1988	current
Smar, Michael	1990	1998
Solonen, Nicholas	1937	1938
Sonee, Manisha	2000	current
Strain, Joe	2003	current
Van Dyke, Lora	1987	1987
Van Riper, Gary	1972	current
Wallenberg, Bradford	1986	1994
Webb, Norval	1952	1962
Whitehead, Bower	1896	1917
Whitehill, Dawn	2002	current
Wightkin, William	1980	1983

Appendix D

Distinguished Service Awards, Bowl of Hygeia Awards, and Honorary Presidents Awards

	Distinguished Service Award	Bowl of Hygeia Award	Honorary President Award
1958	Started 1977	None	R. E. Trumm
1959		Floyd Cornwell	John Kent
1960		Thomas K. Haggar	Clark Eidsmoe & Floyd LeBlanc
1961		C. L. "Roy" Doherty	John Burke
1962		M. C. Beckers	Fred Vilas
1963		Harold W. Mills	T. C. Rutherford
1964		Neil Fuller	Guilford Gross
1965		Ted Hustead	Harry Lee
1966		Otto Tommeraason	Murray Widdis
1967		Kenneth Redman	Edgar Schmiedt
1968		Harold L. Tisher	George Minard
1969		Tom Mills	Martin Osterhaus
1970		Vere Larsen	Dean Hockett
1971		Roger Eastman	L. H. McKenna
1972		Martin Osterhaus	Clifford Shannon
1973		Robert Ehrke	Kenneth Redman
1974		Carveth Thompson	Lawrence Stelzer
1975		Milton Swenson	Shirley Vail
1976		Lloyd Wagner	Mike Otterberg
1977	Harvey Jewett III & Dick Brown	Earle Crissman	Raymond Meyer
1978	None	Cliff Thomas	R. T. Westre
1979	John Bibby	George Tibbs	Les Heilman
1980	Shirley Heitland	Ephriam Sieler	Art Hurst
1981	Glenn Velau	Garvin Bertsch	Madalyn Winner
1982	Dennis Pierson	Jack Bailey	Don Turgeon
1983	None	Wiley Vogt	Maurice Hiatt
1984	None	Jack Dady	Stanford Schmiedt
1985	Harold H. Schuler	Dale Stroschein	Ray Hopponen
1986	None	John Nelson	Dallas Butterbrodt
1987	Dennis Kasmingk	Ken Jones	Burdette C. Anderson
1988	Glady Pugh	Ron Schwans	Laura Fritz
1989	Gene Van Pelt	Bob Wik	Jack Bailey

1990	James Abdnor	Stan Schmiedt	Carveth Thompson
1991	Matt Mathison	Ron Huether	Garvin Bertsch
1992	Jeanine Icenogle	Robert Gregg	Dale Auchampach
1993	Chuck Brau	James Schmidt	James White
1994	Sharon Casey	Terry Casey	Bernard Hietbrink
1995	Frank Kloucek	Arvid Liebe	Bernie Shroll
1996	Joan Hogan	Stan Petrik	Pat Lynn
1997	Pam Stotz	Al Pfeifle	Ron Park
1998	None	Margaret Zard	Ephriam Sieler
1999	Marilyn Eighmy	Kevin Wurtz	Ann Jordre
2000	Robert Riter	Linda Pierson	Harlan Meier
2001	Linda Bartholomew & Rogene Dutton	Jack Burns	Doug Berkley
2002	Sharon Van Riper	Jo Prang	Everett Randall
2003	Mark Griffin	Philip Dohn	Gary Karel

Appendix E
Hustead Awards, Young Pharmacist Awards, Innovative Practice Awards

	Hustead Awards	Young Pharmacist Awards	Innovative Practice Awards
1987	None	Mark Zwaska	Started 1993
1988	Ted Hustead	Renee Sutton	
1989	Bernard Hietbrink	Kari Shanard	
1990	Mark Zwaska	James Bregel	
1991	Roger Eastman	Stacey Fristad	
1992	Cliff Thomas	Paula Stotz	
1993	Galen Jordre	Loma Jennings	Yee-Lai Chiu
1994	Pamela Harris-Oines	Tim Gallagher	Brian Dressing
1995	Linda Pierson	Hugh Mack	Mark Kantack
1996	Robert Gregg	Steve Aamot	Lynn Greff
1997	Robert Wik	Kathy Mulner-Keiner	Jocelyn Prang
1998	Gary Van Riper	Karla Overland-Janssen	Anne Nopens
1999	Lloyd Jones	Shelly Pulscher	William Ladwig
2000	Terry Casey	Chad Scholten	Rodney Marchiando
2001	Brian Kaatz	Kendall Goetz	Heather Kruse
2002	Margaret Zard	Jodi Johnson	Cheri Kraemer
2003	Arvid Liebe	Anne Nopens	Kendall Goetz

Appendix F
South Dakota Society Health-System Pharmacists

	Presidents	Pharmacists of the Year
1977-1978	Galen Jordre	
1978-1979	Holly McKillop	
1979-1980	Chuck Reinders	
1980-1981	Robert Lewis	
1981-1982	Gary Karel	Don Strahl
1982-1983	Ron Nelson	Ron Huether
1983-1984	Dan Somsen	Gary Karel
1984-1985	Ron Huether	Chuck Reinders
1985-1986	Rosemary Hooten	Dave Kuper
1986-1987	Mark Zwaska	Bill Bradfeldt
1987-1988	Mark O'Brien	Diane Pecheny
1988-1989	Brian Kaatz	Gary Van Riper
1989-1990	Tom Wolff	Laurie Garry
1990-1991	Jerome Kappes	Kim Messerschmidt
1991-1992	Dana Darger	Dan Somsen
1992-1993	Michael Duncan	Mark O'Brien
1993-1994	Kari Shanard-Koenders	Mark Zwaska
1994-1995	Ron Johnson	Deb Dees
1995-1996	Terri McEntaffer	Brian Kaatz
1996-1997	James Clem	Janet Fischer
1997-1998	Pam Harris-Oines	Jerome Kappes
1998-1999	Debra Dees	Ronald Johnson
1999-2000	Dennis Hedge	Linda Oyen
2000-2001	Vince Reilly	Deb Pritchett
2001-2002	Thomas Johnson	Dennis Hedge
2002-2003	Misty Jensen	Glenn Voss

A History of Pharmacy in South Dakota

Appendix G
Leadership, SDSU College of Pharmacy

Chemistry Department
        1888-1895 Professor James H. Shepard

Department of Pharmacy
        1895-1896 Head, David Franklin Jones
        1896-1917 Head, Bower T. Whitehead
        1917-1918 Head, Earl R. Serles
        1918-1919 Head, Charles A. Locke
        1919-1923 Head, Earl R. Serles

Division of Pharmacy
        1923-1940 Dean, Earl R. Serles
        1940-1964 Dean, Floyd J. LeBlanc

College of Pharmacy
        1964-1965 Dean, Guilford C. Gross
        1966-1986 Dean, Raymond E. Hopponen
        1987-1994 Dean, Bernard E. Hietbrink
        1995-2002 Dean, Danny L. Lattin
        2003-   Dean, Brian L. Kaatz

Appendix H

Association and Board of Pharmacy Secretaries
1886-1887 W. S. Branch, Parker
1887-1897 I. A. Keith, Lake Preston
1897-1923 E. C. Bent, Dell Rapids
1923-1925 D. F. Dexter, Canton
1925-1929 W. P. Loesch, Oldham
1929-1934 Rowland G. Jones, Jr., Gettysburg
1935-1942 Kenneth Jones, Gettysburg
1942-1963 Bliss C. Wilson, Letcher
1964-1986 Harold H. Schuler, Pierre
1986-1997 Galen Jordre, Gettysburg
(Separation of Association from Board of Pharmacy)

Association Executive Directors
1997-1999 Terri McEntaffer,
2000-2002 Robert Coolidge, Pierre
2002-2003 Tobi Lyon, Meadow
2003-   Robert Overturf, Rapid City

Board of Pharmacy Executive Secretary
1997-   Dennis M. Jones, Sioux Falls

A History of Pharmacy in South Dakota

Appendix I
Presidents, Ladies' Auxiliary, SDPhA
(Auxiliary to SDPhA after 1980) Disbanded 2001

1902	Mrs. W. A. Simpson, Flandreau
1903	Mrs. W. A. Simpson, Flandreau
1904	Mrs. G. C. Bradley, De Smet
1905	Mrs. George Sabin, Redfield
1906	Mrs. F. G. Stickles, Mellette
1907	Mrs. J. E. Heisler, Huron
1908	Mrs. W. F. Michel, Willow Lake
1909	Mrs. D. F. Jones, Watertown
1910	Mrs. L. E. Highley, Hot Springs
1911	Mrs. H. A. Sasse, Henry
1912	Mrs. R. O. Grover, Huron
1913	Mrs. F. D. Kriebs, Beresford
1914	Mrs. W. P. Hagerty, Avon
1915	Mrs. Sig F. Sampson, Yankton
1916	Mrs. C. F. Hanson, Woonsocket
1917	Mrs. E. M. Jones, Clark
1918	WW I
1919	WW I
1920	WW I
1921	Mrs. E. R. Serles, Brookings
1922	Mrs. J. A. Pool, Redfield
1923	Mrs. H. A. Perriton, Huron
1924	Mrs. L. F. Chladek, Tyndall
1925	Mrs. R. B. Syverson, Madison
1926	Mrs. A. Duffner, Watertown
1927	Mrs. Swen Amundson, Mobridge
1928	Mrs. George Sherman, Huron
1929	Mrs. J. J. McKay, Pierre
1930	Mrs. H. J. Werner, Ramona
1931	Mrs. H. J. Werner, Ramona
1932	Mrs. O. C. Nicolls, Mitchell
1933	Mrs. N. B. Porter, Madison
1934	Mrs. Lloyd Daniels, Aberdeen
1935	Mrs. Bliss C. Wilson, Letcher
1936	Mrs. George Lloyd, Spencer
1937	Mrs. J. H. Sidle, Alexandria

1938	Mrs. Herbert S. Crissman, Ipswich
1939	Mrs. Kenneth Jones, Gettysburg
1940	Mrs. M. T. Wilkins, Clark
1941	Mrs, S. A. Amunson, Mobridge
1942	Mrs. R. L. Overholser, Selby
1943	Mrs. Carl Moe, Huron
1944	WWII
1945	WWII
1946	WWII
1947	Mrs. Roy Doherty, Pierre
1948	Mrs. Richard Kendall, Brookings
1949	Mrs. Harold Tisher, Yankton
1950	Mrs. Lloyd Wagner, Marion
1951	Mrs. Neil Fuller, Chamberlain
1952	Mrs. Roger Eastman, Tripp
1953	Mrs. Vere Larsen, Alcester
1954	Mrs. J. C. Shirley, Brookings
1955	Mrs. Fred Scallin, Mitchell
1956	Mrs. Murray Widdis, Sioux Falls
1957	Mrs. Harold Mills, Rapid City
1958	Mrs. Al Knutson, Clark
1959	Mrs. George Lehr, Rapid City
1960	Mrs. Willis Hodson, Aberdeen
1961	Mrs. Bud Fullenkamp, Hudson
1962	Mrs. Linus Werner, Sioux Falls
1963	Mrs. Philip Case, Parker
1964	Mrs. Wayne Shanholtz, Mitchell
1965	Mrs. Lester Hetager, Sioux Falls
1966	Mrs. Carveth Thompson, Faith
1967	Mrs. Arden Rohde, Mitchell
1968	Mrs. Charles Crutchett, Armour
1969	Mrs. Clayton Scott, Sioux Falls
1970	Mrs. James Rogers, Watertown
1971	Mrs. Patrick Lynn, Huron
1972	Mrs. George Tibbs, Rapid City
1973	Mrs. Lloyd Jones, Aberdeen
1974	Mrs. Don Schmitt, Sioux Falls
1975	Mrs. Marcine Thomas, Belle Fourche
1976	Mrs. Ray Meyer, Lennox
1977	Mrs. Sharon Casey, Chamberlain
1978	Mrs. Dorothy Huether, Sioux Falls
1979	Mrs. Sandy Swanson, Madison
1980	Mrs. Mary Ann Stroschein, Sturgis
1981	Mrs. Sharon Van Riper, Brookings
1982	Mrs. Sue Reinders, Sioux Falls
1983	Mrs. Mary Halbkat, Webster

A History of Pharmacy in South Dakota

1984	Mrs. Lynnette Hatch, Bridgewater
1985	Mrs. Karen Jones, Huron
1986	Mrs. Pat Lewis, Sioux Falls
1987	Mrs. Julie Gregg, Chamberlain
1988	Mrs. Rona Stephens, Pierre
1989	Mrs. Janet Liebe, Milbank
1990	Mrs. Jeanne Sinclair, Milbank
1991	Mrs. Beth Uken, Springfield
1992	Mrs. Nina Kappes, Sioux Falls
1993	Mrs. Joanne Carter, Watertown
1994	Mrs. Carol Dingman, Sioux Falls
1995	Mrs. Pat Buechler, Mitchell
1996	Mrs. Maggie Nelson, Mitchell
1997	Mrs. Maggie Nelson, Mitchell
1998	Mrs. Karen Jones, Sioux Falls
1999	Mrs. Janelle McKinstry, Piedmont
2000	Mrs. Pat Lewis, Sioux Falls
2001	Disbanded

Appendix J
Retail Drug Stores in the South Dakota
Part of the Dakota Territory, 1882
(All names following cities are names of the drug stores.
There were 75 drug stores in 45 cities and towns.)

Aberdeen: R. A. Mills
Alexandria: J. Laidlaw
Aurora: Rexford Bros.
Big Stone: John Munro & Co.
Bridgewater: O.K. Ballard; A Wettergreen
Brookings: C. W. Higgins; Smith and Tidball
Cavour: N. C. Estey
Central City: Dillon & Co.; Mann & Bass
Chamberlain: H. W. Le Blond; Robert Sturgeon
Clark: Frank Hoskins
Custer: Wheeler & Crushing
Deadwood: E.C. Bent and Deetken; Knowles & Marshman; Kirk G.
    Phillips; H. Stem & Co.
Dell Rapids: Henry A. Cadd; Henry Cobb
De Smet: G.C. Bradley
Egan: J. E. Schneider.
Flandreau: James Bray; D. S. White
Galena: W. L. Gardner
Gary: Richmond and Merideth
Goodwin: R. Phillips
Groton: J. M. Bennet, Jr.
Huron: Blount & Hood; A. J. Stoel
Kimball: J. P. Vreeland
Lead: Alexander Larvie
Lennox: J. M. Macomber
Madison: A. A. Broadie; Clough & Howe
Marion: Ernest Reiff; Reiff & Nagel
Milbank: F. W. A. Poppe; W. W. Wilson
Mitchell: L. O. Gale; Hammer & Hammer
Parker: W. S. Branch; J. E. Kendall
Pierre: Richardson & Hollemback; J. A. McArthur; M. J. Shubert
Plankinton: J. J. Kibbe
Rapid City: J. W. Cole; Haxby & Son
Redfield: Clark & Alvord

Salem: Pendar & White
Scotland: J. F. Weber
Sioux Falls: L. T. Dunning; N. E. Phillips & Co.
Spearfish: Ledboer & Co.
Sturgis: H. P. Lynch; C. W. Pratt
Tyndall: D. W. Currier
Vermillion: C. C. Eves; A. Helgeson; M. Kerst; G. T. Salmer
Volga: C. H. Drinker; A. C. Porter
Watertown: O. E. Dewey & Co.; Charles Goss; O. H. Tarbell
Webster: J. L. Harris
Worthing: G. Gerber
Yankton: E. M. Coates; Mills & Purdy; George Tammen; G. W.
    Vanderhule; E. Weber.

Source: Polk Directory, Minnesota & Dakota Territory, 1882-1883, Vol.3.
    Courtesy Robert Kolbe Collections, 1301 S. Duluth, Sioux Falls, SD
    57105.

Appendix K
Bibliography

Bender, George A. *A History of Arizona Pharmacy*. Tucson, AZ: Arizona Historical Foundation, 1985.

Board of Pharmacy, SD. Minute Book, 1941-1975. Location 2250 Box 82-15. South Dakota Archives, Pierre, SD.

Board of Pharmacy Office, Executive Secretary Dennis M. Jones, 4305 S. Louise Ave. Suite 104, Sioux Falls, SD 57106.

Cowen, David L. and Helfand, William H. *Pharmacy, An Illustrated History*. New York: Harry N. Abrams, Inc., 1990.

College of Pharmacy, A Centennial Celebration, 1888-1988. Brookings, SD: College of Pharmacy, SDSU.

College of Pharmacy Office, Dean Brian Kaatz. College of Pharmacy, SDSU, Brookings, SD 57007-0099.

Crissman, Herbert S., 1938 Scrapbook. SDPhA office, Pierre, SD 57501.

Eidsmoe, Clark T. *A History of Pharmacy at SDSU 1887-1974*. Brookings, SD: College of Pharmacy, SDSU, 1974.

Fox, Lawrence K. *Who's Who Among South Dakotans*. Vol. 1. Pierre, SD:Statewide Service Co., 1924.

Focus on Pharmacy. Gary C. Van Riper, Ed. Brookings, SD:College of Pharmacy, SDSU.

Grogan, F. James, Pharm.D. *Pharmacy Simplified:A Glossary of Terms*. Canada: Delmar, Thomson Learning, 2001.

Keith, I. H. *Historical Reminiscences, 1886-1905*. SDPhA 1907, p. 70-79.

National Pharmacy Compliance News. South Dakota Board of Pharmacy Newsletter. Park Ridge, Illinois, 60068: NABP Foundation, Inc.

Pharmacists, SD, Chronological List Certificates No. 1 to No. 2841, October 1, 1890 to June 3, 1943. SDPhA Annual Proceedings, 1943, p. 87-129.

Polk Directory. Minnesota and Dakota Territory, Vol. 3, 1882-1883. R. L. Polk. Co. Chicago, Ill.

Polk Directory. Minnesota, Dakota, & Montana, Gazetteer, 1886-1887. R. L. Polk, Co. Chicago, Ill.

Redman, Kenneth. History of the SDSU College of Pharmacy, A Chronology, 1975-1982. Brookings, SD: College of Pharmacy, SDSU. 1983.

Robinson, Doane. *Encyclopedia of South Dakota*. Sioux Falls, SD:Will A. Beach Printing Co., 1925.

Schell, Herbert S. *South Dakota, Its Beginnings and Growth*. New York: American Book Company, 1942.

Schuler, Harold H. *The South Dakota Capitol in Pierre*. Madison: Karl E. Mundt Foundation, 1985.

————-*A Bridge Apart, History of Early Pierre and Fort Pierre*. Pierre: State Publishing Co., 1987.

————-*Pierre Since 1910*. Freeman, SD, Pine Hill Press, 1998.

SDPhA Office, Executive Director Robert Overturf. PO Box 518, Pierre, SD 57501.

SDPhA Annual Convention Proceedings, surviving issues 1891-1973. SDPhA Office, Pierre, SD.

SDPhA Minute Books, SDPhA Office, Pierre, SD.

SD Pharmacy Newsletter, 1964-1986. SDPhA Office, Pierre, SD.

South Dakota Pharmacist, 1986-2002. SDPhA Office, Pierre, SD.

South Dakota Legislative Manual (Blue book) 1963. Pierre, SD.

South Dakota Pharmacy Law and Information, SDPhA Office, Pierre, SD. 2000.

Stat-Gram, 1996-2002. SDPhA Office, Pierre, SD.

Technicians, Pharmacy. Sesquicentennial Stepping Stone Summits. Summit Two. Baltimore, MD, May 2002.

The College of Pharmacy, Gary C. Van Riper, Ed. Brookings, SD: College of Pharmacy, SDSU.

Thomas, Cliff. *Humor In Pharmacy*. Nemo, SD: Nemo Publishing Co., 1998.

To order extra copies of
A History of Pharmacy in South Dakota

Contact SD Pharmacists Association
PO Box 518, Pierre, SD 57501
605-224-2338

Index

Davis Bros. Inc.: 153
Deadwood pharmacists: 1876, 1, 2
Dean's Club: 231
Dees, Deb.: 256
Deetken, Julius: early Deadwood, 2; 1882 and 1886 drug stores, 7,8, 300
Degrees, College of Pharmacy: 1893-1994, 231
Denholm, Congressman Frank: 152
Denver College of Pharmacy: 136
Department of Commerce & Consumer Affairs—Board of Pharmacy: 158, 159
Department of Pharmacy, changed name to Division of Pharmacy: 79
Depression, Dust, Hard times: 90, 91
Dewald, Carol A.: 193
Dexter, D.F.: 71
Discriminatory Pricing: 154, 185
Dispensary: 79
Distinguished Alumnus Award, College of Pharmacy: 198
Distinguished Service Awards: 291
Distinguished Young Pharmacist Awards: 180, 293
District: resolutions, agenda, nominees, presidents 139-141, 153, 154, 180
Division of Pharmacy: summary 1888-1934, 98
Doctor of Pharmacy (P.D.): SDPhA, 187, 188
Doherty, C.L. "Roy": 73, 109
Dow, Harry L.: 111
Drug Garden: 63, 64, 81, ended 1984
Drug Inspector: 94, 95, 111, 112, 123, 144, 166, 189
Drug Product Selection: 161, 162
Drug samples: 185
Drug store ownership limited: 94, 124-129
Drug stores: 1881 store, 3; early Yankton and Deadwood, 2; 1882-1886 drug stores, 300
Drug store sidelines: 1917, 59
Drug store laboratory vs. manufacturers laboratory: 58
Druggist: name, 18
Druggists' Mutual Fire Insurance Co.: 73
Drury, Jay: 172
Dual line prescription form: 161, 218
Duncan, Michael: 255
Dunning, L. T.: 10
Dutton, Rogene: 206

Dwivedi, Chandrahar: 230, 237

E
Eastman, Roger: 133, 139, 142, 211
Eastman, Mrs. Roger: 120
Economic Survey by College of Pharmacy: 1987, 189
Educational and Legislative Section: 73
Eernisse, Welles C.: 119
Ehrke, Robert W.: 137, 138, 142, 153, 155, 157, 165
Eidsmoe, Clark T.: depression, graduates 101, 170, 193, 198
Eighmy, Marilyn: 238
Electronic Licensure Transfer Program: 225
Enrollments, grads: 1980-1988, 191
Examinations, Board: 20-24, 40-42, 75
Externship program: 233

F
Fair Trade Act: 91
Farrar, Governor Frank: 136
Farver, Debra K.: 230
Fifty-Year Membership Certificates: 119
Finances, Association, 1992-1999: 208
Fischer, Janet R.: 230
Five-year degree: 128,147
Flu shots, pharmacists: 227
Focus on Pharmacy, magazine: 235
France, L. G.: 94
Frary, G. G.: 56
Free choice of pharmacy: 142
French, Jennie: 8
Freier, Garry: 209
Fuller, Neil E.: 119
Fuller, Mrs. Neil E.: 120

G
Gackstetter, Dean: 140
Gallup Poll, 1994: ranking pharmacists, 213
Gamble, US Senator Robert J.: 52
Gangelhoff, Jaime: 207
Generic Drug: 161
Garry, Laurie: 255
Gerdes, Mark: 205, 216
Gifford, Congressman and Mrs. Oscar S.:38
Goetz, Edane M.: 193
Goeden, Galen: 210
Graduates, College of Pharmacy: 1884-1917, 64
Graham, Mark: 220

Great Moments in Pharmacy, painting: 90
Great Sioux Reservation: 1, 9
Greater University System, 1931: 99
Gregg, Robert: 152, 180, 190
Gross, Dean Guilford: 121, 128, 129, 140, 146, 168, 228
Grover, R. D.: 54
Guan, Xiangming: 230
Gubbrud, Governor and Mrs. Archie: 136
Guthmiller, Shirley: 212

H
Haggar, Don: 138, 141
Haggar, Tom: 89, 119, 140, 142
Halbkat, F. W.: 56, 61, 62
Halbkat Jr., Jack: 180
Hall, Nettie C.: first woman officer, 16
Harrison Narcotic Law: 56
Health Professional Assistance Program (HPAP): 227
Health Maintenance Organization (HMO): 151
Hedge, Dennis: 233, 258
Hegg, Annie: 258
Heida, Gerrit: 185
Heisler, Mrs. John E.: 39
Heitland, Shirley: 166, 170, 190, 191
Helgeland, David: 182, 185, 229, 230, 236
Helmey, Isaac M.: 43
Hendricks, Bernard: 174, 233
Herreid, Governor Charles E.: 40
Hersrud, James: 155, 190
Hetager, Les: 172, 180, 189
Hietbrink, Dean Bernard: 192, 198, 227-229; scholarship fund, 238
High School requirement: 42, 45, 46, 63
Highley, L. E.: 32, 33, 94
Hilson, Ann: 258
Historical Committee: 181
Hobo Day: 80, 169, 237
Hoch, Bill: 139
Hodson, Willis: 120, 160
Hooding Ceremony: 232
Hogan, Joan: 190, 219
Hogstad Jr., Anton: 63, 64
Holm, Melvin C.: 138, 142
Honorary President's Awards: 120, list 291
Hopkins, Cyril G.: 26
Hopponen, Dean Raymond E.: 146, 168, 191, 192, 196, 197, 228, 230, 238
Hospital Pharmacy: 252-260

Household Remedy Law: 110, 111, 220, 221
Huether, Ron: 172, 180, 253
Humphrey Jr., Vice-President Hubert H.: 136
Humor In Pharmacy, Cliff Thomas: 153
Hussey, Nora: 220
Hustead Pharmacist of the Year Awards: 181, list Appendix E, 293
Hustead, Bill: 137, 184, 198, 211
Hustead, Dorothy: 211
Hustead, Marjorie: 211
Hustead, Rick: 211
Hustead, Ted E.: 106, 178, 184, 211,
Hustead, Ted H.: 211

I
Icenogle, Jeanine: 267
Income, prescriptions: 87, 89
Industrial Collegian: magazine, 80, 193, 235
Influenza shots: 227
Innovative Practice Awards: 209, list Appendix E, 293
Institutional Pharmacy Committee: 153, 253
Institutes, pharmaceutical by SDSU: 115
Insurance cards: 218
Intern name replaced apprentice: 165
Intern rule change: 225, 233, 234
Interprofessional agreement 1958: 119
Issak, LaVonne: 265

J
Janklow, Governor William: 155, 184, 212, 218
Jarratt, A. A.: 106
Jensen, Governor Leslie: 92
Jensen, Misty J.: 258
Jensen, Wendy: 232, 257
Jewett III, Harvey: 153
Jewett Drug: 31, 38, 72, 120; start scholarship, 100; 153, 180, 239, 314
Johnson, Annette M.: 258
Johnson, Ron: 231, 257
Johnson, Thomas J.: 229, 258
Johnson, U. S. Senator Tim: 229
Jones, David F.: 27, 36, 40, 43, 45, 72, 74
Jones, Mrs. D. F.: 38
Jones, Secretary Dennis M.:190, 216, 217, 219, 220, 223, 226
Jones, E.M.: 45
Jones, Mrs. E. M.: 38, 39
Jones, James "Jack": 140, 189, 223
Jones, Secretary Kenneth: 88, 92, 107, 103

A History of Pharmacy in South Dakota

McKay, J. J.: 72, 86, 96
McKennan Hospital: 234, 261
McKesson Drug: 72, 316
McKesson & Robbins: 107, 120, 151, 180, 316
McKinstry, Earl: 205, 212, 257, 262, 263
McMaster, Governor W.H.: 77
McMurdy, Walter: 111
Medicine development: 1940-1950, 134
Medicine Shoppe, Yankton: 234
Meierhenry, Mark: 186
Meintsma, Julia: 210
Mellette, Governor Arthur: 12
Memorial Hour: 71, 210, 211
Messerschmidt, Kim: 230
Meyer, Dave: 256
Michel, Mr. and Mrs. W. F.: 39, 73
Mickelson, Governor George S.: 190, 255
Mickelson, State Rep. George T.: 92, 112
Miller, Callie: 8
Mills, Harold W.: 105, 124
Mills, Tom: 90, 119, 154
Mills & Purdy Drug: 1
Milwaukee Railroad: 4
Modernization of pharmacies: 135
Moriatry, John: 172
Morstad, Anne: 258
Mowell, LaVerne J. 118, 121
Mundt, U. S. Senator Karl E.: 87, 89, 121
Murdy, Duncan: 220, 226

N
NABP: 42, 62, 76, 164, 165, 170, 191
NABPLEX, NAPLEX: 224, 225
Narcotics, early laws: 55,56
National Association of Retail Druggists (NARD): 17, 34, 87, 88, 90
National Community Pharmacists Association: (NCPA) [Formerly NARD], 205, 231, 265
National Formulary (NF): 110, 190
National Guard Army ambulance: 54
National Pharmacy Compliance News: Board newsletter, 227
National Pharmacy Week: 1991-2000, 211, 212
National Practitioner Data Bank— Healthcare Integrity & Protection Data Bank: (NPDB-HIPDB), 227
Nelson, Deborah K.: 193
Nelson, John: 113, 153, 190

Nelson, Ron: 172, 174, 253
Neumayer, B. H.: 71
Newsletters: 30, 73, 80, 121, 139, 192, 193, 208, 213, 235
Nicolls, Mrs. O. C.: 93
Non-pharmacist owners: 124, 125
Non-Prescription Drugs, license: 220
Nonresident pharmacies, license: 221
Norbeck, Governor Peter: 54, 57
Northwestern Drug: 72, 153, 180
Northwestern Druggist: 30, 89, 109
Nursing Department attached to Division of Pharmacy: 101
Nye, Mrs. W. A.: 12, 38

O
Old Central: 25
Omodt, Gary: 139, 140, 147, 154
Opportunities night: 239
Overland-Janssen, Karla: 210, 213
Overholser, R.L.: 108
Overturf, Robert: 207
Ownership: limited to pharmacist, unconstitutional, 110

P
Page, Warren J.: 1881 drug store, 3
Part-time pharmacies in hospitals and nursing homes: 145
Patient Counseling: 215, 222
Patent Medicine License: 96, 110, 220, 221
Patient Package Inserts: 184
Patient Records: 215, 222
Peaslee, C. W.: 37
Peddler medicine wagons: 37, 38, 54-55
Perisho, President E. C.: 57, 63
Perriton, Mrs. H. A.: 70
Peterson, Edward W.: 119
Petrik, Stan: 184
Pettigrew, H. P.: 13-15
Pfeifle, Allen: 144, 165, 166, 180, 191, 217, 264
Pharm-Assist Committee: 180
Pharmaceutical Association: 1886, 4, 5
Pharmacia: 182, 183
Pharmacies 1931: non-pharmacist ownership, 94, 95, 109; ownership 1954; 123
Pharmacies: western SD, 1898, 12
Pharmacist's Charity Day: 183
Pharmacist degrees: 1898, 20

A History of Pharmacy in South Dakota

Register as pharmacist: in 1890, 19
Reilly, Vince: 258
Reinders, Charles: 155
Reiswig, Robert: 210
Rennich, Judy: 262, 266
Remington, Professor: 52
Restricted drug area in pharmacy: 126
Rho Chi Society: 100, 169, 194, 196, 237
Riter, Robert Jr.: 186, 214
Rogers, James: 151
Rogers, Mrs. James: 151
Rosenau, Susan: 212
Rotations, intern training: 234
Rutherford, T.C.: 165

S
Sabin, Mrs. George C.: 38
Salary Survey, 1998-1999: 213, 231
Sales tax: 88, 158
Sasse, H. A.: 32
Shanholtz, Wayne: 133, 138
Scallin, S.F.: 73
Schmiedt, Stan: 265
Schnaidt, H. G.: 53
Scholarship, first: 99
Scholarship & Dinner Dance: Awards, 195, 238
Schuler, Harold H.: 8; Air Force School, 114; secretary, 133, 152, 154, 159, 166, 178, 188; published books, 179, 207; About the Author, 318
Schuler, Herman & Freida: 8
Schumacher, Jody L.: 193
Schutz, J. Chris: 76
Schwans, Marilyn: 187
Schwans, Ron: 154, 184
Schwartz, Milford L.: 124
Schwartz Sectional System: 79
Score Transfer Program: 224
Scott, Clayton: 138, 151
Searle Drug Co.: 182
Seefeldt, Teresa: 236
Self-service drug store license: 109
Separation of Board and Association: 159, 186, 203-206
Serles, C.M.: 71
Serles, Earl R.: 64, 75, 79, 97 Scholarship fund, 130, 168, 196; pres. of AACP 1938-1939, 113; pres. APHA 1946-1947, 113
Sevareid, Eric: 104
Skancke, Pat: 262

Shepard, James H.: 26
Shepard Hall, 26, 147, pharmacy addition and dedicated, 168
Shirley, J. C.: 119
Shoenhard, Leslie: 212
Sidle, John H.: 107
Simpson, Mrs. W. A. first Ladies' Auxiliary president: 38
Slagle, President Robert L.: 45
Smith, Doug: 255
Smith, F. C.: 38
SD Society of Health-System Pharmacists: 252-258, presidents and pharmacists of the year, Appendix F; 294
SD Association of Pharmacy Technicians, (SDAPT): 261-267. list of charter members and presidents, 267;
SD Medical Association: 119, 161, 227, 236
SD Pharmacy Newsletter: 139, 182
South Dakota Pharmacist: 119, 182, 206, 208, 213,
Stat-Gram: 208, 213, 266
Split exams by Board of Pharmacy: 124
State Fair: 32, 39, 155, 212
Statz, Joseph F.; 184
Statz, Joseph H.: 184
Statz, Joseph M.: 184
Statz, Stephen R.: 184, 220, 226
Stephens, James: 155, 180, 196
Stickles, Mr. and Mrs. Fred. G.: 39, 71
Stites, A. H.: 12, 14, 20, 21, 22, 53
Stotz, Pam: 205
Stotz, Paula: 212
Strahl, Donald: 172, 198
Stroschein, Dale: 180, 219
Stroschein, Mary Ann: 180
Student Membership, SDPhA: 205, 209
Student Loan Fund: 99, 100, 129
Substitution of drugs: 127, 161, 218
Surveys: 164, 188, 213
Sutton, Renee: 212
Swanson, Ed: 154, 181
Swenson, Milton: 152

T
Tammen, George: 207
Tarbell, O.H.: 20
Technicians, pharmacy: 261-268
Tel-Drug: 184
Television outreach program: 146
Territorial, pharmacist certificates: 7, 8

Jewett Drug Company

Aberdeen, SD

a subsidiary of

D&K Healthcare Resources Inc.

is proud to be
Partners with Independent Pharmacies for over 120 years

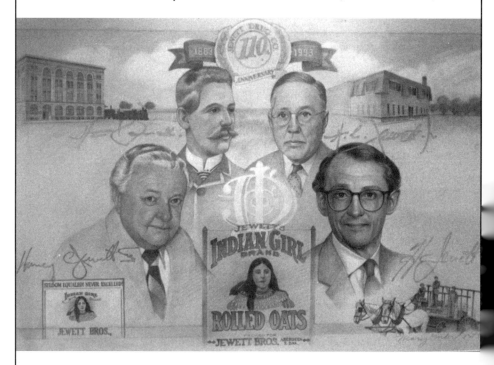

We thank you for your support!

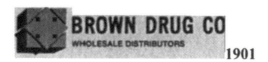

1901

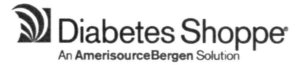

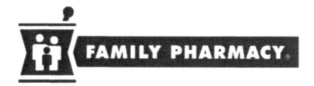

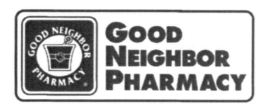

2004

Serving the *independent* retail pharmacy since 1901

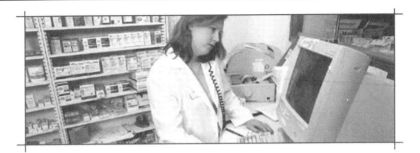

PARTNERING WITH
SOUTH DAKOTA PHARMACY

The Retail Druggists Mutual Insurance Association of Iowa was organized in October 1909 by members of the Iowa Pharmaceutical Association. In 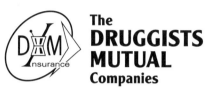 January 1916, the name was changed to Druggists Mutual Insurance Association of Iowa. This name was later revised to Druggists Mutual Insurance Company. In 1992, the company name was again changed and remains today as Pharmacists Mutual Insurance Company.

Pharmacists Mutual became licensed to provide insurance in South Dakota in 1951. Larry Higinbotham served as the first salesperson from 1956 until his retirement in 1975. Lee Ann Fiala is the current sales representative.

Pharmacists Mutual continues to serve the South Dakota pharmacy profession providing individual professional liability for pharmacists and pharmacy technicians, businessowners coverage, workers compensation, auto, homeowners, student protection, life, health, disability and financial planning services. Pharmacists Mutual pledges to continue to provide you the best service and best products at fair rates, as we have done since 1909.

Pharmacists *Mutual*Companies

- Pharmacists Mutual Insurance Company
- Pharmacsts Life Insurance Company
- Pharmacists National® Insurance Corp.
- PMC Quality Commitment, Inc.
- Pro Advantage Services, Inc.

800-247-5930 • P.O. Box 370, Algona, Iowa 50511 • www.phmic.com

Notice: This is not a claims reporting site. You cannot electronically report a claim to us. To report a claim, call 800-247-5930.

About the Author

Harold H. Schuler was born and raised on a farm near Tripp, S.D. After graduation from Tripp High School, he served in World War II as a member of the 20th Army Air Force in Guam. He graduated from the University of South Dakota with a B.A. in 1950 and a M.Ed. in 1951. That year he was named Director of the S.D. School Lunch program in the State Department of Public Instruction in Pierre, and served three years.

He served as an assistant to United States Senator Francis Case in the United States Senate, Washington, D.C., 1954-1962. Following the death of Senator Case in 1962, he purchased the Hughes County Abstract Company in Pierre, S. D. In 1964, he was appointed as Executive Secretary of the S.D. Board of Pharmacy and the S.D. Pharmaceutical Association. He sold the abstract company in 1979, but continued working for the Board of Pharmacy and Pharmaceutical Association until his retirement in 1986. Since retirement, he and his wife Leona, a former Pierre High School English teacher, spend their winters in Arizona and their summers in Pierre. They have three children, Lynda, Debra, and Mark.

Harold, who wrote his first book, *South Dakota Government* in 1966, continued his interest in historical writing. Since 1985, he has authored the following published books on South Dakota history:

The South Dakota Capitol in Pierre, 1985
A Bridge Apart, History of Early Pierre and Fort Pierre, 1987
Fort Pierre Chouteau, 1990
Fort Sully: Guns at Sunset, 1992
Camp Rapid, 1995
South Dakota Armories, 1996
Fort Sisseton, 1996
Adjutant Generals of the South Dakota National Guard, 1997
Pierre Since 1910, 1998
Lewis and Clark in the Pierre and Fort Pierre Area, 2001
The Lighted Cross, History of the First United Methodist Church in Pierre, 2002

He also had two articles printed in the *South Dakota History* magazine: *A Photographic Essay on the Capitol of South Dakota, 1989*; and *Patriotic Pageantry: Presidential Visits to South Dakota, 2000*. His article on Custer's First Venture into the Black Hills appeared in The Tombstone Epitaph, Tombstone, Arizona, June 1995.

Schuler was a past director of the Pierre S.D. Chamber of Commerce; past chairman of the City of Pierre Golf Board; chairman of the 1963 Governor Archie Gubbrud Inaugural Committee; and past president of the Pierre Elks Lodge. He is a member of the United Methodist Church, American Legion, Veterans of Foreign Wars. He is a member of the Society of Southwest Authors, and both the South Dakota and Arizona Historical Societies. He is also a past member of Western Writer's of America. During the winter months in Tucson, he serves as a docent at Fort Lowell Military Museum. His booklet, *Surgeons and Sabers at Fort Lowell, Arizona* was released by the museum in 2003.